Design for Dementia, Mental Health and Wellbeing

I0131192

This edited volume offers the first overview and reflective discussion of how design can contribute to people's wellbeing and mental health in the context of dementia, mental illness and neurodiversity.

This book explores and promotes holistic, salutogenic and preventive strategies that recognise and respond to people's needs, wants, wishes and rights to further health, wellbeing and equality. Bringing together years of experience as designers and clinicians, the contributors to the book emphasise how design can be a collaborative, creative process as well as an outcome of this process, and they reveal how this is guided by mental health and design policy. Through its three parts, the book explores themes of ethics, citizenship and power relationships in co-design, providing an overview of current developments and approaches in co-design; of the culturally and value sensitive adaptation of design interventions and their applications, many of which are a result of co-design; and of policy and related standards in and for design and mental health. In this way, the book demonstrates how design can help to support people, their care partners and care professionals in promoting mental health and wellbeing, and it offers a rich resource on how to create a sustainable future for care in this domain.

The book provides a unique and holistic overview and resource for designers, researchers, students, policy providers and health and care professionals to help support the development and adoption of person-centred design processes and interventions.

Kristina Niedderer is Professor of Design at Manchester Metropolitan University, UK.

Geke Ludden is Professor of Interaction Design at the University of Twente, the Netherlands.

Tom Dening is Professor of Dementia Research in the School of Medicine, University of Nottingham, UK.

Vjera Holthoff-Detto is Professor of Old Age Psychiatry at the Faculty of Medicine Carl Gustav Carus, Technische Universität Dresden, Germany.

Design for Social Responsibility

Series Editor: Rachel Cooper

Social responsibility, in various disguises, has been a recurring theme in design for many years. Since the 1960s several more or less commercial approaches have evolved. In the 1970s designers were encouraged to abandon 'design for profit' in favour of a more compassionate approach inspired by Papanek. In the 1980s and 1990s profit and ethical issues were no longer considered mutually exclusive and more market-oriented concepts emerged, such as the 'green consumer' and ethical investment. The purchase of socially responsible, 'ethical' products and services has been stimulated by the dissemination of research into sustainability issues in consumer publications. Accessibility and inclusivity have also attracted a great deal of design interest and recently designers have turned to solving social and crime-related problems. Organisations supporting and funding such projects have recently included the NHS (research into design for patient safety); the Home Office has (design against crime); Engineering and Physical Sciences Research Council (design decision-making for urban sustainability).

Businesses are encouraged (and increasingly forced by legislation) to set their own socially responsible agendas that depend on design to be realised. Design decisions all have environmental, social and ethical impacts, so there is a pressing need to provide guidelines for designers and design students within an overarching framework that takes a holistic approach to socially responsible design. This edited series of guides is aimed at students of design, product development, architecture and marketing and design and management professionals working in the sectors covered by each title. Each volume includes: The background and history of the topic, its significance in social and commercial contexts and trends in the field. Exemplar design case studies. Guidelines for the designer and advice on tools, techniques and resources available.

9. Design for Healthcare
Edited by Emmanuel Tsekleves and Rachel Cooper

10. Design for Personalisation
Edited by Iryna Kuksa and Tom Fisher

11. Design for Behaviour Change
Edited by Kristina Niedderer, Stephen Clune and Geke Ludden

12. Design for Wellbeing
An Applied Approach
Edited by Ann Petermans and Rebecca Cain

13. Design for Global Challenges and Goals
Edited by Emmanuel Tsekleves, Rachel Cooper and Jak Spencer

14. Design for People Living with Dementia
Interactions and Innovations
Emmanuel Tsekleves and John Keady

15. Design for Transformative Learning
A Practical Approach to Memory-Making and Perspective-Shifting
Lisa Grocott

16. Design for Dementia, Mental Health and Wellbeing
Co-Design, Interventions and Policy
Edited by Kristina Niedderer, Geke Ludden, Tom Dening and Vjera Holthoff-Detto

For more information about this series, please visit: www.routledge.com/Design-for-Social-Responsibility /book-series/DSR

Design for Dementia, Mental Health and Wellbeing

Co-Design, Interventions and Policy

Edited by Kristina Niedderer, Geke Ludden, Tom Dening and Vjera Holthoff-Detto

Routledge
Taylor & Francis Group

LONDON AND NEW YORK

Designed cover image: © Getty Images

First published 2025
by Routledge
4 Park Square, Milton Park, Abingdon, Oxon OX14 4RN

and by Routledge
605 Third Avenue, New York, NY 10158

Routledge is an imprint of the Taylor & Francis Group, an informa business

© 2025 selection and editorial matter, Kristina Niedderer, Geke Ludden, Tom Dening and Vjera Holthoff-Detto; individual chapters, the contributors

British Library Cataloguing-in-Publication Data
A catalogue record for this book is available from the British Library

Library of Congress Cataloging-in-Publication Data
Names: Niedderer, Kristina, editor. | Ludden, Geke, editor. | Dening, Tom, editor. | Holthoff-Detto, Vjera, editor. Title:
Design for dementia, mental health and wellbeing: co-design, interventions and policy / edited by Kristina Niedderer, Geke Ludden, Tom Dening, and Vjera Holthoff-Detto.
Description: Abingdon, Oxon: Routledge, 2024. | Includes bibliographical references and index.
Identifiers: LCCN 2023055400 (print) | LCCN 2023055401 (ebook) | ISBN 9781032331188 (hardback) | ISBN 9781032331171 (paperback) | ISBN 9781003318262 (ebook)
Subjects: LCSH: Design--Human factors. | Well-being. | People with mental disabilities--Mental health.
Classification: LCC NK1520 .D465325 2024 (print) | LCC NK1520 (ebook) | DDC 744.087/4--dc23/eng/20240327
LC record available at https://lccn.loc.gov/2023055400
LC ebook record available at https://lccn.loc.gov/2023055401

ISBN: 978-1-032-33118-8 (hbk)
ISBN: 978-1-032-33117-1 (pbk)
ISBN: 978-1-003-31826-2 (ebk)

DOI: 10.4324/9781003318262

Typeset in Times New Roman
by Deanta Global Publishing Services, Chennai, India

Contents

List of figures

x *List of figures*

List of tables

Contributor biographies

Rosa Almeida is the Participatory Design Manager at Fundación INTRAS Living Lab, holding an MSc in Third Generation Therapies with a technology application emphasis and a gerontology background. She has managed various RDI EU projects since 2012 dedicated to the co-development of innovative solutions for health, wellbeing and integrated care.

Manish Asthana is a cognitive psychologist, and his ongoing research aims to understand the role of psychological, physiological, affective and cognitive aspects in ergonomics (i.e. human factor design). His current research focuses on understanding the role of human cognitive abilities in product usage. He is also interested in investigating human cognitive limitations in problem-solving strategies and decision-making concerning design research methods.

Nienke Beerlage-de Jong is an Assistant Professor at the Health Technology and Services Research section of the University of Twente. Her research focuses on participatory development, implementation and evaluation of eHealth technology for wicked health(care) challenges, in which she brings together stakeholders from academia, business and healthcare.

Andy Bell has been with Centre for Mental Health since 2002 and became Chief Executive in 2023. He has worked for more than 25 years in the voluntary sector, striving for equality and social justice through research, communicating evidence, influencing policy and informing debate.

Elena Bellini is an architect and co-founder of DU IT, an engineering company based in Florence, Italy, specialising in multi-sensory environments. She has a PhD in Architectural Technology in the field of sensory design for autism. She works on the design of spaces for care and living, to offer spaces for regulation and re-balancing of one's senses, especially for people with cognitive disability, dementia or autism. She is a post-doctoral Research Fellow, studying health and active ageing, and Adjunct Professor, Department of Architecture, University of Florence.

Jill Bennett is Scientia Professor and Australian Research Council Laureate Fellow and founding Director of the Big Anxiety Research Centre (BARC). Jill's ARC Laureate supports the transdisciplinary Felt Experience & Empathy Lab [fEEL] at UNSW. fEEL brings together psychosocial and creative practitioners, specialising in trauma/mental health engagement, and in the use of experiential media, such as virtual reality, to communicate embodied experience.

Michaelle Bosse obtained her PhD on the subject of 'Mindful Design as an Approach to Promote Mindfulness'. Her professional experience focuses on usability and user experience for Information Systems. She has a research assistant position at the Chair for Information Systems, esp. Business Information Management at Martin Luther University

Halle-Wittenberg. There, she works on an applied and collaborative research project called ELISE (Relieving the Load on the Care Infrastructure through IT-based Integration of Spontaneous Civic Engagement).

Camilla Buchanan, co-Head, UK *Policy Lab*, is a policymaker and strategic designer focused on bringing creative and caring techniques to policy-making. She has worked in lots of different contexts in the UK and around the world on social policy issues ranging from recidivism to school attendance, and more technical areas of policy like social investment. The *Policy Lab* is a highly innovative government team looking at new ways to make policy better for the people it affects.

Jane Cannon, MBE, qualified as an electrical engineer and had a career in technology starting in her family's engineering business then various management and leadership roles in industry. She was also a Partner in Ernst & Young and a Director in the Home Office. More recently Jane has been working on improving young people's mental health including with NHS England on the Quality Improvement Taskforce for inpatient services and also working with the Royal College of Psychiatrists.

Donna Maria Coleston-Shields is a Consultant Clinical Psychologist and Neuropsychologist with specialist skills in the neuropsychology of dementia and later life, in addition to her broader therapy and systemic skills. Drawing on extensive clinical experience in dementia and neurosciences, her wider interests include managing clinical complexity to prevent hospital admission and facilitate discharge, promoting therapeutic environments and carer support. She continues to work clinically across a range of older adult services when opportunity arises.

Jill Corbyn is the founder and director of Neurodiverse Connection CIC and an associate with NDTi. Jill was the lead author on NHSE's Sensory Friendly Ward Principles, the 'It's Not Rocket Science' report into meeting sensory needs in mental health inpatient environments, and on the 'Supporting Autistic Flourishing at Home and Beyond' paper for the LGA. Jill co-produces all documents with other autistic people and specialises in neurodivergent experiences of sensory environments.

Michael P. Craven, PhD, is a Principal Research Fellow at the NIHR MindTech HealthTech Research Centre, Institute of Mental Health, University of Nottingham, specialising in methodology and applied research in the co-design and evaluation of digital health and medical devices. He is also a member of the Faculty of Engineering's Human Factors Research Group, the Centre for Dementia and the European INTERDEM Assistive Technologies Taskforce and is trustee of the Trent Dementia charity.

Jennifer E. Cross, PhD, is the Director of the Institute for Research in the Social Sciences and Professor of Sociology at Colorado State University. She works with community partners in applied research to promote public health, community attachment and social sustainability. Her research focuses on community approaches to regenerative development, processes of social change and capacity building for transformational change.

Deana Davalos, PhD, is a Professor in the Cognitive Neuroscience programme in the Department of Psychology at Colorado State University. She is also the director of the Aging Clinic of the Rockies and the associate director of the Columbine Health Systems Center for Healthy Aging. Her work focuses on developing methods to better understand pathological ageing and strategies for improving healthy ageing and preventing or reducing cognitive decline.

Aaron Davis is a lecturer in architecture with a teaching and research focus on co-design and community engagement processes, interdisciplinary collaboration and the intersection between social and environmental sustainability from the University of South Australia.

Jeroen Deenik is a psychomotor therapist, health psychologist and epidemiologist. He is the head of the psychotic disorders research line at GGz Central, a large mental healthcare organisation in the middle of the Netherlands. He is leading research on sedentary behaviour, physical activity and lifestyle in people with (severe) mental illness.

Tessa Dekkers is an Assistant Professor in the section of Psychology, Health and Technology at the University of Twente. Her research focuses on co-design with people in vulnerable situations and is informed by her interdisciplinary background in both health psychology and industrial design engineering.

Tom Dening is Professor of Dementia Research in the School of Medicine, University of Nottingham, UK. He is also an Honorary Consultant in Old Age Psychiatry at Nottinghamshire Healthcare NHS Foundation Trust. His interests include a wide range of clinical topics and psychosocial aspects of dementia. He is one of the editors of the Oxford Textbook of Old Age Psychiatry, the leading international work in this field, with the 4th edition to be published in 2025.

Jason A. Dibbs is an associate lecturer and doctoral candidate in architecture at the University of Sydney. He is the project officer for the Brain, Mind and Mallett Street research collaboration. His work focuses on aesthetics and ethics in spatial histories.

Raquel Losada Durán is the Director of Applied Research and Knowledge at Fundación INTRAS. Holding an MSc in Social Psychology and Organisational Anthropology, she is an expert in Organisational Intelligence. She has directed over 30 European and Spanish-funded Research and Innovation projects in technologies for Health and Wellbeing.

Thomas Engelsma is an Assistant Professor and PhD candidate at Amsterdam UMC, NL, focusing on the design and implementation of digital health technology for vulnerable older adults.

Meara Faw, PhD, is an associate professor of Communication Studies at Colorado State University. Her research explores the intersections of interpersonal communication and health, with specific interests in understanding how relationships with close friends and family impact well-being. In particular, she focuses on how supportive communication, conflict management and caregiving communication affect people's experiences of stress and social belonging.

Alexia Gkika is an accomplished lighting designer working for Buro Happold. Her focus on sustainability and inclusivity is driven by the advancing LED technology offering notable benefits on energy optimisation and product longevity. Her keen interest has led her to dedicate time in collaborations with academic/research bodies and organisations with the aim of deepening her knowledge range on aspects related to sensorial stimulation and visual comfort for neurodivergent people.

Ian Gwilt is a Professor of Design in UniSA: Creative, University of South Australia. His current areas of research include practice and theory in visual communication design in the context of healthcare and wellbeing, the development of novel information visualisation techniques to facilitate the understanding of data for non-specialist audiences and the design of hybrid environments and experiences; interactive installations, augmented reality artefacts and locations that shape the experience of public spaces.

Tahnee Heirbaut is a researcher and lecturer at the University of Twente. She conducts and coordinates projects on the evaluation of eHealth, implementation and qualitative research in the (forensic) mental health sector.

Leigh-Anne Hepburn is an Associate Professor of Design at the University of Sydney. Her research explores co-design and participatory design for innovation and changes across communities, organisations and government. She has a particular interest in design for health and wellbeing.

Vjera Holthoff-Detto is a Professor of Old Age Psychiatry at the Faculty of Medicine Carl Gustav Carus, Technische Universität Dresden, Germany. She is a board-certified neurologist, psychiatrist and clinical geriatrician. Her interests include geriatric depression, cognitive disorders, non-pharmacological interventions and psychotherapy in old age.

Cathy Hope is the Engagement and Impact Director and Coordinator of the Play, Creativity and Wellbeing Project in the Centre for Creative and Cultural Research in the Faculty of Arts and Design at the University of Canberra. Cathy's applied research projects seek to improve place and wellbeing outcomes by making more playful, inclusive environments through cross-sector and community collaborations.

Sarah Hughes has been Chief Executive of Mind since 2022. Previously, she was the CEO of the Centre for Mental Health. She has worked in mental health and criminal justice for 34 years. After originally training as a social worker, Sarah has spent the majority of her career in the voluntary sector within both community and secure settings.

Erika Renedo-Illarregi, PhD, founded a social enterprise in 2013 to explore the wellbeing benefits of co-design, working with people with mental health problems and prisoners before formalising her research through a PhD. She is especially interested in understanding how and why designing impacts people psychologically. Her travels through India informed a pluralist approach in her work, nurturing an ongoing interest in alternative belief systems around unusual experiences and deeply acknowledging every person's reality.

Monique W. M. Jaspers is a Professor in Biomedical Informatics and head of the 'Human Factors Engineering in Health Information Technology' research line at the department of Medical Informatics, Amsterdam UMC, Amsterdam, NL. She is also the Director of the Educational Institute for Medical Informatics at the Amsterdam UMC–University of Amsterdam.

Vivek Kant is cross-trained in design, engineering and cognitive/behavioural sciences. His research interests are human–machine interaction, human factors, human systems integration, sociotechnical systems, along with the history and philosophy of design.

Saskia Kelders is an Associate Professor at the University of Twente and an extraordinary professor at North-West University. Her multidisciplinary work uses innovative research to investigate the relationship between technology, engagement and effectiveness of eHealth. She is also the editor of the Centre for eHealth and Wellbeing Research's handbook of eHealth and a lead educator in this field.

Gail Kenning, PhD, is an interdisciplinary researcher, an artist working with socially engaged practices and a designer using psychosocial and participatory approaches to understand, support and explore transformative possibilities in relation to ageing, dementia and trauma. She engages in a range of qualitative, psychosocial methods and phenomenological/deep listening analysis approaches as part of The Big Anxiety Research Centre UNSW Sydney.

Hanneke Kip is an Assistant Professor at the University of Twente and a Researcher at Transfore, an organisation for forensic mental healthcare. Her prolific research focuses on the development, implementation and evaluation of eHealth interventions such as VR, wearables and mobile apps for vulnerable psychiatric patient populations.

Randy Klaassen is an Assistant Professor of Human Media Interaction at the University of Twente.

Christopher Kueh is an Associate Professor of Design at Edith Cowan University, trained as a graphic and information designer with a focus on expanding and applying the ways designers think to improve and innovate businesses, organisations and communities.

Kate Langham is a Senior Co-Design Lead at *Policy Lab* UK. She has extensive design leadership experience in industry, academia and government roles, specialising in creating innovative co-design practices that achieve social and environmental impact. Kate's passion is reimagining policy-making using people-centred approaches to transform policy outcomes for citizens. She has a PhD in co-design and lectures at universities and conferences, sharing her enthusiasm for user-centred design.

Rebecca (Becca) Lassell, PhD, OTR/L is an Assistant Professor in the Department of Health & Wellness Design at Indiana University's School of Public Health. Becca's programme of research focuses on designing community-based interventions to improve brain health and health equity. Her research interests include participatory research, nature-based interventions, Alzheimer's disease and mild cognitive impairment.

Vanessa Lefton, Ethnography Lead, is the co-head of ethnographic research at Policy Lab, and leads complex multidisciplinary projects that experiment with film/experimental ethnography (alongside design, systems change, art) on policy relating to inequality issues.

Jennifer N. W. Lim is a Reader in Health Inequalities and Behavioural Science, University of Wolverhampton, UK. She engages actively with the Chinese community, reducing dementia stigma and promoting brain health using cultural tailoring and public health theoretical frameworks. Current projects include improving dementia research participation in Black communities and culturally appropriate implementation science. She created the first UK-wide project of Chinese communities, building knowledge about dementia and brain health.

Geke Ludden is a full professor of Interaction Design at the University of Twente. In a range of projects, often in multi- and cross-disciplinary teams, she studies how the design of products and services influences people's behaviour and motivation with a specific interest in how products and services can support healthy behaviour and in how technology (interactive devices and wearables) can engage people in therapy at home.

Benedetta Lusi is a PhD candidate at Interaction Design Group at the University of Twente. Bridging HCI, design for care and philosophy of technology, her research focuses on designing compassionate technology for mental health and wellbeing.

Charlotte van Lotringen graduated in applied cognitive psychology and is currently conducting PhD research at the University of Twente on compassionate technology. In a multidisciplinary team, she researches how technology can be used in mental health care to foster compassion. In this project, she works together with clients, professionals and other stakeholders to develop guidelines for compassionate blended treatment that supports the professional in recognising and alleviating suffering.

Alessia Macchi is an architect and independent researcher, based in Florence, Italy, who collaborates with DU IT on projects relating to multi-sensory environments. She has a PhD in Architectural Technology in the field of sensory design for birth environments. She works on participatory and co-design processes to foster user bio-psycho-social wellbeing through built environment design.

Laura Malinin, PhD, is the Inaugural Director of the Nancy Richardson Design Center and an Associate Professor of Interior Architecture and Design at Colorado State University. An environmental designer and cognitive scientist, her work bridges research and co-design practice by examining relationships between human cognition and designed environments, including how socio-physical environments can more effectively support creativity, health and wellbeing.

Jordan McKibbin received a bachelor's with honours in Mechatronics engineering from the University of Wollongong and a Diploma in Design Strategies from the University of Canberra. He has worked as a research assistant for the University of Canberra and the University of South Australia. He is interested in community development, intergenerational programmes and sustainable business practices.

Donald McNeill is a Professor of Urbanism at the University of Sydney. His research is located at the intersection of human geography, economic sociology, spatial planning and urban design and architecture, with a particular interest in the political and cultural economy of globalisation and cities.

Kristina Niedderer, PhD, is a Professor of Design at Manchester Metropolitan University. Niedderer's research focuses on the role of design to engender mindful interaction and behaviour change for health and sustainability. She led the European projects 'Designing for People with Dementia' (2016-2020, MSCA GA No. 691001) and IDoService (2020-2022, MSCA GA No. 895620) and the ICanDo project (2023-24, ES/Y007778/1) funded by UKRI as part of the Healthy Ageing Challenge.

Matthijs Noordzij is a full professor in Health Psychology and Technology at the University of Twente. He studies the scientific basis and design principles for how (sensor) technology (e.g. a smartwatch measuring physiological signals and capable of giving coaching cues) might support and change (mental) healthcare and self-management.

Teresa Orihuela is a clinical psychologist at the psychiatric day hospital in San Telmo, in Palencia. She holds a masters degree in Human Sexuality (1985), Psychotherapy and Psychoanalytic Clinic (2018) and Executive Development from IESE Business School (2020). Her published works focus on mental health, deafness, sexuality, disability and peer support in mental healthcare.

Fanke Peng is an Associate Professor and Enterprise Fellow at the University of South Australia. She is an award-winning educator, designer and researcher in design-led social innovation, co-design for health and wellbeing, design innovation in ageing well and cross-cultural design.

Dr. Linda W. P. Peute (Dr. Linda Dusseljee-Peute) is a senior researcher and Director of the eHealth Living & Learning Lab, Amsterdam UMC, NL. Her expertise is in the application of human-factor methods in biomedical informatics.

Paul A. Rodgers is a Professor of Design at the University of Strathclyde, Department of Design, Manufacturing and Engineering Management (DMEM). He has over 25 years of experience in product design research and is the author of more than 170 papers and 16 books. His current research interests explore the discipline of design and how disruptive design interventions can enact positive change in health and social care and elsewhere.

Stephanie Schouten is a researcher at the University of Twente and Isala Hospital. Her research focuses on the design, development and evaluation of evidence-based eHealth technology via interdisciplinary teamwork and collaboration with end-users.

Chris L. Smith is a Professor of Architectural Theory at the University of Sydney. His research concerns the nexus of architecture and the body, with recent work focusing on the complex intersections of architecture, the biosciences and medical humanities.

Jodi Sturge is an assistant professor with the IxD group at the Department of Design, Production and Management in the Faculty of Engineering Technology at the University of Twente, the Netherlands. Her mixed-method research focuses on mobility, human-building interaction and wellbeing to evaluate and inform the design of healthcare facilities, home environments and social infrastructure.

Rishi Tak is an interaction design professional with a keen interest in design, art and technology. He likes to work across physical and digital spaces to communicate ideas, solve problems and create value-driven solutions across various human endeavours.

Cathy Treadaway is a Professor Emeritus at Cardiff Metropolitan University, Wales, UK, and Research Director of HUG by LAUGH Ltd. She is an experienced designer, writer and researcher. Her work focuses on creativity, sensory touch, design for dementia and wellbeing. Cathy designed HUG with Aidan Taylor in 2017, informed by LAUGH dementia research. HUG was acquired by the Science Museum, London in 2023, for the UK National Collection (Medical).

Isabelle Tournier, PhD, is Maître de Conference (associate professor) at the University of Montpellier in Integrative neuropsychology of adults and older adults. Previously, she was a teaching and research fellow at Toulouse Jean Jaurès University (France) and a research fellow for the Horizon2020 MSCA IDoService project (2020–2022) at Manchester Metropolitan University (UK). She has a background in psychology of ageing, and her research focuses on adaptation, autonomy and wellbeing in ageing.

Lindsey Wilhelm, PhD, is an Associate Professor of Music Therapy at Colorado State University, an affiliate of the Columbine Health Systems Center for Healthy Ageing and a member of the Sound Health Network. As a board-certified music therapist, her research examines how music and music-based approaches support older adults and the ageing process, with specific interests related to the accessibility of music experiences and community music.

Christian Wölfel, PhD, is a trained industrial designer, researcher and lecturer at the Chair of Industrial Design Engineering at Technische Universität Dresden, Germany. His research relates to the design and experience of complex systems in professional domains. It is grounded in cognitive and social sciences and aims for sustainable solutions. He teaches design fundamentals, design theory and design research in interdisciplinary settings. He is a board member of the German Society for Design Theory and Research (DGTF).

Madeline Zabar is a PhD student at the University of South Australia exploring how co-design can improve mental health outcomes for young people and build sustainability in the mental health system. She is a Senior Consultant, with a background in service and system design to improve learner experiences in the Australian Tertiary Education system, and has worked at the forefront of social policy for the Australian Government. .

1 Introduction

Designing for wellbeing in the context of dementia, mental illness and neurodiversity

Kristina Niedderer, Geke Ludden, Tom Dening and Vjera Holthoff-Detto

Setting the scene

This book offers the first collective overview and reflective discussion of how design – as a collaborative creative process as well as an outcome of this process – can contribute to people's wellbeing and mental health in the context of dementia, mental illness and neurodiversity, and how this is guided by mental health and design policy. The aim is to demonstrate how design can help support people, their care partners and care professionals in promoting mental health and wellbeing. For this purpose, the book provides an overview of current developments and approaches in co-design, in the application of design interventions – many of which are a result of co-design – and in policy and related standards in and for design and mental health.

Mental health and wellbeing and its opposite – mental ill-health (sometimes also referred to as ill-being) – have been highlighted by the COVID-19 pandemic. Before the pandemic, discussions of mental health were far less visible. They were broadly focused on mental health in the workplace and stigma, substance abuse, medication and therapy. Since the pandemic, which had a significant impact on people's overall health and wellbeing, the issue of mental health has been openly in the public eye. Existing topics have become emphasised and new issues have emerged, such as remote working and loneliness, telehealth and digital mental health, prevention and resilience, public awareness and stigma and government and policy responses. The pandemic has further highlighted the need for support for vulnerable populations, such as those affected by dementia, mental illness or neurodiversity as well as their care partners, friends and families – whether in their own homes, in public contexts or when seeking support from health and social care.

Especially the confinement to our homes and the increased need for self-care has drawn attention to the immediate environment we live in and to the services we receive face-to-face or remotely, and their design. This has put a spotlight on the design of our homes, how we live and interact with others, how we utilise our surrounding spaces and neighbourhoods, whether it is for shopping, exercise or socialising and has caused a flurry of innovations in these areas relating to analogue and digital services. For example, we have seen a rise in outdoor activities to enable socialising and exercise, and health care services suddenly moved from face-to-face provision to online consultations, expediting the development of e- and m-health services provision – all of which have to be designed. But we have also seen the failure of such developments, especially in care home provision with the isolation of people in care and how this has been detrimental, for example, and perhaps especially to people with dementia, for many of whom the isolation has hastened cognitive decline and caused profound loneliness and ill-health.

DOI: 10.4324/9781003318262-1

In response, many projects and initiatives have sprung up to provide help and support people's wellbeing. A common example was mask-making at the early stages of the pandemic where communities got together online to sew masks to help care services, but which also gave makers a sense of empowerment through being able to do something to help (Martindale et al., 2021; Schnittka, 2021). Also focused on volunteering, although not specifically in response to COVID, the IDoService project co-designed a volunteer service with and for people with early-stage dementia to help them re-focus and consider their aspirations after the diagnosis, stay socially connected and make a contribution to their community. In this way, the service helps to give people a sense of purpose and to feel valued (Tournier et al., 2023; Niedderer et al., 2023).

Such examples and experiences highlight the importance of emotional wellbeing and self-empowerment, social engagement and citizenship. They also raise questions about access and accessibility as well as ethical practice and managing power relationships. This book traces these issues through its triple focus on co-design, design interventions and policy through its three parts. Through exploration from these three perspectives, the book draws a multi-layered picture of the questions and issues raised, in an attempt to provide answers and guidance – to at least some of them – through discussions of collaborative designing, through examples of design interventions aimed at promoting mental health and wellbeing and through exploration of policy for guiding the development of wellbeing-related approaches for design.

The integration of design in the context of mental health and wellbeing positions our book firmly in inter-, cross- and trans-disciplinary areas of practice. As such, we work across different conventions and terminologies and cannot take their meaning for granted. We therefore start by explaining our position and key concepts. Throughout, the book takes a distinct focus on wellbeing, combining salutogenic, mindful and empathic approaches to designing for mental health, aimed at furthering wellbeing and preventive strategies. We believe design, including diverse creative approaches, is an essential – but still largely overlooked – approach to furthering mental health and wellbeing because of its key role in shaping our everyday living as well as the delivery of care, be this through traditional or digital means. This book seeks to demonstrate the significant role of design and the beneficial impact design can have in promoting wellbeing and mental health.

Understanding design as 'changing existing situations into preferred ones' (Simon, 1996, p. 111), we propose that design can be used to embed salutogenic, mindful and empathic approaches to enable and support wellbeing and mental health. In line with Simon's definition, we understand design here as a process which is essentially rooted in creative thinking and whose collaborative application – co-design – is increasingly being recognised and used in health and care contexts to facilitate better outcomes – and by extension wellbeing – through bottom-up change. This means that change is not imposed from above, but that the voice of those concerned – people with lived experience, such as people with dementia, carers and health care professionals – are involved in the development process and are therefore able to direct what problems need addressing and how solutions are developed to make them both relevant and fit for purpose. Furthermore, people's involvement in co-design, and in the related processes of co-creation or co-production, can promote wellbeing in itself (Zeilig et al., 2019) while at the same time helping to develop better interactions, services, products and environments to promote wellbeing through their use.

Wellbeing is a broad term, which has been defined from a number of different perspectives. We essentially adopt a view on wellbeing from positive psychology. Synthesising different key approaches, Niedderer et al. (2022a) have proposed wellbeing as being based on three main aspects and their interconnections, including emotional wellbeing, social wellbeing and (personal) agency. Emotional wellbeing is associated with safety/trust, comfort, feeling well, happiness and joy. Social engagement is related to inclusion, connectedness and attachment. Agency comprises identity, confidence, optimism, meaningful occupation, autonomy and growth. Niedderer et al. (2022a) further explain that positive emotional wellbeing beneficially influences the level and quality of social engagement and vice versa. Emotional wellbeing and social engagement are related to personal agency, defined as meaningful intentional action. The experience of having personal agency in one's life is an important determinant of wellbeing that can improve both confidence and optimism, with examples including learning, starting new activities or decision making (Zeilig et al., 2019).

The salutogenic focus on wellbeing inherent in this understanding derives from Antonovsky's original approach (1996), which is important because it shifts the focus from illness to health, from a focus on disease and risk to one of seeking solutions and quality of life. This focus aligns with our design approach and reflects design's contribution to care rather than medicine. The salutogenic approach is innate to design because of its focus on creating desirable situations and finding solutions. The salutogenic focus on wellbeing also offers the inclusion of empathy and compassion, especially through design's collaborative approach of co-design, which foregrounds working with users to understand and draw upon their personal experiences of, and feelings towards, situations, environments and the use of products or services. In this way, co-design can help to find solutions that are informed by real-world experiences of the people using or delivering a service or intervention, etc. to ensure that solutions meet the expectations, wishes and needs of the user group or, in other words, that any design solutions are relevant, appropriate and fit for purpose (Kouprie & Sleeswijk Visser, 2009; Treadaway et al., 2019).

One of the ways to achieve empathy, compassion and wellbeing, and to include them in design, is through mindful strategies. 'Mindfulness is the basic human ability to be fully present, aware of where we are and what we're doing' (Mindful, 2023). Both meditation-based and cognitive mindfulness include elements such as being in the present moment, non-judgemental acceptance of emotions and events and reflection on these to help engender new views and perspectives (Kabat-Zinn, 2003a, 2003b; Langer, 1989, 2010; Wells et al., 2013). Langer (1989) has shown that being in the present moment and developing new perspectives can improve physical and mental wellbeing. Being mindfully present in the here and now can provide an alternative road to selfhood through creating a sense of identity through sensory awareness. Developing new perspectives, both related to sensory and cognitive insights, can offer choice (Niedderer, 2014), which can afford agency in the sense of meaningful intentional action. A mindful approach is a key component of our salutogenic design approach to wellbeing because it helps to promote empathy, it provides strategies that enable new perspectives to re-envision self and one's context. Therefore, it enables us to see new solutions, and it provides ethical values that can guide our approach to co-design. A salutogenic design approach to wellbeing, incorporating mindfulness and empathy, can further promote resilience and quality of life in the face of adversity by offering approaches at all stages of life and in many everyday situations (e.g. Bethell et al., 2016). Positive emotions, engendered by these approaches, can encourage more reflective and creative thinking, having a broader perspective and, in turn, more flexible coping strategies, as a basis for resilience to adverse situations and conditions (Gloria & Steinhardt, 2016). Such approaches not only further resilience but can also be used preventively.

Our focus in this book is particularly on the wellbeing relating to mental health over the life span, including those with dementia, mental illness and people who identify as neurodivergent. The reason for bringing these three groups together in the discussions of this book – in what might easily be seen as too broad a brush – is twofold: firstly, due to their conditions, all three groups are regularly affected by mental ill-health (WHO, 2022). As a consequence, they share similar experiences and challenges relating to everyday life, health and social care, including the need for emotional support, social inclusion and self-empowerment, which can be facilitated through co-design and through the development of person-centred, psychosocial design-based interventions to provide tailored support. Secondly, design solutions are often inclusive and transferable between similar situations and needs. Therefore, solutions that can help promote wellbeing for one group may well be transferable to another. For example, when developing the *This is Me* game (Niedderer et al., 2022a), participants regularly commented on its potential use for other groups. While the game was developed to support people diagnosed with dementia to (re-)focus on their aspirations, suggestions were that the game could also be used for cancer or trauma survivors, or those with depression, who struggle with similar issues and could benefit from refocusing from their difficult experience onto their aspirations for the present and future.

Through its threefold focus and approach, this book addresses key national and international priorities regarding mental health and wellbeing for people affected by dementia and mental illness as well as those considering themselves neurodivergent, such as the UN Sustainable Development Goals 3 and 10 (United Nations, 2023), the WHO Mental Health Action Programme (WHO, 2021a), the WHO Dementia Plan (WHO, 2018) and A UK Framework for Mental Health Research (Department of Health, 2017).

Focus and terminology: mental health in the context of dementia, mental illness and neurodiversity

Focusing on mental health in relation to dementia, mental illness and neurodiversity, with its considerable breadth, we believe our focus and use of terminology need some explaining. As indicated above, our approach to mental health is strongly driven by our salutogenic design focus on wellbeing. In this vein, we understand mental health in line with the World Health Organisation's (WHO) definition as:

> a state of mental well-being that enables people to cope with the stresses of life, realize their abilities, learn well and work well, and contribute to their community. It is an integral component of health and well-being that underpins our individual and collective abilities to make decisions, build relationships and shape the world we live in. Mental health is a basic human right. And it is crucial to personal, community and socio-economic development. Mental health is more than the absence of mental disorders. It exists on a complex continuum, which is experienced differently from one person to the next, with varying degrees of difficulty and distress and potentially very different social and clinical outcomes.
>
> (WHO, 2022)

In relation to this definition of mental health (also termed mental wellbeing and used interchangeably here), we use the term mental ill-health to denote the absence and opposite of mental health and wellbeing. The WHO further explains that '[p]eople with mental health conditions are more likely to experience lower levels of mental well-being, but this is not always or necessarily the case' whereby '[m]ental health conditions include mental disorders and psychosocial disabilities as well as other mental states associated with significant distress, impairment in functioning, or risk of self-harm' (WHO, 2022). In addition to this definition, we here use the terms 'mental disorder' interchangeably with the term 'mental illness'.

Mental health and wellbeing are an essential foundation for all people, from childhood into old age, and a human right in many countries worldwide. This book therefore includes contributions relating to mental health and wellbeing across the life span. Furthermore, over the last decade or so, there has been a significant rise in cases of dementia and mental illness and an increased recognition of neurodiversity.

Neurodiversity describes the variation in the human experience of the world, in school, at work, and through social relationships. Driven by both genetic and environmental factors, an estimated 15-20 percent of the world's population exhibits some form of neurodivergence.
(National Cancer Institute, 2022; Doyle, 2020)

Dwyer (2022) reviews the discussions of neurodiversity in the aim to provide a balanced perspective. He finds that neurodiversity can be related to mental ill-health, especially where this is being hidden by people in an attempt to 'normalise' their condition. He concludes that 'the optimal neurodiversity approach should take a middle ground between the social and medical models' and that this approach considers 'disability as emerging from an interaction of individual and context', allowing 'interventions to either change individuals in limited ways (e.g. teaching skills, using medication to manage difficulties) or to change environments and societies' (p. 86).

In spite of this emerging distinction, neurodiverse conditions are still often counted under mental disorders, such as in the Global Burden of Disease (GBD) 2019 study. Mental disorders also affect people across the lifespan. Globally, 970 million people were diagnosed with a mental disorder in 2019, with anxiety and depression being the leading illnesses (GBD 2019 Mental Disorders Collaborators, 2022). The GBD 2019 further includes bipolar disorder, autism spectrum disorder, attention-deficit hyperactivity disorder and eating disorders, among others. The GBD 2019 showed that mental disorders remained among the top ten leading causes of burden worldwide, with no evidence of global reduction in the burden since 1990, and with an estimated global cost of US$5 trillion per year (Arias et al., 2022).

Anxiety and depression are also closely associated with dementia. Dementia arises from neurological degenerative disease, which predominantly, but not exclusively, affects older adults. About 55 million people are living with dementia worldwide, and this figure is expected to rise to 132 million by 2050 (World Health Organization, 2023). People living with different types of dementia experience similar symptoms, such as memory loss, language problems and mood change, which affect their wellbeing. With currently no medical cure, the focus is on care and quality of life, because people with dementia can live for more than 15 years after being diagnosed (Wolters et al., 2018). About 5% of cases of dementia have onset younger than age 65, and this can have an especially devastating effect upon individuals and their families (Ray & Dening, 2021).

These developments mean that there has been a growing demand for health and care services, which in turn feel under increasing pressure (Al-Haboubi & Oladimeji, 2022), and there is a need to provide cost-effective alleviation for these pressures. Non-pharmacological interventions, e.g. psychological or social approaches, are now usually recommended as a first line of response (Alcove, 2013). However, in health and care, much of mental health provision still relies on a medical model of disability and a predominantly pharmacological approach to treatment (Chapman, 2020). Therefore, one of the aims of this book is to foreground the benefits and effectiveness of non-pharmacological interventions and, in particular, through Part 2, to provide a snapshot of the increasing work relating to the development of psychosocial interventions in design. The Committee on Developing Evidence-Based Standards for Psychosocial Interventions for Mental Disorders et al. (2015) has arrived at the following definition, which we shall broadly follow here:

Psychosocial interventions for mental health [...] disorders are interpersonal or informational activities, techniques, or strategies that target biological, behavioral, cognitive, emotional, interpersonal, social, or environmental factors with the aim of improving health functioning and well-being.

Psychosocial interventions are predominantly used outside of stationary care to promote living well in the community. In this regard, in the context of dementia studies, Oyebode and Parveen (2019) observe a need for developing psychosocial interventions that focus less on controlling behaviours and more on wider aspects of life. They indicate the need for a more holistic approach to the development and evaluation of psychosocial interventions that includes a focus on human values, wellbeing and quality of life. They further suggest the need to provide solid theoretical foundations for such developments to connect the development and the evaluation of interventions and, by doing so, enhance their evidence-base and, ultimately, their effectiveness.

In addition to the theoretical evidence base, we propose that design development should be carried out with, rather than just for, people with mental health conditions to give people a voice in what support they feel is needed and what shape or form it should take. This proposition is based on an emerging body of co-design studies, which is largely overlooked by standard systematic reviews on interventions, a number of which are reported in this book. Next, we introduce the idea of design in more detail to explain its potential for supporting wellbeing.

The role of design in changing care

Today, it is widely recognised that design can have a significant impact on, and support for, people's mental health and wellbeing (Brankaert & Kenning, 2020; Crafts Council, 2021; Design Council, 2020; Malmberg et al., 2019; Niedderer et al., 2020; Tsekleves & Keady, 2021; WHO, 2021b). Design has a plethora of manifestations, including products, environments, interactions, services and systems and we shall refer to them here collectively as 'things'. Design also has a plethora of applications and uses in the health and care context. It can, for example, help with better wayfinding and care in hospitals for people with dementia (Löhr et al., 2019) or with creating relaxing spaces for children with autism in airports (Bellini, 2019), with developing technologies, devices or apps to support or self-administer mental health training or services (e.g. Brankaert & Kenning, 2020; Cittaro & Vianello, 2014), or with delivering and guiding interactions for mental health services (Neuhoff et al., 2022) to name just a few. This gives design a significant and powerful role.

Design has such an important role because it surrounds us in our daily life and affects all areas of it. While design can offer support in therapeutic and clinical contexts, importantly, it can also offer support in everyday contexts, including at home, at work and in the community, where the majority of people spend their time. In these contexts, design can help with emotional as well as social needs, or it can act as an enabler for prevention or self-care, giving people a choice of how to live their lives. Design has the capability to affect and offer support in any setting, any situation and at any stage of life because of its affordances.

Affordances were originally defined as the actionable properties and relationship between the world (thing) and an actor (person) (Gibson, 1977, 1979). Later they were refined and explained in the context of design as functional or perceptual affordances (Norman, 1990), i.e. as those that allow the user to action physical change, and those that are imagined or performative, both intended and unintended. For example, a pencil affords writing or drawing with it (functional, intended). But it can also be used to pin up someone's long hair (functional, unintended). It may also be given as a gift (perceptual, performative), or perhaps be used as a symbol for freedom of speech (perceptual, imaginative).

Affordances allow us to design things to affect people's emotions (Tromp et al, 2011), their social interactions (Ilstedt-Hjelm, 2003) and to create a sense of agency in that they allow us to take deliberate action through choice (Niedderer, 2014). This makes design a powerful tool, and therefore it has to be considered carefully to understand its consequences. Too often, design is used for commercial gain, to make things visually beautiful and hence attractive to a buyer, without considering the human or natural costs, such as pretty shoes manufactured cheaply that do not fit and deform the foot, or that do not last, and – when thrown away quickly – add to the mountain of waste and pollution. All aspects of design – its visual qualities (aesthetics), its emotional affordances, its social, cultural and societal aspects as well as its material and environmental impacts, among others – therefore have to be considered, especially when designing for mental health and wellbeing.

But back to the affective qualities of designing for people's wellbeing, especially emotions, social interactions and sense of agency. Being able to design for these qualities also means design is not a neutral agent. The affective qualities of designing for people's wellbeing mean that we need to consider the perspective and the in-the-moment experience of the end users. Hence, it is important to be aware of and acknowledge the values imbued in design and through design in people's lives. This is why the integration of relevant values, such as mindfulness and compassion, is important.

Besides design as things, design also encompasses the creative process by which such things are derived, by which affordances and values are embedded in things, and through which they are embedded in people's lives. The design process is therefore of utmost significance. The idea of the design process has changed over time from that of the individual genius who mysteriously develops novel ideas and devices – Leonardo da Vinci might arguably be one of the first – to an understanding that people who will use the designed outcome need to be involved to make the design relevant and fit for purpose (Sanders & Stappers, 2008). Earlier approaches, such as user-centred design, used focus groups to gain user feedback on the designers' developments, the Ford Focus being an example, whose name was derived from the focus group process then pioneered (Mnemonic AI, 2023).

Since then, the design process has developed greatly and the inclusion of all stakeholders in the development process is widely recognised. Due to its collaborative nature, it has aptly been called 'participatory design' or 'co-design' and was brought to prominence by Sanders and Stappers (2008). Over time and in different contexts, co-design has been understood in a number of different ways, and many approaches to co-design have developed, which is reflected in the discussions of this book. Niedderer et al. (2022b) have usefully defined co-design in this context as 'the methodological aspect of the collaborative and joint process of designing' (p. 3) and observe that it is important to include participant stakeholders from the beginning to ensure they are included in defining the design problem as well as developing a solution, and any decision-making along the way. This enables identifying relevant starting points and developing design suitable solutions (McDougall, 2012). A key related term is co-production, which we understand as facilitating the collaborative space that enables successful co-design. In addition, we use the term co-creation to refer to 'the active participation of end users in [the] different phases of the creation process in general' (Dening et al., 2020, p. 4).

By now, co-design has become an established process both for design generally and for healthcare design especially, because of its benefits to creating services that are fit for purpose. Co-design has also been recognised for the benefits it offers participants through involvement in the creative process. For example, co-design can enhance trust and empathy, as shown by Neuhoff et al. (2022) in a study with family caregivers of people with dementia using storytelling–focused co-design methods. Its inclusive and equalising approach, as well as respectful sharing of stories, can give people a voice and nurture trust, thus increasing confidence, agency and wellness (Zeilig et al., 2019). Rodgers (2018) echoes this with additional emphasis on the benefits of social engagement ('being part of something') and of the satisfaction of achieving something (pp. 11–12).

In addition, and complementarily to the bottom-up reformation of design through co-design, guidance through a top-level approach in the form of policy is also of importance to provide a high-level overview of interventions and to guard the quality of design outcomes. Policy can offer guidance here in providing the broader direction of travel as to where interventions may be needed, through promoting the use of co-design, or through incentivising certain changes. Policy in this regard can address and guide health and care as well as design. Therefore, we distinguish design policy from policy design: whereas design policy is policy concerning design, policy design refers here to the development of policy whether in design, health, care or any other area.

In addition to the high-level guidance through policy, and derivative of it, is the establishment of regulations and standards to guarantee the quality of design outcomes. This applies both to tangible outcomes, such as products, as well as intangible outcomes, such as interactions and services. Design generally has not been well regulated, and certainly much less so than, for example, healthcare or architecture where standards are required to avoid failures that may have fatal consequences. There are some regulations for design products, for example regarding health and safety (e.g. CE mark, European Commission, 2023a) and for repair and recycling (e.g. PolyCert Europe, 2023). There is also some (commercial) certification of services, for example with regard to accessibility in response to the European Accessibility Act (European Commission, 2023b) and regulations for the design of medical devices are increasingly present (EU MDR, 2021). However, some parts of design are still unregulated. While this is perhaps in the nature of design as a creative and ever-changing and developing field, there are some areas, such as user experience in terms of noise, light levels etc., where guidance through standards and regulation might be helpful or needed.

We propose that these three areas of design – its process (co-design), its outcomes in the form of design-based interventions and their application, and the guidance of design policy, standards and regulations – all have to come together to develop design for mental health and wellbeing. In addition, they need to be guided by the salutogenic values of wellbeing to effect a change in attitudes and facilitate effective implementation of novel approaches. Therefore, this volume, uniquely, looks at the values and principles which could, and should, guide the design for mental health and wellbeing, and the strategies needed to translate these values into practice. This is reflected in the three parts of the book: co-design, design interventions and policy.

The book

The book comprises three parts: it first discusses co-design and related concepts, including other participatory practices, underpinning ethics, issues around citizenship and power relationships within the process. The second part covers design interventions, many of which are the outcomes of such collaborative design processes, including issues relating to the evidence-based development of design interventions, their application and evaluating such interventions appropriately. The third part brings together voices from different audiences reflecting on the role and development of policy and standards relating to both mental health and design, discussing vision, advisory and regulatory considerations as key for the recognition of design and its regulation in mental health care contexts.

The three parts are framed by this introduction as well as a conclusion chapter that seeks to contextualise the contributions in the three parts and to draw out the overall insights and way forward for the field. Our review and conclusions are guided by our particular focus on the values, principles and practices that underpin our understanding of the co-design processes, development of design interventions and policy perspectives, and that we offer with this book to help develop a responsible and empathic approach for design for mental health and wellbeing. In this way, the book aims to provide a unique and holistic overview and resource for designers, researchers, policy providers and health and care professionals to help support the development and adoption of person-centred processes and interventions.

How the book was developed

Perhaps at this point, it is also useful to acknowledge where this book started and how it was developed. Essentially, the idea for this book arose from the work of the European-funded MinD project 'Designing for People with Dementia' (2016-2020),[1]which investigated the use of design for supporting people with early-stage dementia through design and mindfulness.

During the project, co-design and co-production processes were explored theoretically and in practice to understand better the ins and outs of the process in the dementia context and across different cultures. These processes were used to develop a number of design ideas and to progress them into design concepts and, finally, prototypes that could be tested. Along the way, issues around integrating the different approaches from the various disciplines arose, as well as questions around the ethics of participant involvement and evaluation tools. Exploration of these issues was later published in a series of scientific publications. In addition, the designs and design tools developed were made available as far as possible.[1] The insights and enthusiasm generated by the Mind project led key partners to stay together to progress the work through the MinD network and through this book.

Of course, along the way, changes happened. First of all, there was the insight that the MinD team could never possibly know and cover everything about the book's topic, and therefore we wanted this to be an edited book with an international, open call to reach out to like-minded people to contribute their knowledge and insights. Second, informed by the comments we received from participants during the project on the applicability of designs across different health conditions, and the overlap in cognate health and care service provision of dementia, mental illness and neurodiversity, we decided to broaden the book's scope to include these three areas.

Following the internationally publicised open call for extended abstracts in autumn 2021, complemented by invitation of some key contributors identified through the MinD project work, the editors reviewed all submissions and invited those most relevant for development into draft chapters. In line with our values, we made the development of chapters a collaborative process, and invited all contributors to participate in an online workshop to meet fellow contributors, and to introduce and discuss their proposals. The purpose was for contributors to get to know each other and their mutual contributions, and to get a sense of the context and community, to help everyone to develop their work with that knowledge of the other contributions to promote cohesion. Once full chapter drafts were submitted in spring 2022, chapters were peer reviewed by fellow contributors and by the editors. A second set of contributor workshops was held in summer 2022. All contributors received access to the other chapters, and they were invited to introduce their own chapter and comment on the other chapters in their section. The online meetings lasted two to three hours and were held across several time zones. The sessions were very fruitful, allowing contributors to connect and get insights into each other's work as well as feedback. Following the submissions of full draft chapters in autumn 2022, a rigorous editorial process commenced, reviewing chapters from both design and health perspectives, drawing on the dual expertise of the editorial team.

As a result of prior planning, and of the responses to our open call and invitations, the book was divided into three parts, on co-design, on design interventions and on policy. Within and across those three parts with their overarching themes, there are a number of further strands, which merit a mention: While Part 1 looks at the different approaches and applications of co-design, co-production, co-creation and other cognate terms, they appear across Parts 2 and 3 also in some form or shape from the lens of developing interventions and from a policy angle. The discussions around co-design raise underpinning queries and considerations regarding ethics, agency and citizenship; power relations and empowerment, ranging from the mode of involvement within and through the co-design process to how design evaluation and policy development could or should be informed by it. As indicated above, across the book, the chapters address three broad groups of people with lived experience, which includes people with dementia, people with mental illness (both young and severe), as well as a small number of chapters that are concerned with neurodiversity, especially autism. In addition, the chapters span different contexts, including interventions for the home, for public spaces, for care homes and for other health and care-related facilities. With those different contexts also come different design approaches and different types of design interventions. Case studies, which underpin many of the chapters, are therefore necessarily somewhat case-specific, but, together, provide an immensely valuable overview of examples of the developments and applications of design. Due to the complexity of the subject matter, there is also an overlap within the chapters of the three parts regarding the three main themes, and, as editors, we had to make a decision about what a chapter's main contribution is and, therefore, in which part to place it. Once those decisions were made, within the different parts, we have grouped chapters together led by the main theme, but mindful of these sub-themes, to ensure as clear a structure and flow for the reader as possible. Let's look at the different parts a little more closely.

Co-designing with people with lived experience

Part 1 of the book covers innovative co-design approaches, the values and principles underpinning them, complemented by a series of examples that demonstrate their application in practice. Co-design, co-production and other cognate approaches are increasingly recognised as essential tools for the involvement and empowerment of people in their own health and care decisions and the development of products and services supporting health and care. Part of this recognition is driven by developments regarding social and disability rights to foster wellbeing and equality in the community. This includes ethical considerations about who is involved, how, in what and when, about personhood, identity, self-value and empowerment within the context of, and to facilitate, social engagement, collaboration and partnership with a sense of equality, respect and trust. Frameworks and approaches which encompass these principles and values are explored with regard to different purposes, settings and applications. These, in turn, govern and have led to the development of core co-design processes for implementing co-design in practices, including available co-design toolkits, and which are demonstrated by a variety of examples of co-design practice across a range of settings.

Design interventions for mental health and wellbeing

Part 2 brings together an overview of how design can offer novel approaches and innovations in psychosocial and other non-pharmacological interventions to support people's wellbeing, health and care. These novel approaches include a range of applications including services and systems, analogue and digital products and environments. They can complement traditional approaches to support those living with dementia and mental illness as well as those offering support. Therefore, it is important to recognise that, for the development of interventions, the starting point should not be with a product but with identifying people's needs, wants, wishes, dreams and aspirations identified by, or jointly with, people through the co-design process at the beginning of any development. Furthermore, it is important that design interventions should be evidence-based in their development as well as their evaluation and that they should be informed by both people's experiences and relevant policy and legislation to ensure relevance, appropriateness as well as health and safety, but also to ensure that design interventions offer a delighting factor, which makes them an enjoyable experience to use. If we are to develop innovative design interventions using co-design processes, we need empathic designers and stakeholders who are competent in delivering co-design processes and developing people- and care-related interventions that are practical, safe, as well as delightful to use. This means we have to have approaches fit for equipping designers and everyone else involved in the design process with the relevant tools. This is even more important where people are involved who may have a vulnerability to be able to include them in the development, application and evaluation of design interventions.

Policy and regulations

Vision, advisory and regulatory considerations are an important factor in recognising and guiding the power of design and its application in the mental health and dementia care context. A key is to recognise the importance of design in support of people with dementia and their families in all aspects of their lives in order to incorporate relevant considerations in decision-making related to mental health and dementia. Part 3 explores the availability and accessibility of policy, guidance, regulations and specifications for the development of user-friendly designs in this context, and the work of relevant bodies in this regard. It explores the role and recognition of design in the mental health and care context and how specifications or standards may support the development of dementia/mental health-friendly products and services, taking into account such guidance and criteria within a compassionate co-design process. Associated with this is the exploration of the potential transferability and availability of designs for specific and wider user groups.

Contribution of this book

This book responds to the current state of health and care approaches by exploring and promoting holistic, salutogenic and preventive strategies that recognise and respond to people's needs, wants, wishes and rights to further health, wellbeing and equality, and design is a key factor in achieving this mission. The book therefore explores, and aims to offer insights into and guidance towards, using design to create a more responsible, mindful and empathic approach to supporting and empowering people with dementia, mental illness and neurodiversity and to support their mental health and wellbeing. This book adds to existing literature in several respects in that it draws out the universal and inclusive nature of design to address complex problems. In order to do so, it emphasises the potential of design to contribute to wellbeing and mental health, and it details recent research in and through co-design to illustrate how this can be done. No volume to date that we are aware of seeks to combine experience regarding the impact of design, especially co-design, with the broader field of mental health and wellbeing, and none of the works we have cited above applies theoretical constructs such as mindfulness to their area of interest, or embed current knowledge within policy, or address design regulatory frameworks to promote a salutogenic design approach to mental health and wellbeing. In this way, this book seeks to offer contemporary insights and guidance for designers and all stakeholders involved, including people with dementia, mental illness and those identifying as neurodivergent, their care partners, health and social care professionals, policy providers in design as well as health and social care, third-sector organisations, students in design, health and care and interested members of the public.

Note

1 MinD (2016-2020), a Horizon 2020 MSCA RISE project, GA 691001, www.designingfordementia.eu

References

Alcove. (2013). *The European joint action on dementia: Synthesis report 2013*. Alcove.
Al-Haboubi, Y., & Oladimeji, K. (2022). Awareness, loneliness, and demand for mental health services in the NHS. *BMJ, 377.* https://doi.org/10.1136/bmj.o1178
Antonovsky, A. (1996). The salutogenic model as a theory to guide health promotion. *Health Promotion International, 11*(1), 11–18.
Arias, D., Saxena, S., & Verguet, S. (2022). Quantifying the global burden of mental disorders and their economic value. *EClinicalmedicine, 54,* 101675. https://doi.org/10.1016/j. eclinm.2022.101675
Bellini, E. (2019). *Ambienti sensoriali terapeutici che rendano Abili: Un progetto integrato di vita per persone con Disturbi dello Spettro Autistico.* Firenze University Press. ISBN: 9788864539874 - http://digital.casalini.it/9788864539874
Bethell, C., Gombojav, N., Solloway, M., & Wissow, L. (2016). Adverse childhood experiences, resilience and mindfulness-based approaches: Common denominator issues for children with emotional, mental, or behavioral problems. *Child and Adolescent Psychiatric Clinics of North America, 25*(2), 139–156. https://doi.org/10.1016/j.chc.2015.12.001
Brankaert, R., & Kenning, G. (2020). *HCI and design in the context of dementia.* Springer.
Chapman, R. (2020). Neurodiversity, disability, wellbeing. In H. Bertilsdotter Rosqvist, N. Chown, & A. Stenning (Eds.), *Neurodiversity studies: A new critical paradigm* (pp. 57–72). Routledge.
Chittaro, L., & Vianello, A. (2014). Computer-supported mindfulness: Evaluation of a mobile thought distancing application on naive meditators. *International Journal of Human-Computer Studies, 72*(3), 337–348.
Crafts Council. (2021). *Craft and wellbeing.* Retrieved August 7, 2023, from https://www.craftscouncil .org.uk/topics/craft-and-wellbeing
Dening, T., Gosling, J., Craven, M., & Niedderer, K. (2020). *Guidelines for designing with and for people with dementia, MinD.* Retrieved August 7, 2023 https://designingfordementia.eu/wp-content/uploads /2020/02/Design-Guidelines-v3.pdf
Department of Health. (2017). *A framework for mental health research.* Retrieved August 7, 2023 https:// assets.publishing.service.gov.uk/government/uploads/system/uploads/attachment_data/file/665576/A _framework_for_mental_health_research.pdf
Design Council. (2020). *Design for health & wellbeing.* Retrieved August 7, 2023, from. https://www .designcouncil.org.uk/news-opinion/design-health-wellbeing
Doyle, N. (2020). Neurodiversity at work: A biopsychosocial model and the impact on working adults. *British Medical Bulletin.* https://doi.org/10.1093/bmb/ldaa021
Dwyer, P. (2022). The neurodiversity approach(es): What are they and what do they mean for researchers? *Human Development, 66*(2), 73–92. https://doi.org/10.1159/000523723
PolyCert Europe. (2023). *Certification schemes.* Retrieved August 7, 2023 https://www.polycerteurope.eu /certification-schemes
European Commission. (2023a). *CE marking.* Retrieved August 7, 2023, https://europa.eu/youreurope/ business/product-requirements/labels-markings/ce-marking/index_en.htm
European Commission. (2023b). *European accessibility act.* Retrieved August 7, 2023, http://www .inclusion-europe.eu/european-accessibility-act/
EU MDR. (2021). *The EU MDR entered into application on 26 May 2021.* Retrieved January 28, 2024, from https://eumdr.com
Mnemonic AI. (2023). *Ford's consumer-centric approach.* Retrieved August 7, 2023, https://mnemonic .ai/focus-groups/#:~:text=Ford%20Focus%20Success%3A%20The%20Ford,%2C%20fuel%20effic iency%2C%20and%20styling
GBD 2019 Mental Disorders Collaborators. (2022). Global, regional, and national burden of 12 mental disorders in 204 countries and territories, 1990–2019: A systematic analysis for the global

burden of disease study 2019. *The Lancet Psychiatry, 9*(2), 137–150. https://doi.org/10.1016/S2215 -0366(21)00395-3

Gibson, J. J. (1977). The theory of affordances. In R. E. Shaw & J. Bransford (Eds.), *Perceiving, acting, and knowing.* (pp. 67-82). Lawrence Erlbaum Associates.

Gibson, J. J. (1979). *The ecological approach to visual perception.* Houghton Mifflin.

Gloria, C. T., & Steinhardt, M. A. (2016). Relationships among positive emotions, coping, resilience and mental health. *Stress and Health, 32*(2), 145–156. https://doi.org/10.1002/smi.2589

Ilstedt-Hjelm, S. (2003). Research + design: The making of Brainball. *Interactions, 10*(1), 26–34. ACM Press.

Kabat-Zinn, J. (2003a). Mindfulness-based stress reduction (MBSR). *Constructivism in the Human Sciences, 8*(2), 73–83.

Kabat-Zinn, J. (2003b). Mindfulness-based interventions in context: Past, present, and future. *Clinical Psychology: Science and Practice, 10*(2), 144–156. https://doi.org/10.1093/clipsy.bpg016

Kouprie, M., & Sleeswijk Visser, F. (2009). A framework for empathy in design: Stepping into and out of the user's life. *Journal of Engineering Design, 20*(5), 437–448. https://doi.org/10.1080/09544820902875033

Langer, E. (1989). *Mindfulness.* Da Capo Press.

Langer, E. J. (2010). *Counterclockwise.* Hodder & Stoughton.

Löhr, M., Meißnest, B., & Volmar, B. (2019). *Menschen mit Demenz im Allgemeinkrankenhaus.* Kohlhammer Verlag.

Malmberg, L., Rodrigues, V., Lännerström, L., Wetter-Edman, K., Vink, J., & Holmlid, S. (2019). Service design as a transformational driver toward person-centered care in healthcare. In M. A. Pfannstiel & C. Rasche (Eds.), *Service design and service thinking in healthcare and hospital management.* Springer. https://doi.org/10.1007/978-3-030-00749-2_1

Martindale, A. K., Armstead, C., & McKinney, E. (2021). "I'm not a doctor, but I can sew a mask": The face mask home sewing movement as a means of control during the COVID-19 pandemic of 2020. *Craft Research, 12*(2), 205–222. https://doi.org/10.1386/crre_00050_1

Mindful. (2023). *Getting started with mindfulness.* Retrieved August 3, 2023, https://www.mindful.org/ meditation/mindfulness-getting-started/

National Cancer Institute. (2022, April 25). *Neurodiversity.* National Cancer Institute, Division of Cancer Epidemiology & Genetics. Retrieved August 4, 2023, from https://dceg.cancer.gov/about/ diversity-inclusion/inclusivity-minute/2022/neurodiversity#:~:text=Driven%20by%20both%20 genetic%20and,exhibits%20some%20form%20of%20neurodivergence.&text=Neurodivergent%20 conditions%2C%20including%20attention%20deficit,are%20overrepresented%20in%20STEM%20 fields

Neuhoff, R., Johansen, N. D., & Simeone, L. (2022). Story-centered co-creative methods: A means for relational service design and healthcare innovation. In M. A. Pfannstiel, N. Brehmer, & C. Rasche (Eds.), *Service design practices for healthcare innovation: Paradigms, principles, prospects* (pp. 1–18). Springer. https://doi.org/10.1007/978-3-030-87273-1_25

Niedderer, K., Harrison, D., Gosling, J., Craven, M., Blackler, A., Losada, R., & Cid, T. (2020). Working with experts with experience: Charting co-production and co-design in the development of HCI based design. In G. Kenning & R. Braenkert (Eds.), *HCI and design in the context of dementia* (pp. 303–320). Springer. https://doi.org/10.1007/978-3-030-32835-1_19

Niedderer, K., Holthoff-Detto, V., van Rompay, T. J. L., Karahanoğlu, A., Ludden, G. D. S., Almeida, R., Losada Durán, R., Bueno Aguado, Y., Lim, J. N. W., Smith, T., et al. (2022a). This is Me: Evaluation of a board game to promote social engagement, wellbeing and agency in people with dementia through mindful life-storytelling. *Journal of Aging Studies, 60*. https://doi.org/10.1016/j.jaging.2021.100995

Niedderer, K., Orton, L., & Tournier, I. (2022b). An overview of current practices and approaches to co-designing services with and for people with dementia towards developing a framework for best practice. In D. Lockton, S. Lenzi, P. Hekkert, A. Oak, J. Sádaba, & P. Lloyd (Eds.), *DRS2022: Bilbao, Spain.* DRS. https://doi.org/10.21606/drs.2022.463

Niedderer, K., Tournier, I., Orton, L., & Threlfall, S. (2023). I can do: Co-designing a service with and for people with dementia to engage with volunteering. *Social Sciences, 12*(6), 364. https://doi.org/10 .3390/socsci12060364

Niedderer, K. (2014). Mediating mindful social interactions through design. In C. T. Ngnoumen & E. Langer (Eds.), *The Wiley. Blackwell handbook of mindfulness* (Vol. 1, pp. 345–366). Wiley.

Norman, D. A. (1990). *The design of everyday things*. Doubleday.

Oyebode, J. R., & Parveen, S. (2019). Psychosocial interventions for people with dementia: An overview and commentary on recent developments. *Dementia, 18*(1), 8–35. https://doi.org/10.1177/1471301216656096

Ray, M., & Dening, T. (2021). Understanding the causes, symptoms and effects of young-onset dementia. *Nursing Standard, 36*(1), 43–50. https://pubmed.ncbi.nlm.nih.gov/33314810/

Rodgers, P. A. (2018). Co-designing with people living with dementia. *Co-Design, 14*, 188–202. https://doi.org/10.1080/15710882.2017.1282527

Sanders, E. B.-N., & Stappers, J. P. (2008). Co-creation and the new landscapes of design. *Co-Design, 4*, 5–18. https://doi.org/10.1080/15710880701875068

Schnittka, C. G. (2021). Older adults' philanthropic crafting of face masks during COVID-19. *Craft Research, 12*(2), 223–245. https://doi.org/10.1386/crre_00051_1

Simon, H. A. (1996). *The sciences of the artificial* (3rd ed.). MIT.

Tournier, I., Orton, L., Dening, T., Ahmed, A., Holthoff-Detto, V., & Niedderer, K. (2023). An investigation of the wishes, needs, opportunities and challenges of accessing meaningful activities for people living with mild to moderate dementia. *International Journal of Environmental Research and Public Health, 20*(7), 5358. https://doi.org/10.3390/ijerph20075358

Treadaway, C., Taylor, A., & Fennell, J. (2019). Compassionate design for dementia care. *International Journal of Design Creativity and Innovation, 7*(3), 144–157. https://doi.org/10.1080/21650349.2018.1501280

Tromp, N., Hekkert, P., & Verbeek, P. P. (2011). Design for socially responsible behaviour: A classification of influence based on intended user experience. *Design Issues, 27*(3), 3–19.

Tsekleves, E., & Keady, J. (2021). *Design for people living with dementia: Interactions and innovations*. Routledge.

United Nations. (2023). *The 17 goals*. Retrieved August 7, 2023, https://sdgs.un.org/goals

Wells, R. E., Yeh, G. Y., Kerr, C. E., Wolkin, J., Davis, R. B., Tan, Y., Spaeth, R., Wall, R. B., Walsh, J., Kaptchuk, T. J., Press, D., Phillips, R. S., & Kong, J. (2013). Meditation's impact on default mode network and hippocampus in mild cognitive impairment: A pilot study. *Neuroscience Letters*. https://doi.org/10.1016/j.neulet.2013.10.001

Wolters, F. J., Tinga, L. M., Dhana, K., Koudstaal, P. J., Hofman, A., Bos, D., Franco, O. H., & Ikram, M. A. (2018). Life expectancy with and without dementia: A population-based study of dementia burden and preventive potential. *American Journal of Epidemiology, 188*(2), 372–381. https://doi.org/10.1093/aje/kwy234

WHO. (2018). *Towards a dementia plan: A WHO guide*. Retrieved August 9, 2023, https://apps.who.int/iris/bitstream/handle/10665/272642/9789241514132-eng.pdf?ua=1

WHO. (2021a). *Mental health action plan 2013–2020*. Retrieved August 9, 2023, https://www.who.int/publications/i/item/9789241506021

WHO. (2021b). *WHO launches new platform for knowledge exchange on dementia*. Retrieved March 3, 2024, https://www.who.int/news/item/05-05-2021-who-launches-new-platform-for-knowledge-exchange-on-dementia

WHO. (2022). *Mental health*. Retrieved August 4, 2023, from https://www.who.int/news-room/fact-sheets/detail/mental-health-strengthening-our-response

World Health Organization. (2023, March 13). *Dementia*. Retrieved April 11, 2023, from https://www.who.int/news-room/fact-sheets/detail/dementia#:~:text=Key%20facts,nearly%2010%20million%20new%20cases

Zeilig, H., Tischler, V., van der Byl Williams, M., West, J., & Strohmaier, S. (2019). Co-creativity, well-being and agency: A case study analysis of a co-creative arts group for people with dementia. *Journal of Aging Studies, 49*, 16–24. https://doi.org/10.1016/j.jaging.2019.03.002

Part 1
Co-designing for wellbeing

Introduction

Co-designing with people with lived experience

Kristina Niedderer, Geke Ludden, Tom Dening and Vjera Holthoff-Detto

Setting the scene for Part 1

A recurring theme in health care, which many of us will have experienced, is that we are often treated based on assumptions about our capabilities. There are some common examples, and we use two anecdotes here to illustrate some core issues.

The first example relates to people with a presumed reduced mental capacity, such as those with a diagnosis of dementia, mental illness or similar. They are normally asked to bring a care partner, such as a relative or friend, to the diagnosis meeting. In this situation, it is very common that the doctor delivering the diagnosis does so speaking with eye contact to the care partner – rather than the person receiving the diagnosis – or that they ask questions about the person as if they weren't there. A similar behaviour can be observed, even where no reduced mental capacity is involved at all, just because a person is, for example, sitting in a wheelchair, perhaps because of some kind of leg injury. In the particular case of one of the editors, the medical assistant was handing the patient paperwork to the care partner pushing the wheelchair, even though they didn't have their hands free, instead of to the patient herself sitting in the wheelchair and who had both hands free with nothing else to do.

These two examples convey a certain attitude towards anyone labelled 'a patient', especially if there are certain mental or physical attributes present (mental illness, wheelchair), and reveal common underlying power relationships and inherent stigma. We suggest that it is important to challenge such attitudes in order to improve health and care services, and related interactions, products and environments. Design has a part to play in enabling people, reducing stigmatising behaviour and addressing power imbalances. Consequently, patients as well as all other stakeholders need to be involved in the process of designing change, and we can do this through co-design practices.

Sifting the terminology: PPI, co-production, co-creation, co-design and experts by experience

Within UK health and care services, involving target groups (patients, other stakeholders) to improve services has been part of policy since at least 1999, termed Patient and Public Involvement (PPI)[1] (Greenhalgh, 2009). PPI activities bring 'lay participants' and their accounts of lived experiences to the centre of health services development and delivery (Jones & Pietila, 2020), p. 809). The involvement of stakeholders in the development of health and care services has become common since, usually in a consultation and advisory function and closely related to co-production. In their critical review of co-production and participatory action research (PAR) approaches, Locock and Boaz (2019) explain that the origins of co-production 'are in community-based service planning and quality improvement' (Ostrom et al., 1978).

DOI: 10.4324/9781003318262-3

Despite these attempts to involve patients and the public in improving existing health and care services and a supportive policy context, involvement remains low and there are persistent calls 'to better involve patients and the public and to place them at the centre of healthcare' (Ocloo & Matthews, 2016, p. 626). They explain that uncertainty persists with the methodology and practical conduct as well as the evaluation of user involvement, especially 'how to involve and support a diversity of individuals, and in ways that allow them to work in partnership to genuinely influence decision-making' (p. 626). Their criticisms include that 'models of PPI are too narrow, and few organisations mention empowerment or address equality and diversity in their involvement strategies' (p. 626). In response, they call for 'the adoption of models and frameworks that enable power and decision-making to be shared more equitably with patients and the public in designing, planning and co-producing healthcare' (p. 626). This sentiment is echoed by Locock and Boaz (2019), raising the question of 'How can we avoid constructing people as vulnerable participants rather than partners, with agency?' (p. 416).

There have been attempts to address these issues for some time. To signify the value of lay participants and a change in power relations, the term 'expert by experience' has been introduced (McLaughlin, 2009). McLaughlin explains that the adoption of the term 'experts by experience' is an important reclassification of the social worker–service user relationship, as it, unlike 'service user', 'client', 'consumer' or 'customer' before it, makes a claim for a specialist knowledge base rooted in an individual's experience of using services (p. 1111). Jones and Pietilä (2020, p. 809) explain further that the experiences shared by participants should not be regarded as 'lay accounts' or 'ad hoc tales', but as valuable insights regarding specific issues or purposes, and this is certainly becoming more and more acknowledged today. In addition to PPI and co-production, a range of participatory action research (PAR) approaches (Locock & Boaz, 2019) have emerged over the last 15 to 20 years, developed by or adopted from the creative disciplines. Masterson et al. (2022, p. 980) have reviewed these different concepts, including co-production, co-creation and co-design, from a health and social care perspective. Their review highlights that even a single concept such as co-design is interpreted in different ways with different understandings and approaches. Drawing on Osborne et al. (2016), Locock and Boaz (2019, p. 414) define co-design 'as an active, voluntary process of producers and users working together to redesign individual services'. They propose that if co-design is underpinned by participatory action research methods, it has the potential to offer 'genuine involvement; a focus on understanding many perspectives; an iterative and investigatory style; and a commitment to changing things in the interest of those who have to live and work with the results' (p. 414). They propose that the distinguishing feature of all co-design processes is 'the way they can bring together multiple stakeholders, not just researchers and patients' (Locock & Boaz, 2019, p. 414). This is a useful understanding of co-design for this book and able to encompass the further interpretations used in the following chapters. In addition, we broadly understand the related term of co-production as facilitating the collaborative space that enables successful co-design. We use the term co-creation to refer to 'the active participation of end users in [the] different phases of the creation process in general' (Dening et al., 2020, p. 4).

Looking further into the concept of co-design, the dominant co-design approach used in health currently is experience-based co-design (EBCD) (Robert et al., 2015). EBCD is described by Robert et al. (2015) to include the following steps:

Setting up the project.
Gathering staff experiences through observation and in-depth interviews.
Gathering patient and carer experiences through 12 to 15 filmed narrative-based interviews

Bringing staff, patients and carers together to share their experiences of a service and identify their shared priorities for improvement, prompted by an edited 30-minute 'trigger' film of patient narratives.
Small groups of patients and staff work on the identified priorities (typically 4–6) over three or four months.
Celebration and review event.

(Robert et al., 2015, p. 1)

The key co-design approach in the field of design is rooted in Sanders and Stappers' work (2008, 2014), which involves users in the development process, including creative and decision-making processes from beginning to end. It is important to include participant stakeholders from the beginning to ensure they are included in defining the design problem as well as developing a solution, and any decision-making along the way. This enables identifying relevant starting points and developing suitable design solutions (McDougall, 2012; Niedderer et al., 2022). By comparison with EBCD, creative co-design approaches from design are much less structured than the clearly defined EBCD approach. While in principle following the same steps as EBCD, the tools of creative co-design are far more varied and far less prescriptive. Tools may include, for example, storytelling around objects to elicit experiences, storyboarding to elicit emotions, role-play to better understand existing situations or to try out potential future solutions (Wang et al., 2019). The key here is that the creative methods involved are not only used to elicit experiences and insights but to brainstorm, envisage and develop future solutions together with experts by experience. Therefore, while EBCD is close to the creative co-design approach by Sanders and Stappers (2008, 2014), EBCD focuses more on participants' experiences while creative co-design also includes a strong focus on creative processes to find solutions. We argue that this is essential for a salutogenic approach that aims to include full and equitable involvement but is also able to create the desired change.

One further point of discussion emerges from the review of collaborative frameworks by Greenhalgh et al. (2019) who have identified five categories of frameworks, including 'power-focused; priority-setting; study-focused; report-focused; and partnership-focused' (p. 785). They found that these frameworks were very specific to the individual groups developing them and therefore had limited transferability. Therefore, they propose that instead of a fixed framework, 'a menu of evidence-based resources which stakeholders can use to co-design their own frameworks' may be more useful (Greenhalgh et al., 2019, p. 785). This situation can certainly be seen in practice and is reflected in the chapters of this part of our book, which demonstrate cohesion in their aspirations of working with participants by experience, but which at the same time are drawing on specifically formulated co-design methodologies with their unique set of co-design approaches and tools.

The values and ethics of working together

Shifting the focus back onto the people involved in the process, we want to dwell a little more on the role and inclusion of experts by experience. Whether PPI, co-creation, co-production or co-design, the inclusion of experts by experience is by now very much recognised for all of them, although – as discussed above – the role might differ from consultation and advice at specific stages to full inclusion throughout research and development, including in creative and decision-making processes.

The increasing work with experts by experience has raised a number of issues relating to the working ethos and conduct within multi-stakeholder teams, such as the need to manage power-relations and to protect experts by experience who are seen by the state for one reason or another as 'vulnerable'. This has resulted in a plethora of legal frameworks and practices for protection, such as ethics frameworks, ethics applications, consent procedures, etc.

This leads back to our initial mention of the concept of mental capacity as applied to choice and decision-making, with many countries now having specific legislation in this area, e.g. the England and Wales Mental Capacity Act 2005 (Crown, 2024). There is a presumption that individuals, even if 'vulnerable', have the ability to make choices and agree to participate, and there is an obligation on others to try to overcome barriers that may interfere with capacity. Obvious examples of this are easy-read documents for people with limited literacy. Arguably, participation should be seen as a human right rather than a privilege dependent upon capacity (Cahill, 2018), but most law is not that progressive.

The focus on protection in itself has received criticism as being paternalistic, as often not fit for purpose, and as not recognising the agency of experts by experience. The focus is therefore on developing shared values, which are often unique to specific projects (Greenhalgh et al., 2019). Nevertheless, there are common denominators for such values, although with local interpretations and ways of putting them into practice to enable and empower all participants. Key values mentioned regularly include collaboration in the spirit of partnership, foregrounding the importance of a sense of equality, respect and trust to promote equitable involvement and collaboration (e.g. Dening et al., 2020; Page, 2022; Vargas et al., 2022). If the process is done well, it tends to produce a sense of empowerment and citizenship for all involved.

Another impact of successful involvement in co-design, or related approaches, is the wellbeing benefit for the individual from being involved in such processes. Not only do experts by experience have a lot to offer to society through their involvement, but this involvement in co-design or co-creation activities can in turn help people, for example with a diagnosis of dementia, to stay socially connected and build self-esteem (Rodgers, 2018; Zeilig et al., 2019). Successful involvement can directly promote aspects of wellbeing, such as social engagement (Zeilig et al., 2019) as well as helping 'to re-contextualise past experiences and support the rediscovery of skills and expertise, leading experts by experience to construct both professionalised and politicised identities' (Jones & Pietilä, 2020, p. 809).

Chapter overview

Together, the chapters in Part 1 explore co-design and related approaches and their key role for the creative involvement and empowerment of people in the development of their own health and care provision. The chapters examine the ethical and social values and principles underpinning collaborative creative practices theoretically, supported by a series of examples that demonstrate their application in practice across a range of settings.

As always when looking at the real world, there is significant complexity, and this part integrates multiple themes, which we have organised into five strands: as is to be expected, strand one covers the discussion and examples of co-design, co-production or co-creation in some form or shape, their different approaches and applications. The second strand considers the ethics of collaborating with experts with experience, including agency and citizenship as well as power relations and empowerment. The third strand concerns the application context: the two framing chapters – Chapter 2 and Chapter 8 – offer considerations within the dementia care context, whereas Chapters 3–7 focus on mental health and mental illness, covering young and severe mental illness, as well as mental health services, also embracing neurodiversity. Strand four concerns the different health and care contexts, including public and private providers, research and community projects as well as e-health provision. Strand five is the location contexts, covering examples from North America, Australia and Europe. This allows for an overview, comparison and integration of knowledge, views and approaches across these three continents.

The order of the chapters moves from the broader conceptual approaches and framework considerations relating to ethics, co-production and co-design towards methods and applications of co-design in specific design and arts contexts framed around situated case studies.

In Chapter 2, the first contribution in Part 1, colleagues from INTRAS in Spain offer a review by their own expert-by-experience group of ethics regulations and requirements. Their review reveals contradictions and tensions with the aims of inclusion, empowerment and equality of co-production approaches, leading them to offer a value framework for future work. In Chapter 3, Peng and colleagues from Australia follow on with a literature review of co-design models and frameworks in the context of youth mental health to develop and offer their own, overarching, integrated framework and model for co-design across design applications. In Chapter 4, Hepburn and colleagues explore and build co-design in action, focusing on the co-design in health spaces for The Brain and Mind Centre, Sydney, Australia. While the Centre covers all aspects of mental health, the work reported here has focused specifically on spaces for youth mental health, and hence youth groups as experts by experience. The insights from their project add another methodological building block to the arsenal of co-design, which this part of the book is developing, in that Hepburn and colleagues have identified and distinguished generative approaches from evidence-based approaches, with the latter relating to intentional co-design activity, as is common in planned design activity, whereas the former relates to emergent co-design activities, which might emerge from everyday life scenarios. This work re-affirms the importance of the creative and generative power of design.

With Chapter 5, we move towards more detailed case studies. Dekkers and colleagues from the Netherlands provide a set of 23 detailed co-design guidelines in the context of e-health for severe mental illness. Their guidelines are derived from a literature review, and their application is then illustrated through four case studies. In this way, Dekkers and colleagues provide a further layer of detail on what to consider and how to approach the co-design process. In Chapter 6, Illaregi offers an auto-ethnographic case study on the co-creation process in the context of mental health services provision in the UK. It foregrounds the voice of the designer, complemented by the voices of experts by experience involved in the creative processes of the study. This chapter offers an unusual and detailed collation of insights into the role of the co-designer-facilitator and the range of considerations, learning, self-doubt and breakthroughs in facilitating the process of co-design. In Chapter 7, Kenning and Bennett take us back to Australia with two case studies: one from The Big Anxiety festival reporting on co-creation with young people, especially from indigenous communities, to address high rates of youth suicide. The second is the exhibition 'Spaces Between People' that reports on the co-creation of two projects from the Melbourne festival – *We're just gonna call it all BPD* and *A Safer Place? Stories from the Emergency Department* – to promote engagement of the public with the lived experience of the healthcare system. Kenning and Bennett's work continues the thread from Illaregi's work of co-design, here in the form of 'psychosocial engagement design', which is conceived as a 'radically bottom up, emergent and responsive practice that entails the designer "letting go" rather than maintaining full control of design'. With Chapter 8 by Malinin and colleagues from the United States, we return to the focus on people with dementia. Their chapter illustrates the iterative collaborative development of the 'B Sharp' community performing arts music programme, which sought to expand the programme's access for people with dementia and their informal care partners. Through a grassroots co-design process, drawing on an empathy-focused human-centred design approach, the programme has been gradually expanded and its different parts evaluated with people with dementia and their care partners.

Summary

Looking over the collection of chapters brought together in the first part of this book, we can say that there are two key foci: co-creation for wellbeing and co-design for change. Co-creation for wellbeing acknowledges the positive impact on the individual and their wellbeing through involvement in the process, which promotes the three aspects of wellbeing: a sense of emotional wellbeing through social engagement and inclusion, due to the recognition of one's own abilities giving a heightened sense of self as well as of agency through being able to make a change towards 'a preferred situation' for oneself or for others. This includes the values introduced and developed through the co-production process, while co-design encapsulates the tangible change beyond one's own sense of wellbeing. This change can be functional, making things work better in practical ways to increase accessibility and usefulness. Or it can be cultural, changing perceptions and reducing stigma, for example, to increase inclusion through making provisions more appropriate and acceptable.

The current recognition of the value of co-design is based on a development over time, which creates a continuum that reaches from the traditional inclusion of participants as passive research subjects, to becoming advisors, to becoming active collaborators in the design process, the decision-making and even the research process overall. This change is based on the shift from seeing people as passive, whether as 'patients' or 'research subjects', to seeing them as active experts who hold valuable knowledge in their own right. An important part of this shift is the recognition of the importance of creating a balanced and equitable working relationship within the collaborative process. This needs to include the mutual valuing of all collaborators through building respect and trust, and through seeing each other's strengths to establish balanced power relationships. While this is the ideal scenario, the realisation of this scenario is yet to be achieved as many outstanding issues remain. The chapters collectively address these and seek to offer ways forward across the continuum of collaborative and co-design processes. They demonstrate how these issues can and need to be acknowledged and negotiated for each individual project while sharing a wider ethos.

Note

1 Or sometimes PPIE, including the term "engagement".

References

Cahill, S. (2018). *Dementia and human rights*. Policy Press.
Crown. (2024). *Mental capacity act 2005*. Retrieved January 29, 2024, from https://www.legislation.gov .uk/ukpga/2005/9/contents
Dening, T., Gosling, J., Craven, M., & Niedderer, K. (2020). Guidelines for designing with and for people with dementia. *Mind*. https://designingfordementia.eu/wp-content/uploads/2020/02/Design-Guidelines -v3.pdf
Greenhalgh, T. (2009). Patient and public involvement in chronic illness: Beyond the expert patient. *BMJ*, *338*, b49. https://doi.org/10.1136/bmj.b49
Greenhalgh, T., Hinton, L., Finlay, T., et al. (2019). Frameworks for supporting patient and public involvement in research: Systematic review and co-design pilot. *Health Expectations*, *22*(4), 785–801. https://doi.org/10.1111/hex.12888
Jones, M., & Pietilä, I. (2020). Personal perspectives on patient and public involvement – Stories about becoming and being an expert by experience. *Sociology of Health and Illness*, *42*(4), 809–824. https:// doi.org/10.1111/1467-9566.13064

Locock, L., & Boaz, A. (2019). Drawing straight lines along blurred boundaries: Qualitative research, patient and public involvement in medical research, co-production and co-design. *Evidence and Policy*, *15*(3), 409–421. https://doi.org/10.1332/174426419X15552999451313

Masterson, D., Areskoug Josefsson, K., Robert, G., Nylander, E., & Kjellström, S. (2022). Mapping definitions of co-production and co-design in health and social care: A systematic scoping review providing lessons for the future. *Health Expectations*, *25*(3), 902–913. https://doi.org/10.1111/hex.13470

McDougall, S. (2012). *Co-production, co-design and co-creation: What is the difference?* Retrieved October 22, 2023, from https://www.stakeholderdesign.com/co-production-versus-co-design-what-is-the-difference/

McLaughlin, H. (2009). What's in a name: 'client', 'patient', 'customer', 'consumer', 'expert by experience', 'service user' – What's Next? *British Journal of Social Work*, *39*(6), 1101–1117.

Niedderer, K., Orton, L., & Tournier, I. (2022). An overview of current practices and approaches to co-designing services with and for people with dementia towards developing a framework for best practice. In D. Lockton, S. Lenzi, P. Hekkert, A. Oak, J. Sádaba, & P. Lloyd (Eds.), *DRS2022: Bilbao*. DRS. https://doi.org/10.21606/drs.2022.463

Ocloo, J., & Matthews, R. (2016). From tokenism to empowerment: Progressing patient and public involvement in healthcare improvement. *BMJ Quality and Safety*, *25*(8), 626–632. https://doi.org/10.1136/bmjqs-2015-004839

Osborne, S., Radnor, Z., & Strokosch, K. (2016). Co-production and the co-creation of value in public services: A suitable case for treatment? *Public Management Review*, *18*(5), 639–653. http://doi.org/10.1080/14719037.2015.1111927

Ostrom, E., Parks, R. B., Whitaker, G. P., & Percy, S. L. (1978). The public service production process: A framework for analyzing police services. *Policy Studies Journal*, *7*(1), 381–389. https://doi.org/10.1111/j.1541-0072.1978.tb01782.x

Page, K. (2022). Ethics and the co-production of knowledge. *Public Health Research and Practice*, *32*(2). https://doi.org/10.17061/phrp3222213

Robert, G., Cornwell, J., Locock, L., Purushotham, A., Sturmey, G., & Gager, M. (2015). Patients and staff as codesigners of healthcare services. *BMJ*, *350*, g7714. https://doi.org/10.1136/bmj.g7714

Rodgers, P. A. (2018). Co-designing with people living with dementia. *CoDesign*, *14*(3), 188–202. https://doi.org/10.1080/15710882.2017.1282527

Sanders, E. B.-N., & Stappers, J. P. (2008). Co-creation and the new landscapes of design. *Co-Design*, *4*(1), 5–18. https://doi.org/10.1080/15710880701875068

Sanders, E. B.-N., & Stappers, P. J. (2014). Probes, toolkits and prototypes: Three approaches to making in codesigning. *CoDesign*, *10*(1), 5–14. https://doi.org/10.1080/15710882.2014.888183

Vargas, C., Whelan, J., Brimblecombe, J., & Allender, S. (2022). Co-creation, co-design and co-production for public health: A perspective on definitions and distinctions. *Public Health Research and Practice*, *32*(2). https://doi.org/10.17061/phrp322221

Wang, G., Marradi, C., Albayrak, A., & van der Cammen, T. J. M. (2019). Co-designing with people with dementia: A scoping review of involving people with dementia in design research. *Maturitas*, *127*, 55–63. https://doi.org/10.1016/j.maturitas.2019.06.003

Zeilig, H., Tischler, V., van der Byl Williams, M., West, J., & Strohmaier, S. (2019). Co-creativity, well-being and agency: A case study analysis of a co-creative arts group for people with dementia. *Journal of Aging Studies*, *49*, 16–24. https://doi.org/10.1016/j.jaging.2019.03.002

2 A moral compass for co-creation challenges involving experts by experience in research and innovation projects in mental health and wellbeing in later life

Raquel Losada Durán, Rosa Almeida and Teresa Orihuela

Introduction

In Europe, there has been a significant increase in the use of co-creative practices that encourage the involvement of users of care services, patients and citizens in the development and conduct of social and health Research and Innovation (R&I) in mental health and wellbeing in later life. Co-creative practices are understood in this chapter as processes where a designer and one or more communities of practice (Cattaneo, 2020) participate in creating new designer futures (Holmlid et al., 2015). The increase in the use of co-creation is reflected in the large number of projects concerning the design and development of innovative products, services and care processes in areas such as the promotion, self-management and prevention of, and intervention in, mental health issues in older adults. Likewise, other promising domains with regard to co-creation are active ageing, independent living and assisted-living supported by technology to improve the quality of life and wellbeing of those affected by mental illness, cognitive decline or other chronic diseases[1]. Nonetheless, despite the widespread use of the concept of 'co-creation', there is a 'need for models that lead to an effective integration of co-design and bottom-up co-creation initiatives for encouraging/stimulating scientific and technological advancement as the result of a synergic, inclusive cooperation among actors that usually work autonomously' (Deserti et al., 2021, p. v).

In order to achieve such an integration, and for co-creation to lead to this advancement in R&I in mental health and wellbeing in ageing, this chapter first examines the proposition that R&I constitute a moral and public good and that its development therefore requires reflection on the ethics of public participation and how to ensure genuine, full and impactful involvement. Second, it investigates the values attributed to co-creation as a moral compass for addressing some of the challenges inherent in this form of participation.

In the second part, the chapter illustrates these suppositions through an emic case study of the INTRAS Foundation's Group of Experts by Experience (EbE). It presents the content analysis of the verbal contributions from a co-creation session dedicated to the development of a code of conduct based on shared values to guide the future participation sessions in which this group is involved. The emic perspective studies phenomena from within a cultural context to understand their unique aspects (Pike, K. L. 1967; Fetvadjiev et al., 2015). In this case, the focus is on the individual representations and understandings of members of the EbE group in relation to the co-creation values, as they have experienced them in different R&I projects in which they have taken part. The common themes addressed in these projects have been the ageing process, coping with psychological distress, loss of autonomy, informal care and some difficult life experiences (e.g. loneliness). The extensive involvement of this group in R&I initiatives provides an *ex post facto* opportunity for investigating the lived experience of the values and ethics of co-creation and for determining its function as a moral compass in achieving genuine involvement.

DOI: 10.4324/9781003318262-4

At the end of the chapter, we contrast the results with findings from previous research. We outline the principles towards a code of conduct to guide co-creation practices to ensure the full and meaningful involvement of EbE, and we propose future avenues for research.

Research and innovation for the public good: investigating the ethical foundations for effective, genuine and full participation in research for mental health and wellbeing in later life

'Research has traditionally been seen as an extension of human knowledge and thus as a moral and public good' (Stahl, 2013, p.708). Recent history, however, shows how human knowledge and the growing power of technology can move away from the sphere of the common good and respect for people's dignity. Therefore, preventing risks and harmful outcomes of research, especially in the social and health field where vulnerable people are at stake, is a necessary first step, but it is also important to pay attention to the nature and quality of the process, particularly participation (Strand & Kaiser, 2015).

Following this understanding of R&I as a means for creating moral and public good, the participation of EbE takes on new importance for bringing greater relevance, representativeness and legitimacy to R&I, including those experiencing mental health issues. To safeguard the quality of the involvement process, it is necessary to examine the ethical and normative basis. We first approach this from a human rights perspective: Article 27 of the Declaration of Human Rights (United Nations General Assembly, 1948) states that 'Everyone has the right freely to participate in the cultural life of the community, to enjoy the arts and to share in scientific advancement and its benefits.' Furthermore, it states that 'Everyone has the right to the protection of the moral and material interests resulting from any scientific, literary or artistic production of which he is the author.' These two articles determine the right of the public to take active part in R&I, but they do not specify the nature of their role in participatory R&I activity, or the nature of the benefit.

Since R&I in mental health, wellbeing and ageing often involves people with disabilities, the Convention on the Rights of Persons with Disabilities (United Nations General Assembly, 2006) also needs to be examined. It refers effectively to the right to full and effective participation in society on equal terms with others. It refers to the concept of 'universal design' (Art. 2) understood as the design of products, environments, programmes and services that can be used by all people, to the greatest extent possible, without the need for adaptation or specialised design. However, the role that people with disabilities might have in the development of these designs, not only as consumers but also as active researchers or research participants, is not made explicit and needs investigation. The full participation of people with disabilities in all aspects of society arises from the general principles of the convention, but references to effective participation in R&I relating to the experiential knowledge of their disability are missing. The closest pronouncement is that of Article 30 referring to the right to participation in cultural life on equal terms with others, which includes the right to participate and to use 'their creative, artistic, and intellectual potential, not only for their own benefit but also for the enrichment of society' (United Nations General Assembly, 2006).

Moving beyond the recognition of the right to participation of all people in scientific activity, potential ethical challenges become evident when working with the public in R&I: inadequate allocation of time, tokenism, not considering issues such as diversity and inclusion (Pandya-Wood et al., 2017) as well as a lack of involvement in all the different phases of research (White, 2020). Therefore, it is essential to understand better how people with disabilities and functional diversity can be included equitably, even as active co-researchers.

Cortina makes this imperative clear by pointing out that 'there are experts in means, but the ends can only be determined by those affected by the implementation of a science, because they are the ones who know best what that good consists of' (Cortina, 1993, p. 260, as cited in Fernández-Beltrán et al., 2017, p. 1044). Therefore, the role of expert professionals is to give advice, but the decision should lie in the hands of those affected (O'Donnell & Entwistle 2004). This can be done by ensuring that older adults with cognitive impairment or mental health issues have access to active participation. But it is also essential to educate individuals about their responsibility when making decisions, especially those that affect humankind as a whole, such as health research or health policy decisions (Fernández-Beltrán et al., 2017, p. 1044).

Since Cortina's research, concepts such as Responsible Research and Innovation (RRI) have been gaining momentum and are moving towards a broader approach in innovation policy, focusing on the processes and products of innovation to achieve acceptable and desirable results (Stahl, 2013). RRI in Europe is defined as 'the joint work of social agents throughout the entire research and innovation process in order to align processes and their results more effectively with the values, needs and expectations of European society' (European Commission, 2015). It has been, since its earliest formulation about stakeholder participation, referencing the need for involving stakeholders in the development of solutions that benefit the common good (Sutcliffe, 2011). In response, the recent involvement of EbE is improving research quality and relevance by incorporating the unique perspectives that patients, service users and their carers can contribute (Brett et al., 2014).

The Rome Declaration on RRI in Europe (Italian Presidency of the Council of the European Union, 2014) called for the adoption by all European institutions, European Union Member States and their organisations, businesses and civil societies to place RRI as a central objective of all policies and activities, with the aim of including RRI principles in research and innovation programmes. According to the European Commission[2], RRI encompasses six fundamental principles, including first and foremost the broad involvement of society in the research process as well as ethical principles and respect for fundamental rights (Karner et al., 2016; ORBIT, 2023). European RRI is a general approach to R&I, but its emphasis on responding to society's values and expectations of integrating it into its research process clearly marks a direction that favours research which promotes the public good. It also provides an ethical reference point, covering aspects such as accountability, policy framework, participation and citizenship to provide the ethical basis for involving EbE in R&I in mental health and wellbeing in later life.

The Valencia School's model of Corporate Social Responsibility (CSR), which is based on dialogical ethics, provides a further pertinent framework for RRI by offering foundations of moral validity for its approach. Dialogical ethics makes it possible to link the development of more responsible research and innovation to stakeholder theory, so as to act in a responsive and respectful way to the legitimate interests of the people concerned (Sánchez Pachón, J. 2014). In dialogical ethics, the moral consensus is reached through critical and inclusive communication. Accordingly, R&I can be considered responsible if decisions on the acceptability and desirability of the process and its results have been reached by all those potentially affected in an open dialogue under equitable conditions of participation (Fernández-Beltrán et al., 2017).

The involvement of EbE is more frequent in public organisations, especially in the field of health and welfare, but companies also increasingly involve EbE in the R&I of future products or services because people who have experience of a health condition or disability can be very creative in finding solutions to the challenges presented by the environment relating to all aspects, including usability, aesthetics, emotional experience or application of designs. EbE involvement also promotes their social inclusion, equality and empowerment. Hiring EbE in research and development practices is an example of sustainability and corporate social responsibility (Jacobson, 2021).

However, as pointed out previously, the participation of EbE can sometimes unintentionally lead to a disregard for ethical principles and a violation of respect and dignity of individuals. Some common practices in research can jeopardise the physical and mental safety of participants or fail to promote real accessibility, such as allocating insufficient time and resources for public involvement, tokenistic participation, late involvement in the R&I process, not being present at the stage of defining the aims and designing the research, or not giving everyone an equal opportunity to participate. Further, unclear communication early on in the research, difficulties for participants to freely withdraw from participation, inappropriate or insensitive treatment of people, a lack of confidentiality and respect for privacy of participants as well as a lack of appreciation and recognition, among others, are practices that call into question a meaningful and ethical involvement (Pandya-Wood et al., 2017). It is, therefore, necessary to reflect on these aspects to establish ethical participation guidelines that allow the contribution by EbE to the R&I process to be valuable and meaningful and the R&I process to be respectful of the people who participate in it. This means understanding what the strengths and challenges of conducting participatory research with EbE are (Mann & Hung, 2019) and what 'good' looks like in practice (Liabo et al., 2020). In this sense, a possible way forward is to make explicit the values attributed to public involvement (PI) in general, and co-creation in R&I in particular, with the aim of managing possible tensions and of maximising the benefits for researchers and lay experts within research (Gradinger et al., 2015). Such values represent mutually shared considerations about how to interact with the environment and direct human behaviour in a way that is considered moral, thus providing a moral compass.

Co-creation in the field of mental health and wellbeing in later life: value-based participation as a moral compass in the face of public engagement challenges

The growing rise of co-creation as a tool for innovating with and for citizens is recognised by the European Commission as of crucial importance to ensure that the results and impacts of R&I are respectful and representative of society's values. This approach has been promoted across Horizon 2020 and Horizon Europe programmes respectively. Although co-creation does not constitute a pillar within the European RRI (European Commission, 2012), it falls under the concept of public involvement, referring to a set of participatory practices that place citizens, patients or service users at the centre of actions or interventions, ensuring their ability to decide and influence the future of Science and Technology. Within the values of RRI, social inclusion is implemented within and through participatory practices in line with the founding principles of the European Union, that trace back to the Treaty of Rome in 1957[3].

However, within social and health R&I, there is a lack of understanding of the dynamic and implications of such participation. This includes i) the criteria to decide whether participation is beneficial or not in a given context; ii) the rights, duties and roles of those who participate; iii) mechanisms of participation and the power relations between all stakeholders; iv) the impact and whether involvement is worth the effort; v) the relationship/tensions between the lived experience approach and the scientific and expert knowledge paradigm. These issues are largely influenced by the form and level of participation (White, 1996). For example, consulting the public, as a one-way form of transmitting knowledge, is not the same as a genuine co-creation that involves the sharing and co-production of knowledge (Smallman & Patel, 2018).

There are a number of empirical studies that have tried to address these issues in social and health research and in human services provision, especially in the UK and the Netherlands. They also report positive impacts and significant contributions of involvement (Brett et al.,

2014; Graaf et al., 2019; Gubrium, 2016; Mockford et al., 2012). Public and Patient Involvement (PPI) has become a key feature in the UK, helping to promote person-centred research (Pandya-Wood, 2017). The knowledge generated from such research can have an important influence on the development of health policies and services, which is why efforts have been made to involve diverse stakeholders in health-related research and decisions, engaging them from the very beginning, including the funding phase. Involving patients and users in this way helps to make research relevant and important for patients and service-user communities (O'Donnell & Entwistle, 2004) and gives it greater credibility.

Complementary conceptual frameworks of participation focus on experiential expertise, such as the lived experience movement, peer-to-peer support, experts by experience, lay experts, service users and carers involvement[4] (Castro et al., 2019; Mazanderani et al., 2020). Involvement of end-users or patients is seen as valuable and generates value in care, service evaluation, training and research (Parr, 2022) – value being defined here not only in economic terms, but also in ethical, welfare and social terms. The aforementioned studies provide evidence of the benefits of co-creation on an individual level, such as greater empowerment of the people involved, increased self-esteem, creation of meaning and personal legacy, greater significance and relevance of R&I including diversity, accessibility, usefulness, adoption, alignment with the values and priorities of a community, and on a social level, such as more inclusive, horizontal and destigmatising policies and contributions to related rights of participation, equality and inclusion. These benefits occur at different levels of research and for different stakeholders, including at micro-system level (patients and their family or social support network), meso-system level (professionals, service providers, policymakers) and macro-system level (policy, social impact) (Nickel et al., 2016).

Clarifying these values for research, both qualitative and quantitative, through collaborative reflection before starting co-participation in research helps to mitigate problems and reduce malpractice. The benefit of making explicit the underpinning values of co-creation for both research approaches lies in providing a moral compass, because 'acting in a way that is considered "moral" by the group, secures inclusion and elicits respect from others' (Ellemers & Toorn, 2015, p. 189). Gradinger et al. (2015) sought to ascertain these values to support the successful application of co-creation. They identified three overarching value systems, each containing five value clusters: i) normative values concerned with ethical and/or political issues including value clusters associated with empowerment; change/action; accountability, rights and ethics; ii) substantive values encompassing consequences of public involvement in research and effectiveness, such as quality/relevance, validity/reliability, representativeness/objectivity and generalisability of evidence and iii) process values relating to the realisation of participation, including equality/partnership, respect/trust, openness and honesty, independence and clarity (process) (Gradinger et al., 2015). Gradinger's values are used as a starting point and reference for comparison in the emic case study described in the next section, aimed at refining the ethics of co-creation.

An emic approach to understanding the values of Experts by Experience in Spain

Group of Experts by Experience (GEE) Foundation for Active Ageing

This is the first GEE established in the region of Castilla y León, and one of only three in Spain in the social-health field. It may also be the only one in Spain to date, which is aligned in its form and operation to the GEEs of the UK and Central Europe where this practice is more common. It was established under the auspices of INTRAS Foundation in 2016. It was created as a space for discussion and promotion of co-creation activities for a healthy life, mental health and active ageing in a framework of co-research and social innovation. The first sessions of the GEE explored the motivations that drive participation (Almeida, R. et al., 2020), and since then it has been collecting insights from participants.

From 2016 to 2023, more than 70 people with the following profiles have been part of the GEE for at least 18 months: i) older adults with mild cognitive impairment; ii) older adults with mild to moderate dementia; iii) older adults from active and healthy ageing programmes with subjective memory complaints and/or psychological distress; iv) adults and older adults in the role of family caregivers.

The group's research has made valuable contributions to numerous projects of scientific and technical excellence, such as the projects MinD (2016-2020), CAPTAIN (2017–2021), MOAI Labs (2021–2023) and Hosmartai (2021–2024). Likewise, in social projects such as MIND INCLUSION 2.0 (2018–2020), in innovation projects in terms of welfare policies such as PROCURA (2018-2021), or Integr@tención (2018–2021), and in projects aimed at the co-creation of innovative assisted technologies for independent living.

At present, the group consists of older adults who are concerned about unwanted loneliness and isolation, even if they have a good social network, and who have experienced subjective memory complaints with further concerns about memory loss with a special interest in preventive actions. More generally, they are interested in giving meaning to their lives and in an active search for mental, physical and social wellbeing.

Purpose, design and participation of the study

A review session was proposed (May 2022) about the participation in the Group of Experts by Experience up to the present to identify and characterise the different values associated with collaborative activities. This included the process of co-creating a code of conduct for improving the functioning of the group morally, relationally and productively (experiential knowledge contribution to ongoing research). From the current group of 14 GEE members invited to the session, eight participants attended, four women and four men, with an average age of 75 years (W=74.5; M=76.8).

Data collection and analysis

A content analysis was carried out of the meaning of the oral or written productions on values and judgements from this session with the GEE. An audio recording during the session ensured a confirmatory resource. Two researchers independently derived themes from the audio recording using a template with an initial coding frame, in which they recorded all value statements and judgements. They then proceeded to categorise the values in a structured Excel sheet for the creation of value clusters, which were organised according to the value system by Gradinger et al. (2015). The inter-rater agreement among observers was 95%. Gradinger et al's (2015) definitions, including their three-value systems structure, were used to facilitate the comparability of results: how values and beliefs act as guiding principles for attitudes and behaviours, for what is important and what is not important for each person.

Results

The results of the analysis were organised in a conceptual map to provide an overview of the relationships between value statements with elements of shared meaning. Following the coding, the number of times a certain keyword or convergent statement was mentioned was counted.

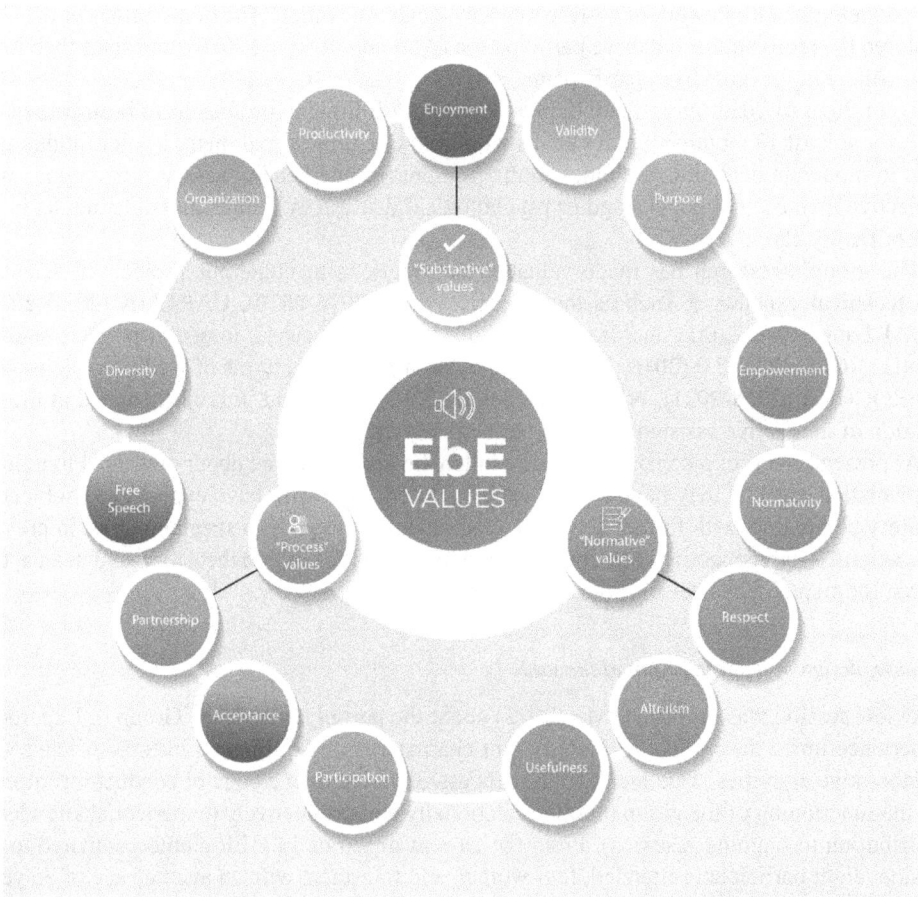

Figure 2.1 Data synthesis: mapping of the value-coding groups assigned to the three value systems

Individual and group value codings were identified according to the adopted value definition and these were grouped into clusters of related values as shown in Figure 2.1.

A summary of the values organised as normative values, substantive values and process values according to Gradinger et al. (2015) is presented in Table 2.1.

Although Gradinger et al. present a different grouping of values, these are closely related to our findings (respect for diversity and individual experience, openness, flexibility and compromise). With regard to the differences, it is worth highlighting that our study is based on participants' direct verbal production analysis, whilst Gradinger et al. considered public-involvement–related statements as expressed in scientific literature. Therefore, one of the main contributions of the present study is that it corroborates a significant part of the values constellation of Gradinger et al. through real co-creative participation, which offers promising grounds for further studies.

Comparing both studies regarding the normative value system, our results suggest that the EbE statements align, mainly in the importance given to, and understanding of, the value of 'empowerment'. Our study provides more concrete statements on rights and ethics, focusing on 'altruistic' actions and the importance of 'respect'. In a previous analysis of the group's motivations (Almeida et al., 2020), it has become evident that such values stem from motivational

Table 2.1 Value systems and value clusters

Normative value system: focused on moral, ethical and/or political concerns associated with PI in research.	*Substantive value system: focused on concerns about the consequences of PI in research.*	*Process value system: focused on concerns about the conduct of PI in research.*
Empowerment: Participants as informers of GEE actions, greater sense of ownership, leadership and boldness (user-led change). Focus on **positive communication**.	**Purpose:** Clear **purpose** of the group and its actions, with an incremental perspective towards even greater group autonomy. Results-focused thinking.	**Partnership:** Broad **connection** and **cohesion**, welcome in the group as a fundamental concern, and to act in the group as an engine to combat isolation.
Altruism: Focus on the common good/ solidarity, self-assigning a mission to be bridges to others for their **inclusion**.	**Productivity:** Evaluate through indicators of success for a sense of compliance. Perception of **independence** of institutions in terms of GEE output.	**Participation:** **Commitment** to attendance and frequency, **motivation** and **optimism** in participation.
Respect: Promotion of **tolerance** and **dialectics**, without judging or imposing criteria, avoiding prejudices and conflicts.	**Validity:** **Validity of results** including good communication of results, with a high perception of **experiential value**.	**Diversity:** **Heterogeneity** understood as complementarity, **openness** and perceived and encouraged **flexibility**.
Usefulness: Concern about the usefulness of their **contributions** and of the group activity in turning knowledge into action.	**Enjoyment:** Wellbeing resulting from participation, individual and group and increased **creativity** in dynamic and joyful environments with a balanced formula between co-creation and playful and social activities.	**Acceptance:** Acceptance and **understanding** of the richness of individual expectations and experiences.
Normativity: Consolidating the group's identity, creating a vision and values and guiding norms (marking the direction of the group) and promoting **exemplariness**.	**Organisation:** Clear but flexible roles (logistics facilitated by the guide, and participants perceived as equals), with a tendency towards accompanied self-management.	**Free speech:** Including **active listening**, an attitude of **empathy** and **trust** among members.

sources for participation, both intrinsic (esteem building, self-realisation, self-improvement) and extrinsic (the desire to contribute to the common good). The sense value of 'utility' is related to Gradinger et al.'s Change/Action value although it focuses on a more personal view of value. Similarly, our value of 'normativity' partly corresponds to that of 'accountability/trans-parency', although this has been assigned in Gradinger's review to the substantive value system.

In the substantive value system, the EbE statements highlighted the value of a 'clear pur-pose' as a group, connected to the value of 'productivity', which highlighted the importance of evaluation measures of success for that purpose. This is in line with, and complements, the values of efficiency, quality and relevance of Gradinger et al.'s review. The 'validity' referred to in both papers relates them through the sense of appropriateness and credibility, which in the Spanish EbE group was equated to the 'validity' of results and perceived experiential value. Two new values of 'enjoyment' and 'flexible organisation' emerged in this study. Related to enjoyment, participants highlighted how individual and collective participation in lively environments boosts wellbeing and creativity, blending co-creation with playful activities. With regard to organization, they emphasised the blend of clear yet adaptable roles in an environment where all participants are seen as equals, pointing towards a model of guided autonomy.

Finally, as far as the process value system is concerned, the EbE referred to the importance of 'ownership' as an encompassing aspect that promotes belonging to the group. This is reflected in the value of 'participation' as the behaviour they favour and the inclusion of which they want to improve as a group with regard to the values of 'diversity', 'acceptance' and 'freedom of expression'.

Conclusions and future avenues for research

Based on our results, the compass function of the values to overcome co-creation challenges in working with EbE's groups can be summarised as follows.

The respect for substantive values such as diversity, individual experience, flexibility and acceptance, freedom of expression, etc., is key to creating a space for safe relationships, such as a space that fosters valid *outcomes* and facilitates productivity; that favours equal relationships between all stakeholders, be they professionals or experts by experience, without harming anyone; and that allows for mutual exchange. Research organisations are in a position to facilitate the creation of these conditions through initiating activities or discussions within this framework of rights and duties of the parties. This has been shown to lead to a high level of motivation on the part of the participants, which in turn will lead to high-value results.

Group membership and participation are essential for intrinsic motivation. They must allow for personal growth and the construction of meaning in life. Moreover, a shift is noticeable in their relationship with the organisation's professionals (in this case INTRAS') arising from being endowed with the mission of being guides for the professionals. GEE members commented that life is 'a path with many stumbling blocks and I am excited to think that it can facilitate the paths for others' and 'we bring a multifaceted, holistic vision of reality that is incomplete without us'. They also take on a commitment to others: 'we have to make the mission of EbE known so that other people in need can participate'.

In terms of the relationship between expert knowledge and experiential knowledge, the group was very clear about the separation of roles and that its mission was 'to enlighten professionals [engineers, healthcare professionals] with our ideas', ideas that in their view 'are of high value' as the 'organisation entrusts us with a mission as brains'. EbE participants felt that the analysis and evaluation of their ideas by the organisation towards inclusion in their policy and practices had to be possible and should be promoted. Therefore, the resolution to the traditional tension between the two knowledge paradigms (expert vs. experiential knowledge), which this group contributes, is that EbEs inspire, stimulate, guide, discover and encourage serendipity, with a high degree of commitment and acceptance that they can be evaluated on their productivity, but with no desire to proto-professionalise, as this would be a perversion of their true value.

Norms must exist, and this EbE group has defined them as a framework for co-habitation between stakeholders whose meaning and significance is to act as a guarantee of interpersonal safe space. However, values adopted must not be universal but functional, belonging to the group that develops them and to the 'here and now'.

In understanding social behaviour in co-creation practices, emic and ethical perspectives cannot be clearly separated but must be understood in relation to each other. These are approaches that can be useful and complementary (Harris, 1976). This study has addressed the lack of studies taking an emic perspective with a view to reduce the tension between experiential and expert knowledge and to help overcome the challenges encountered by EbE groups. Future research from an emic perspective could help to understand the intentions, motivations, goals and attitudes, thoughts and feelings that derive from the environment, actions and experiences as EbE under the lens of the researched group.

It is evident that everyone has their personal and nuanced understanding of the co-creation experience since we all have our own subjectivity that leads to unique ways of making meaning. Combining individual meanings together for creative collective understandings can provide the 'wider picture', the ideal but reachable end of a process of collaboration that draws on different forms of knowledge, expertise and perspectives, guided by the moral compass of the principles and values that belong to the 'here and now' of each group. In this sense, it is extremely important to continue shaping legitimate practices that make the most of lived experience in research and innovation in mental health, wellbeing and later life, and to conduct research on the participatory journeys of EbEs to understand negative and positive influences of relational transactions that modulate inner experience (and vice versa) integral to their world, in order to make participatory processes more humane, more empathetic and more cohesive.

This brief study of the values associated with EbE activity marks the beginning of a line of research that seeks to co-create a code of conduct (moral compass) to improve the functioning of the group at an emotional, relational and productive level. The approach we have implemented suggests the analysis of individuals' values within an expert-by-experience group as a cornerstone for co-creation of ethical guidelines, since it is crucial to align individuals' values with normative, substantive and process co-creation values to promote adherence and consistent behaviour with these values. Taking it further, the importance of delving deeper into this approach can furnish an ethical bedrock to other recent works addressing normative guidelines or standards for engaging EbEs in participatory and co-creative approaches in R&I activities, such as the Gold Standards for Ethical Research (Deep, 2020), the Co-creation Guide (Fisher et al., 2022) and the Co-creating in Mental Health Toolkit (Mental Health Europe, 2023). Through illuminating the perspectives of the main actors, rather than a viewpoint solely anchored in the external vision of researchers or a strictly normative stance, our work seeks to offer an example of good practice in the process of establishing or bolstering the work of other EbEs. As suggested by our findings, designing an ethical framework and/or a code of conduct for EbE groups is intrinsically connected to an exploration of the inner world of participants and the myriad ways groups can foster mutual capacity-building endeavours, unlocking creative prospects and all-encompassing experiences that embrace the psychosocial facets of participation.

Acknowledgements

The emic approach to the values associated with the activity of the GEE established in Valladolid (Spain) with the support of INTRAS Foundation included the participation of eight members of the group in this research. We extend our thanks to the entire group and to the members who have collaborated as co-researchers since 2016 participating in this collaborative and highly participatory innovation space, focused on unlocking the value of lived experience in the processes of co-creation of innovation for health and social wellbeing.

Notes

1 The European Union Framework for Research and Innovation Horizon 2020 and Horizon Europe has
   funded a large number of projects in this area, such as: SCALINGS (2018–2021), COVAL (2018–
   2021), CASCADE (2021–2024), INDEMAND (2017–2020), INHERIT (2016–2019), VITALISE
   (2021–2024), MIND (2016–2020), CAPTAIN (2017–2020), and HOSMARTAI (2021–2024).
2 The main political entity and public funder of R&I on the European continent.
3 https://ec.europa.eu/archives/emu_history/documents/treaties/rometreaty2.pdf
4 These are as yet unstructured movements that seek to incorporate the knowledge of users or patients
   beyond professional expertise by involving them in co-research, to provide lay training on the experience of their condition, to provide peer support as expert patients or to evaluate and inspect the provision of care, etc.

References

Almeida, R., Losada, R., Bueno, Y., Bamidis, P., Petsani, D., Konstantinidis, E., Hopper, L., Carroll, J.,
   Gabriella, P., Kouyoumdjian, M., & Diaz-Orueta, U. (2020, October 20–22). *Value driven participation
   in co-creation of the virtual coach captain to support independent living at home*. 30th Alzheimer
   Europe Conference, Online Conference.
Brett, J., Staniszewska, S., Mockford, C., Herron-Marx, S., Hughes, J., Tysall, C., & Suleman, R. (2014).
   Mapping the impact of patient and public involvement on health and social care research: A systematic
   review. *Health Expectations: An International Journal of Public Participation in Health Care and
   Health Policy*, *17*(5), 637–650. https://doi.org/10.1111/j.1369-7625.2012.00795.x
CAPTAIN Project. (2023, August 3). *Coach assistant via projected interface*. Horizon, 2020, GA: 769830.
   https://www.captain-eu.org/
Castro, E. M., Van Regenmortel, T., Sermeus, W., & Vanhaecht, K. (2019). Patients' experiential
   knowledge and expertise in health care: A hybrid concept analysis. *Social Theory and Health*, *17*(3),
   307–330. https://doi.org/10.1057/s41285-018-0081-6
Cattaneo, C. (2020). Community of practices. In S. Idowu, R. Schmidpeter, N. Capaldi, L. Zu, M. Del
   Baldo, & R. Abreu (Eds.), *Encyclopedia of sustainable management*. Springer. https://doi.org/10.1007
   /978-3-030-02006-4_921-1
DEEP (2020). *The DEEP-ethics gold standards for dementia research*. https://www.dementiavoices.org
   .uk/wp-content/uploads/2020/07/The-DEEP-Ethics-Gold-Standards-for-Dementia-Research.pdf
Deserti, A., Real, M., & Schmittinger, F. (2021). *Co-creation for responsible research and innovation:
   Experimenting with design methods and tools*. Springer Series in Design and Innovation. https://doi.org
   /10.1007/978-3-030-78733-2.
Ellemers, N., & Van der Toorn, J. (2015). Groups as moral anchors. *Current Opinion in Psychology*, *6*,
   189–194. https://doi.org/10.1016/j.copsyc.2015.08.018
European Commission. (2012). *Responsible research and innovation: Europe's ability to respond to
   societal challenges*. Publications Office: Directorate-General for Research and Innovation. https://data
   .europa.eu/doi/10.2777/11739
European Commission. (2015). *Eco-Innovation at the heart of European policies*. Retrieved April 5, 2023,
   from https://green-business.ec.europa.eu/eco-innovation_en
Fernández-Beltrán, F., García-Marzá, D., Sanahuja Sanahuja, R., Andrés Martínez, A., & Barberá
   Forcadell, F. (2017). La gestión de la comunicación para el impulso de la Investigación e Innovación
   Responsables:propuesta de protocolo desde la ética dialógica. *Revista Latina de Comunicación Social*,
   71, 1040–1062. https://doi.org/10.4185/RLCS-2017-1207
Fetvadjiev, V. H., & van de Vijver, F. J. R. (2015). Measures of personality across cultures. In G. J. Boyle,
   D. H. Saklofske, & G. Matthews (Eds.), *Measures of personality and social psychological constructs*
   (pp. 752–776). Academic Press. https://doi.org/10.1016/B978-0-12-386915-9.00026-7
Fisher, T., Garley, C., & Morgan, N. (2022). *Dementia and co-creation*. Alzheimer's Society. https://www
   .alzheimers.org.uk/research/our-research/practical-guide-designing-products-services-people-affected
   -dementia

Graaff, M. B., Stoopendaal, A., & Leistikow, I. (2019). Transforming clients into experts-by-experience: A pilot in client participation in Dutch long-term elderly care homes inspectorate supervision. *Health Policy*, *123*(3), 275–280. https://doi.org/10.1016/j.healthpol.2018.11.006

Gradinger, F., Britten, N., Wyatt, K., Froggatt, K., Gibson, A., Jacoby, A., Lobban, F., Mayes, D., Snape, D., Rawcliffe, T., & Popay, J. (2015). Values associated with public involvement in health and social care research: A narrative review. *Health Expectations*, *18*(5), 661–675. https://doi.org/10.1111/hex.12158

Gubrium, J. F., Andreassen, P., & Solvang, P. (2016). *Reimagining the human service relationship.* Columbia University Press. https://doi.org/10.7312/gubr17152

Harris, M. (1976). History and significance of the emic/etic distinction. *Annual Review of Anthropology*, *5*(1), 329–350. https://doi.org/10.1146/annurev.an.05.100176.00155

Holmlid, S., Mattelmäki, T., Visser, F. S., & Vaajakallio, K. (2015). Co-creative practices in service innovation. In R. Agarwal, W. Selen, G. Roos, & R. Green (Eds.), *The handbook of service innovation.* Springer. https://doi.org/10.1007/978-1-4471-6590-3_25

HOSMARTAI. (2023 August 3). *Hospital smart development based on AI.* Horizon, 2020, GA: 101016834. https://www.hosmartai.eu/

INTEGR@TENCIÓN. (2023 August 3). *Cross-border platform for scaling-up innovative solutions for social and healthcare.* POCTEP, GA: 0675_INTEGRATENCION_2_E. http://www.integratencion.eu/

Italian Presidency of the Council of the European Union. (2014, November 21). *Rome declaration on responsible research and innovation in Europe, Rome, Italy.* https://digital-strategy.ec.europa.eu/en/library/rome-declaration-responsible-research-and-innovation-europe

Jacobson, S. (2021). Experts by experience as contributors to research and development in a corporate context. *Studies in Health Technology and Informatics*, *282*, 71–86. https://doi.org/10.3233/SHTI210386

Karner, S., Bajmócy, Z., Deblonde, M., Balázs, B., Pataki, G., Racovita, M., Snick, A., Thaler, A., & Wicher, M. (2016). RRI concepts, practices, barriers and potential levers. Deliverable D1.1, Ref. Ares(2016)6743323 - 01/12/2016. *FoTRRIS*. http://www.fotrris-h2020.eu

Liabo, K., Boddy, K., Bortoli, S., Irvine, J., Boult, H., Fredlund, M., Joseph, N., Bjornstad, G., & Morris, C. (2020). Public involvement in health research: What does 'good' look like in practice? *Research Involvement and Engagement*, *6*(11). https://doi.org/10.1186/s40900-020-0183-x

Mann, J., & Hung, L. (2019). Co-research with people living with dementia for change. *Action Research*, *17*(4), 573–590. https://doi.org/10.1177/1476750318787005

Mazanderani, F., Noorani, T., Dudhwala, F., & Kamwendo, Z. T. (2020). Knowledge, evidence, expertise? The epistemics of experience in contemporary healthcare. *Evidence and Policy*, *16*(2), 267–284. https://doi.org/10.1332/174426420X15808912561112

Mental Health Europe. (2023). *Toolkit: Co-creating in mental health.* Mental Health Europe. https://www.mhe-sme.org/wp-content/uploads/2023/05/MHE-Co-Creation-Toolkit-FINAL.pdf

MOAI Labs. (2021–2023). *Collective intelligence and social and health technology laboratories to combat isolation and loneliness of the elderly.* Interreg SUDOE–European Regional Development Fund (ERDF), GA: SOE4/P1/E1078. https://www.moailabs.eu/en/

MinD, (2016–2020). *Designing for people with dementia: Designing for mindful self-empowerment and social engagement, 2020, GA: 691001.* Retrieved July 31, 2023, from https://designingfordementia.eu/

MIND INCLUSION 2.0 (2018–2020), Erasmus KA. (2018). *1-IT02-KA204-048425.* https://www.mindinclusion.eu/

Mockford, C., Staniszewska, S., Griffiths, F., & Herron-Marx, S. (2012). The impact of patient and public involvement on UK NHS health care: A systematic review. *International Journal for Quality in Health Care*, *24*(1), 28–38. https://doi.org/10.1093/intqhc/mzr066r

Nickel, S., Trojan, A., & Kofahl, C. (2016). Involving self-help groups in health-care institutions: The patients' contribution to and their view of "self-help friendliness" as an approach to implement quality criteria of sustainable co-operation. *Health Expectations*, *20*(2). https://doi.org/10.1111/hex.12455

O'Donnell, M., & Entwistle, V. (2004). Consumer involvement in decisions about what health-related research is funded. *Health Policy*, *70*(3), 281–290. https://doi.org/10.1016/j.healthpol.2004.04.004

ORBIT. (2023). *The keys of responsible research and innovation*. De Montfort University. https://www .orbit-rri.org/resources/keys-of-rri/

Pandya-Wood, R., Barron, D. S., & Elliott, J. (2017). A framework for public involvement at the design stage of NHS health and social care research: Time to develop ethically conscious standards. *Research Involvement and Engagement*, *3*(1), 6. https://doi.org/10.1186/s40900-017-0058-y

Parr, S. (2022). 'Navigating' the value of lived experience in support work with multiply disadvantaged adults. *Journal of Social Policy: First View*, 1–18. https://doi.org/10.1017/S0047279421000921

Pike, K. L. (1967). Etic and emic standpoints for the description of behavior. In K. L. Pike (Ed.), *Language in relation to a unified theory of the structure of human behavior* (pp. 37–72). Mouton & Co. https:// doi.org/10.1037/14786-002

PROCURA. (2018–2021). Promotion of innovative public procurement policies for digital transformation and scaling-up, INTERREG SUDOE – European Regional Development Fund (ERDF), GA: SOE2/ P1/E0840. *Twitter*. https://twitter.com/PROCURA_innov

Sánchez Pachón, J. (2014). La Escuela de Valencia: Ética y Hermenéutica. *La Albolafia*, *2*. https://dialnet .unirioja.es/descarga/articulo/5135672.pdf

SCALINGS. (2018). *Scaling-up co-creation*. Horizon, 2020, GA 788359. Retrieved April 5, 2023, from https://scalings.eu/

Smallman, M., & Patel, T. (2018). *Co-design for society in science and innovation: Deliverable 1.1*. RRI Research Landscape. Retrieved September 5, 2023, from https://siscodeproject .eu /wp -content / uploads /2018 /11 /RRI -Research-Landscape D1 .1 .pdf

Stahl, B. C. (2013). Responsible research and innovation: The role of privacy in an emerging framework. *Science and Public Policy*, *40*(6), 708–716. https://doi.org/10.1093/scipol/sct067

Strand, R., & Kaiser, M. (2015). *Report on ethical issues raised by emerging sciences and technologies*. Report written for the Council of Europe. Committee on Bioethics. Retrieved May 16, 2023, from https://rm.coe.int/168030751d https://siscodeproject.eu/resources/

Sutcliffe, H. (2011). *A report on responsible research & innovation, matter*. http://www.apenetwork.it/ application/files/6815/9956/8160/2011_MATTER_HSutcliffe_ReportonRRI.pdf

United Nations General Assembly. (1948, December 10). *Universal declaration of human rights* (General Assembly resolution 217 A). Retrieved July 31, 2023, from https://www.un.org/en/about-us/universal -declaration-of-human-rights

United Nations General Assembly. (2006, December 13). *International convention on the rights of persons with disabilities. Sixty-first session of the general assembly by resolution A/RES/61/106*. Retrieved July 31, 2023, from https://www.ohchr.org/en/instruments-mechanisms/instruments/convention-rights -persons-disabilities

White, M. G. (2020). Why human subjects research protection is important. *Ochsner Journal*, *20*(1), 16– 33. https://doi.org/10.31486/toj.20.5012

White, S. (1996). Depoliticising development: The uses and abuses of participation. *Development in Practice*, *6*(1), 6–15. https://doi.org/10.1080/0961452961000157564

3 Co-design for sustainable youth mental health in Australia

*Madeline Zabar, Fanke Peng, Aaron Davis,
Christopher Kueh and Ian Gwilt*

Introduction

The COVID-19 pandemic has exacerbated the already significant issue of mental health among young people, in Australia and globally (AIHW, 2022). High rates of mental illness and low mental wellbeing, in concert with a limited supply of mental health services (Hall et al., 2019) and low help-seeking behaviours (Ben-David et al., 2017), can negatively impact young people as they navigate the transition from childhood to adulthood (Productivity Commission, 2020, p. 258). This is problematic, as the impacts of poor mental health and mental illness, particularly when compounded over time, can affect social, educational and economic development and outcomes (Bradshaw at al., 2014, p. 5; Keyes, 2002, p. 207), leading to, and often continuing, cycles of disadvantage (Bradshaw et al., 2014).

Co-design is a collaborative approach to design that promotes participation from different stakeholders to shape, respond and create solutions to identified problems (Wallace et al., 2021). The principles and practices of co-design are widely applied in healthcare service design as it provides a framework for embedding the patient voice into the process of developing and redesigning services and interventions (Chamberlain & Patridge, 2017). Co-design has the potential to positively improve the mental health system through collaborative, empathetically led research and design practices, and can help to reshape mental healthcare into a sustainable, patient-centric model that leads to better mental health outcomes. While co-design has been applied in the context of mental health, studies show the focus is largely on the adult population (Lal & Adair, 2014) or older adults, adults with intellectual disabilities, or children (Slattery et al., 2020). This identifies a gap in the literature for youth-specific approaches to design, particularly when considering the complex and dynamic experiences of young people, on top of the vulnerabilities of poor mental health. Creating a youth-friendly model for co-design research that amplifies voices and experiences from diverse, and often disempowered, perspectives will allow for greater insight, better design outcomes, and provide the scaffolding to shape meaningful and sustainable improvements to issues surrounding youth mental health.

The aim of this chapter is to explore the predominant themes, strengths and limitations of co-design studies in youth mental health. This is achieved through a review of the literature, followed by a qualitative analysis through a design thinking lens to identify opportunities to apply co-design in the Australian youth context to create a more patient-centric, salutogenic and sustainable system. Based on this analysis, a model of co-design for youth mental health challenges in Australia is proposed.

A sustainable approach to mental health

Mental health is a complex, multifaceted phenomenon that operates across a continuum. The World Health Organisation (WHO) defines good mental health as:

DOI: 10.4324/9781003318262-5

a state of mental well-being that enables people to cope with the stresses of life, realize their abilities, learn well and work well, and contribute to their community. It is an integral component of health and well-being that underpins our individual and collective abilities to make decisions, build relationships and shape the world we live in.

(WHO, 2022)

This definition is closely aligned with the WHO's definition of good health set out in the preamble of the *Constitution of the World Health Organization*, which is described as 'a state of complete physical, mental and social wellbeing, and not merely the absence of disease or infirmity' (WHO, 1946).

Mental illness is a broad term that refers to a spectrum of conditions and disorders ranging from stress and worry through to clinically diagnosed illnesses such as depression, anxiety disorders, behavioural and aggressive disorders, psychosis and substance abuse (Bradshaw et al., 2014). In the case of Australian youth, the most common mental illnesses are anxiety disorders, depressive disorders and substance abuse (AIHW, 2020, p. 150).

To build on this, the WHO differentiates mental health and mental illness, stating:

Mental health is more than the absence of mental disorders. It exists on a complex continuum, which is experienced differently from one person to the next, with varying degrees of difficulty and distress and potentially very different social and clinical outcomes.

(WHO, 2022)

It is important to highlight the distinction between mental health and mental illness, as mental health is more than being without mental illness. This broader perspective of mental health aligns with Keyes' model (2002) where mental health is marked by effective psychological and social functioning. The model takes a salutogenic orientation (Mjøsund, 2021), which contrasts the traditional pathogenic approach to health and instead focuses on the origin of health and health promotion (Antonovsky, 1996). In Keyes' model of mental health, flourishing is seen as the pinnacle of good mental health (Mjøsund, 2021), which is defined as high subjective wellbeing and positive functioning. Keyes articulates this through the *two continua model*, which defines mental health and illness as two related yet distinct phenomena. Under the *two continua model*, it is possible to enjoy good mental health with mental illness and similarly experience poor mental health without an illness (Westerhof & Keyes, 2010). By separating mental health and mental illness, the perspective opens the door to a more holistic approach to mental health care and personal recovery. To expand on the relationship between mental health and illness, there is consistent longitudinal evidence highlighting that high levels of mental wellbeing reduce the risk of mental illness and disorder (Bohlmeijer & Westerhof, 2021). Wellbeing is here defined as a construct made up of five elements: positive emotion, engagement, meaning, positive relationships and accomplishment, culminating in the ultimate goal of human flourishing (Seligman, 2011, pp. 14–20). People with low psychological wellbeing are seven times more likely to have clinical depression later in life. In contrast, high levels of mental wellbeing reduce the emergence of mood disorders by 28% and anxiety disorders by 53% (Bohlmeijer & Westerhof, 2021, p. 163).

Bohlmeijer and Westerhof (2021) have developed a model for sustainable mental health that articulates the interconnected nature of psychopathology and wellbeing. Their approach highlights the importance of mental illness reduction and a greater presence of mental wellbeing when determining intervention success. This offers great potential in moving towards a more balanced, heuristic and salutogenic approach to mental healthcare, which promotes both positive physiological and psychological outcomes and greater long-term wellbeing (Bohlmeijer & Westerhof, 2021).

Mental health in Australia

Almost half of all Australians experience mental illness in their lifetime (Productivity Commission, 2020), with 75% of illnesses emerging before the age of 25 (Hall et al., 2019, p. 7). Recent studies have identified that 25% of young people aged 15 to 19 experience mental illness in any given year (Hall et al., 2019, p. 7) and more than two thirds of young Australians aged 15 to 24 have struggled with their mental health at some point in their lives (Shipley & Stubley, 2018, p. 13).

Improving and upholding the mental health of citizens has been a point of focus for the Australian Government over the past decade. In 2019–20, the Government spent $11 billion on mental health-related expenditure (AIHW, 2022), which largely focused on subsidised access to psychologists and psychiatrists. In spite of this focus on professional support, as many as two thirds of young people with mental illness do not seek professional help for their conditions (Ben-David et al., 2017, p. 85), and Allen and McKenzie (2015, p. 82) suggest that people wait until later in life to access support.

When it comes to mental health, the research suggests that young people have low treatment and retention rates. Scholten and Granic (2019, p. 1) report that between 64% and 87% of mental illness in youth is undetected or untreated. This is supported by research (Shipley & Stubley, 2018, p. 13), which found that only 29% of young people with mental health challenges sought professional help. While the low uptake of professional support among youth is concerning, so too are the low rates of adherence to, and retention of, professional care. When young people do seek support, the availability of appropriate assistance is limited (Allen & McKenzie, 2015, p. 85). Further, one study found that 45% of patients dropped out of therapy after a month, and another discovered that the retention rate of treatment after three months was as low as 9% (Montague et al., 2015, p. 1). Young people seeking help are therefore likely not to receive an adequate amount of treatment to see meaningful change (Jorm, 2019, p. 1060).

Allen and McKenzie (2015) investigated why help-seeking among Australian youth is so limited. They identified multiple factors that impede help-seeking behaviours, which include embarrassment, low confidence, a lack of mental health literacy and emotional competence, confidentiality concerns, affordability, lack of knowledge of where to find help and a lack of accessibility. Concerningly, the study showed that, in the context of diagnosed mental illness, the more severe an illness is, the less likely the individual is to seek help, despite early intervention being a factor in limiting instances of relapse and recurrence.

As highlighted, mental health is a complex phenomenon that impacts, and is impacted by, diverse and interconnected factors. Poor mental health may limit education and employment opportunities and pathways, diminish social abilities and relationships, increase stigma and lead to a cycle of disadvantage and ill-health (McGorry, 2017, p. 101). Without early and successful intervention, the burden of illness and ill-health can be felt across a lifetime. While there has been significant investment, the current system is not able adequately *to* support, improve and sustain better mental health outcomes for Australian youth. The integration of genuine, authentic and youth-specific co-design as a people-centric approach to understanding complexity in youth mental health may provide an opportunity to reshape the mental health ecosystem so that the system better supports the wellbeing of young Australians.

Co-design for youth mental health

Emergence of co-design in design research

Over the past decade, there has been a growing body of research demonstrating the benefits of the use of co-design within research to improve aspects of mental health and wellbeing (e.g. Mulvale et al., 2019; Orygen: The National Centre of Excellence in Youth Mental Health, 2019). The concept of co-design has links to the Participatory Design movement of the 1970s, centering on people coming together to discuss ideas and generate solutions collectively and collaboratively (Davis et al., 2021, pp. 124–125). Importantly, in designing services and interventions, co-design recognises the role of the designer as a facilitator and partner in the development process (Sanders & Stappers, 2008), seeking to uncover and explore participants' real-world experiences of issues, rather than relying on the designer's external expertise to deliver a top-down approach to innovation (Cockbill et al., 2019).

Although there are varying degrees to which participants are engaged in co-design processes, there is a general ambition to establish a genuine partnership with participants (Hagen et al., 2012). When working in large and complex systems, such as in service design, this commonly includes a variety of different approaches, practices, techniques and stakeholders. This comprises traditional research methods, such as surveys and interviews, to determine touch points and barriers, followed by co-design workshops for ideation and solution design (Cooper et al., 2016; Mulvale et al., 2019). The spectrum of approaches is broad, including, for example, metaphor development, storytelling, personas through empathy mapping, and card-sorting activities to enable meaningful engagement with specific demographics, particularly those with complex health challenges, such as mental illness (Nakarada-Kordic, 2017, p. 229).

An important part of understanding and applying co-design as a process is working with co-design as both a methodology and a set of methods. There is significant flexibility and diversity of methods that can be included within the overarching co-design methodology. This allows researchers to select or develop methods for engagement that are built around the unique requirements of stakeholder groups and proposed project outcomes, rather than being driven by a predetermined formula. This is particularly important when working with vulnerable cohorts, such as young people and those with mental health challenges, as the design methodology can specifically distribute power to enable more meaningful and genuine partnerships with service users (Hagen et al., 2012, p. 6).

Recent developments in co-design have seen the expansion of focus from generating products and tangible or short-term solutions, to longer-term strategies of cultivating positive transformation in social and systemic settings. Deserti et al. (2019) call for co-design in social innovation to focus on the iteration of systemic shifts. Chamberlain and Partridge (2017) encourage designers to approach co-design as the means to generate cultural shifts in healthcare practice. It is critical to understand that highly complex and wicked problems – that is, problems that are unique, have no definitive formulation, and are a symptom of higher order problems (Buchanan, 1992, p. 16) – cannot be solved; they can only be explored through experiments and transformation (Medley & Kueh, 2015). This shift in co-design practice that focuses on transformation is important to youth mental health because challenges that involve social and healthcare systems can be highly complex.

Rationale for co-design

The rationale for drawing on co-design methods for research and design in the mental health context is threefold. Firstly, Hagen et al. (2012) argue that empathetically led research that understands how people act within the specific context will lead to better solutions and greater impact. When the true issues are defined, new understandings and solutions emerge, and credibility is built from the beginning though thoughtful collaboration. Second, participatory design practices can effectively engage with young people and other stakeholders, increasing the likelihood of solution uptake. The methods and tools used throughout the co-design process aim to create shared language, surface tensions and build consensus across different stakeholder groups, with artefacts able to relay abstract and complex concepts in a tangible way to facilitate more robust discussion and idea generation. Third, committing to co-design affirms young peoples' rights in determining their wellbeing journey and participating actively in their care, redistributing power to build more equitable relationships between service-users and service-providers (Hagen et al., 2012, p. 6). This is of particular importance in the mental health space, as the system is traditionally paternalistic in nature (Chamberlin, 2005), with practitioners balancing client autonomy, empowerment and ethics, with duty of care responsibilities, treatment provision and coercion (Jorgensen et al., 2018, p. 1359; Valenti et al., 2015, p1305). Co-design moves the conversation from design 'for' people to design 'with' people (Nakarada-Kordic, 2017, p. 239), which is of significance in the research space, moving traditional 'subjects' to active 'partners' in research and design (Pinfold et al., 2015; Szebeko & Tan, 2010). This promotes meaningful collaboration in service design and delivery, which has the potential to create better, more inclusive solutions that truly empower young people to actively engage in their recovery and healing.

Co-design for youth mental health

When considering the co-design literature, four key concepts emerge with the potential to support and improve youth-specific mental health research. These are: the Young and Well Cooperative Research Centre (YWCRC) co-design framework, experienced-based co-design (EBCD), creative co-design methods and 'low contact co-design' (LCCD).

Australia's YWCRC partners with young people, researchers, practitioners and innovators to explore how technology can improve the mental health and wellbeing of Australian youth. The YWCRC published a framework (the Framework; Hagen et al., 2012) to support collaboration with young people and stakeholders to enable meaningful participatory design. The Framework is focused on the design of interventions, identifying which level of stakeholder involvement is appropriate based on the chosen method. The Framework stipulates three levels of collaboration – 'generate', 'check' and 'listen' – which are assigned to co-design methods to support researchers and designers develop studies that effectively engage with young people. For example, co-design workshops are a space for young people to 'generate' and 'check' concepts, scenarios and prototypes. In contrast, interviews and surveys are methods largely for researchers to 'listen' and recall (Hagen et al., 2012, pp. 11–12). This framework has been successfully utilised, with Realple et al. (2019) drawing on the Framework to design a virtual world for social cognition therapy, and ReachOut Australia[1] redesigning their service offering to better support young people with mental health challenges online (Hagen et al., 2012, p. 19). When applying the Framework, Realpe et al. (2019, p. 37) noted that the genuine partnership with young people was integral to the creation and generation of meaningful, innovative design solutions. Furthermore, the creation of artefacts, such as personas, scenario mapping and user journeys, supports the participation of young people while also facilitating and evaluating user insights throughout the studies (Hagen et al., 2012, p. 19). The Framework offers a practical, flexible guide to research design to support meaningful collaboration and creation with young people and stakeholders.

EBCD is a subset of co-design with theoretical foundations in participatory action research, narrative theory, learning theory and design thinking. Its methodology focuses on equitable collaboration with service users throughout the research and design process, informed by personal narratives and subjective experiences to consider the perspectives of others to co-design and co-create service improvements (Mulvale et al., 2019). EBCD has emerged as an effective co-design methodology that specifically targets the interaction between service users and services, through a focus on experiences and is used in healthcare research. Researchers attribute the emergence of EBCD in part to the paradigm shift toward patient-centred care and the demonstrated positive relationship between patient involvement, satisfaction and empowerment in service users that experience severe and ongoing health challenges (Cooper et al., 2016). The core characteristics of EBCD are:

1. Involve users and professionals throughout the design process as co-designers of services.
2. Focus on service experiences as a whole rather than user satisfaction.
3. Focus on designing improved experiences, not merely processes, systems or the built environment, by identifying the touch points, or the polarizing moments when experiences are powerfully shaped.
4. Use analytic frameworks to understand user experiences within their context.
5. Focus on improving the interface between the user and service by interpreting experiences.
(Mulvale, 2016, p. 119)

The implementation of EBCD in mental health studies follows a four-step process (diagnostic, intervention, implementation and evaluation). The diagnostic stage draws on visual media such as photo-journaling and video to extract experience data, allowing stakeholder control of the narrative and eliciting empathy to humanise the experiences to broader stakeholders. The intervention stage follows, often including a co-design event, bringing together multiple stakeholders to collectively generate interventions that address negative service touchpoints. Some common methods used within this phase include cognitive walkthroughs of the new experiences after design solutions are implemented, organising and prioritising touchpoints through card-sorting activities, experience mapping and storyboarding. The implementation stage then develops and implements design solutions to improve user experience at the identified touchpoints, using methods such as prototyping. The evaluation stage concludes the EBCD process, which includes retrospective interviews, surveys and focus groups to determine the extent to which interventions improved the service experience (Mulvale, 2016, pp. 119–120). The experience focus has the potential to advance the operationalisation of patient-centric healthcare, shifting the power balance in favour of service users and empowering their position in their own health and wellbeing journey (Mulvale et al., 2016).

Embedding creative co-design methods in the context of youth mental health research is seen as a way for researchers to better engage and empower young people in the design process. Research suggests that for people with mental illness and distress, engaging in creative activities and processes can lead to positive outcomes. These creative processes are often used to support recovery for people with mental health challenges (Slattery et al., 2020, p. 1), however researchers identified that drawing on creative methods can also lead to greater engagement in research and design (Nakarada-Kordic et al., 2017). Nakarada-Kordic et al. (2017) advocate for the use of creative methods to engage young people with mental illness better. In a recent publication, Wallace et al. (2021) explored the link between the processes of co-design and attributes of personal wellbeing by reflecting on links between Max-Neef's (1991) matrix of needs and satisfiers and practices of engaging in co-design processes. This initial exploration supports the proposition that participation in co-design processes themselves can be intrinsically valuable to participants' wellbeing, in addition to any benefits from the resultant service or system innovation (Wallace et al., 2021).

Nakarada-Kordic et al. (2017) argue that using storytelling through emojis, developing personas through emotion mapping, card-sorting activities and emotion abstract sketching allows young people with complex health issues to express their unique experiences and perspectives. They found that traditional research methods aimed at adults can be perceived by young people as intimidating or boring, and methods aimed at children as patronising, leading to apathy and discomfort, and limiting participation and idea generation (Nakarada-Kordic et al., 2017). To build on this is an expectation of mass customisation in interactions, as seen in primary, secondary and tertiary education and the increasing shifts toward learner-centred bespoke practices rather than a one-size-fits-all educational approach (Szebeko & Tan, 2010). Drawing on flexible and agile creative methods in co-design helps maintain engagement and motivation, which is of particular importance when mental health is a factor for participation (Nakarada-Kordic et al., 2017).

A more recent emergence in the co-design field is LCCD. LCCD was borne out of necessity due to COVID-19 restricting face-to-face research methods and plots potential research approaches across a spatio-temporal spectrum (Davis et al., 2021). LCCD promotes pluralistic approaches to engagement that provide participants with opportunities to participate in different ways. In the mode of 'different time, different space', it expands the use of cultural probes to focus on their use as dialogic and iterative tools. These approaches have been found to have wide applicability, particularly when collaborating with people from vulnerable backgrounds (Davis et al., 2021). It is assumed these approaches could be successfully deployed in working with young people with mental health challenges.

Shifting away from face-to-face interactions brings a significant number of challenges, not least of which is the loss of the energetic exchange and idea generation from discussion and debate that is at the heart of the co-design process. When analogue techniques are moved to the digital realm without adaptation, there is a danger of creating a lesser experience for participants. However, LCCD encourages practitioners to see this as an opportunity for innovation, drawing on methods, such as 'round robins', to integrate both synchronous and asynchronous ideas and experiences. By working at times and in spaces that better suit stakeholders, greater and more diverse participation becomes possible, particularly from cohorts such as young people and people with disabilities. By developing structures that allow participation without requiring face-to-face attendance at a live event, common barriers, such as time, availability and social stigma can be removed, and new communities of participants can be accessed (Davis et al., 2021). While still an emerging phenomenon, LCCD has the potential to greatly improve youth mental health research and design, meeting people where (and when) they are ready and allowing for greater participation and engagement.

While the Framework, creative co-design, EBCD and LCCD have been successfully applied in the design space and show great promise for adoption in the sustainable youth mental health context, there are limitations and considerations when applying these approaches. In the case of the Framework, it only provides guidance on youth participation within the solution design phase, with young people co-designing inventions and solutions (Hagen et al., 2012, p. 4), which limits its applicability. It also lacks guidance on how to 'generate' ideas and 'check' insights and assumptions in an equitable and accessible manner. While Participatory Design by nature supports a more balanced power dynamic, there is limited discussion on how to navigate challenges when working with diverse stakeholders and guidance on building a research methodology that promotes equity and accessibility. Similarly, in the use of EBCD, Mulvale et al. (2019, p. 3) highlight the lack of attention on the ethical and logistical challenges of EBCD methods when navigating the power imbalances between service providers and young people, the impact of symptoms and stigma on recruitment and participation as well as confidentiality issues through some co-design practices. Finally, EBCD centres on a set of experiences to a specific service or system. While this has translated to benefits within a specific context, most notably within aspects of the healthcare system, the solutions and outcomes do not necessarily lead to more widespread, systematic reform, particularly as there are structural, funding and organisational challenges, which may limit translation and widespread adoption (Mulvale et al., 2019). Co-design and creative methods adopted in studies for youth mental health help to address the complexity and dynamism of the challenges with youth mental health and promote and amplify the experiences and voices of young people. However, similar to the Framework, their novel nature may require further guidance to support successful application. In the case of LCCD, the concept is in its infancy, meaning more needs to be done to demonstrate its value in the youth mental health context. However, it is anticipated that the blended assemblages of methods that sit across the spatiotemporal spectrum of engagement are likely to enable co-design practices to reach new partners and new contributors who may not be willing or able to participate in creative co-design or EBCD processes.

The injection of collaborative, empathetically led, participant-centred research and design methods into youth mental health research offers an excellent opportunity to move to a more preventative, salutogenic, mindful and empathic approach that supports and empowers those experiencing mental illness, as well as those offering support. The literature reviewed above indicates that co-design offers researchers the flexibility to create a research methodology based on the unique requirements of their audience and the ambition of the study, which was demonstrated through the exploration of the Framework, EBCD, creative co-design methods and LCCD. This chapter posits that co-design has a role in improving the mental wellbeing of Australian youth. Accordingly, Table 3.1 provides an overarching framework, articulating the core principles for sustainable youth mental health, coupled with the current reality and the opportunities and frameworks of co-design in this context.

Recommendations for a Youth Mental Health Co-Design Model

When considering youth mental health in Australia, co-design offers methods to engage meaningfully with young people, establish a genuine partnership to generate more effective solutions, and help to shift the dial toward a more sustainable, salutogenic mental healthcare model. Young people with poor mental health experience a unique set of challenges, and co-design, with its adaptive and collaborative nature, can provide a suitable methodology to help solve some of these complex challenges.

Above, this chapter discussed and articulated a methodological co-design framework that integrates key approaches for the youth mental health context. To build on this, we propose a Youth Mental Health Co-design Model that integrates the various co-design approaches discussed in this chapter with relation to the different types of challenges and solutions from specific challenges and object-based solutions to large, complex and 'wicked' problems that require systemic solutions. The Youth Mental Health Co-design Model (the Model) plots the co-design approaches based on the complexity of the youth mental health challenge: creative co-design methods are linked to product and service challenges, experience-based co-design with service, system and cultural challenges, and low-contact co-design with system and cultural challenges (Figure 3.1). The individual categories are discussed in the following.

Table 3.1 Co-design Framework for Sustainable Youth Mental Health

GUIDING PRINCIPLES FOR SUSTAINABLE MENTAL HEALTH					
Underpinned by salutogenic and positive psychology perspectives, the goal of a sustainable mental health system is to support a state of wellbeing and flourishing in which individuals meet their potential, cope with stressors, work productively, fruitfully and meaningfully and contribute to community					
CURRENT YOUTH MENTAL HEALTH CONTEXT	High rates of mental illness and distress	Barriers to accessing services	Low help-seeking behaviours	Low retention and adherence to services	Power imbalances for young people
CO-DESIGN METHODOLOGIES					
EXPERIENCE-BASED CO-DESIGN		CREATIVE CO-DESIGN		LOW-CONTACT CO-DESIGN	
• Focus' on experience to improve the interaction with services • Humanises service interactions and allows stakeholders to control the narrative • Builds toward a patient-centric health care system • Brings multiple stakeholders together to co-create interventions		• Builds genuine partnerships • Adapts to stakeholder and research needs • Includes frameworks specifically designed for the youth mental health field of research (such as the Framework) • Provides creative and novel approaches to meaningfully engage stakeholders		• Allows fluid assemblage of synchronous and asynchronous approaches, in person and remotely • Navigates barriers to support greater participation • Identifies engaging new strategies to build genuine partnerships • Supports greater participation from people from vulnerable backgrounds	

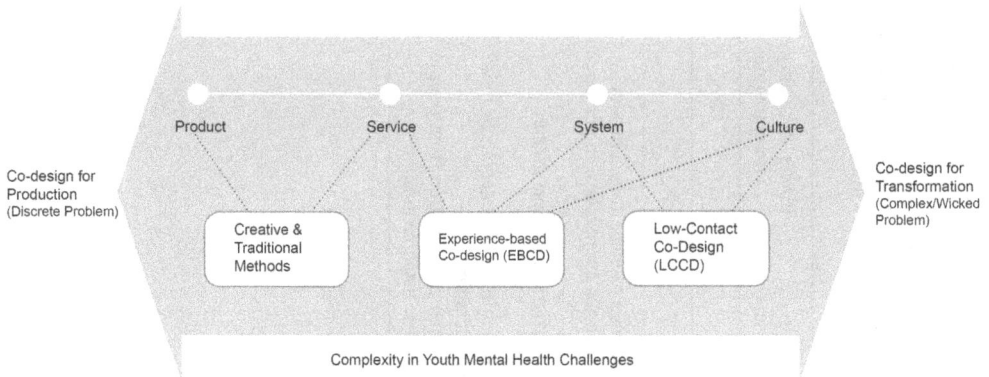

Figure 3.1 Youth Mental Health Co-design Model

Products: Production of objects and digital items engages discrete problems. Creative co-design methods provide an appropriate platform to co-produce these items. It is important to consider both creative methods and traditional research methods for this context, whereby creative design methods can resonate with the youth cohort, which can, in turn, increase engagement with traditional methods, promote more equitable and democratic participation across stakeholder groups and extract greater insight and idea generation from stakeholders (Nakarada-Kordic et al., 2017).

Services: Service-related challenges focus on the improvement of stakeholders' experiences with health and care services. This level of co-design effort engages creative design methods and traditional research methods as well as EBCD. Here, designers provide a creative and collaborative platform for stakeholders to generate suitable service innovations. The use of EBCD helps to address the service touchpoints and barriers that lead to high levels of young people not accessing services, improving the interface between service users and services (Mulvale et al., 2016).

Systems: Systemic challenges are complex, as they involve organisational and government policy and systems. LCCD is an appropriate method for this level because of its flexibility in engaging a broad range of stakeholders. It can be complemented with EBCD to provide insights into experiences that contribute to systemic innovation. Embedding LCCD in studies that focus on whole system and blue-sky reforms removes some of the key barriers to participation, including time, space, stigma and traditional power imbalances. It can thus support greater participation, expression, engagement and diversity to help generate the best possible solutions (Davis et al., 2021). Similarly, EBCD has the potential not only to improve service-related challenges but also support a paradigm shift from paternalism in mental healthcare to a more empathically led, patient-centric healthcare model (Mulvale et al., 2016).

Cultures: Challenges such as stigma surrounding youth mental health are considered as wicked problems that require transformative interventions. Often, the mode of design focuses on shifting mindsets, social and cultural practices and eliminating stigmas surrounding youth mental health. Longer-term transformation can also generate more sustainable strategies to tackle youth mental health challenges. These transformative efforts are highly complex and therefore should involve iterative co-design processes including LCCD and EBCD.

This Model offers a holistic approach to studying youth mental health issues, based on the level of complexity of the design challenge. It can be employed to generate products and services that help young people and the community, with product-driven co-design projects commonly engaging with discrete problems where a certain product is clearly required. It can also contribute to systemic and cultural transformation that engages complex and wicked problems. Like all collaborative design methods, the way in which the approaches are applied, stakeholders engaged and the studies delivered impacts the success of the research outcomes. There are two key limitations of the Model. Firstly, the Model offers a high-level approach to design for mental health studies. The lack of detail may impact the Model's success and the way it is applied in youth mental health research. Furthermore, the Model is based on the available research in the literature and has yet to be tested. As such, further research is required to test and validate the Model, and to provide greater detail and guidance on the methods and approaches applied.

Conclusion

With mental health continuing to impact the wellbeing of Australian youth, novel and collaborative approaches are needed to help solve these complex social issues. Co-design is an effective approach to address youth mental health in Australia. The literature identified the strengths and limitations of traditional and creative co-design methods, the YWCRC Framework, EBCD and LCCD in the context of mental health and design. This led to the proposed Youth Mental Health Co-design Model, presenting the co-design approaches across the spectrum of complexity, from co-design for products (discrete problems) through to co-design for transformation (complex/wicked problems). The Model provides a theoretical framework for youth mental health research and design, drawing on creative and traditional methods, EBCD and LCCD. As these concepts and approaches are still emerging, particularly in the youth mental health context, more research is required to test and validate methodologies, continue to build a body of literature showcasing the fundamental benefits of co-design for youth mental health and shift the dial toward a sustainable, salutogenic mental health system in Australia.

Note

1 ReachOut Australia is a charity supporting young people with mental ill-health to feel better. https://au .reachout.com

References

AIHW (Australian Institute of Health and Welfare). (2020). *Australia's health snapshots.* https://www .aihw.gov.au/getmedia/128856d0-19a0-4841-b5ce-f708fcd62c8c/aihw-aus-234-Australias-health -snapshots-2020.pdf.aspx

AIHW (Australian Institute of Health and Welfare). (2022). *Mental health services in Australia.* https:// www.aihw.gov.au/reports/mental-health-services/mental-health-services-in-australia/report-contents/ covid-19-impact-on-mental-health

Allen, K. A., & Mckenzie, V. L. (2015). Adolescent mental health in an Australian context and future interventions. *International Journal of Mental Health, 44*(1–2), 80–93.

Antonovsky, A. (1996). The salutogenic model as a theory to guide health promotion. *Health Promotion International, 11*(1).11-18

Ben-David, S., Cole, A., Spencer, R., Jaccard, K., & Munson, M. R. (2017). Social context in mental health service use among young adults. *Journal of Social Service Research, 43*(1), 85–99.

Bohlmeijer, E. T., & Westerhof, G. J. (2021). A new model for sustainable mental health. In J. N. Kirby & P. Gilbert (Eds.), *Making an impact on mental health: The applications of psychological research.* (pp154-188).Routledge.

Bradshaw, C., Nguyen, A., Kane, J., & Bass, J. (2014). *Mental health matters: Social inclusion of youth with mental health conditions.* United Nations. https://www.un.org/esa/socdev/documents/youth/youth -mental-health.pdf

Buchanan, R. (1992). Wicked problems in design thinking. *Design Issues, 8*(2), 5–21.

Chamberlain, P., & Partridge, R. (2017). Co-designing co-design: Shifting the culture of practice in healthcare. *The Design Journal, 20*(1), S2010–S2021. https://doi.org/10.1080/14606925.2017.1252720

Chamberlin, J. (2005). User/consumer involvement in mental health service delivery. *Epidemiologia e Psichiatria Sociale,* 14 (1),10–14.

Cockbill, S. A., May, A., & Mitchell, V. (2019). The assessment of meaningful outcomes from co-design: A case study from the energy sector. *She Ji: The Journal of Design, Economics, and Innovation, 5*(3), 187–208.

Cooper, K., Gillmore, C., & Hogg, L. (2016). Experience-based co-design in an adult psychological therapies service. *Journal of Mental Health, 25*(1), 36–40. https://doi.org/10.3109/09638237.2015.1101423

Davis, A., Wallace, N., Langley, J., & Gwilt, I. (2021, January–April). Low-Contact Co-Design: Considering more flexible spatiotemporal models for the co-design workshop. *Strategic Design Research Journal, 14*(1), 124–137. https://doi.org/10.4013/sdrj.2021.141.11

Deserti, A., Eckhardt, J., Kaletka, C., Rizzo, F., & Wascher, E. (2019). Co-design for society in innovation. In J. Howaldt, C. Kaletka, A. Schroder, & M. Zirnbiebl (Eds.), *Atlas of social innovation: A world of new practice* (pp. 90–95). Oekom Verlag.

Hagen, P., Collin, P., Metcalf, A., Nicholas, M., Rahilly, K., & Swainston, N. (2012). *Participatory design of evidence-based online youth mental health promotion, intervention, and treatment. Young and well.* Cooperative Research Centre.

Hall, S., Fildes, J., Perrens, B., Plummer, J., Carlisle, E., Cockayne, N., & Werner-Seidler, A. (2019). *Can we talk? Seven year youth mental health report - 2012–2018.* NSW.

Jørgensen, K., Rendtorff, J. D., & Holen, M. (2018). How patient participation is constructed in mental health care: A grounded theory study. *Scandinavian Journal of Caring Sciences, 32,* 1359–1370. doi:10.1111/scs.12581

Jorm, A. F. (2019). Australia's 'better access' scheme: Has it had an impact on population mental health?' *Australian & New Zealand Journal of Psychiatry, 52*(11), 1057–1062.

Keyes, C. L. M. (2002). The mental health continuum: From languishing to flourishing in life. *Journal of Health and Social Behavior, 43*(2), 207–222. https://doi.org/10.2307/3090197

Lal, S., & Adair, C. (2014). E-mental health: A rapid review of the literature. *Psychiatric Services, 65*(1), 24–32.

Max-Neef, M. A. (1991). *Human scale development: Conception, application and further reflections.* New York: Apex Press.

McGorry, P. (2017). Youth mental health and mental wealth: Reaping the rewards. *Australasian Psychiatry, 25*(2), 101–104.

Medley, S., & Kueh, C. (2015). Beyond problem solving: A framework to teach design as an experiment in the university environment. In L. Noel & M.L. Poy (Eds) *Ministry of Design: From Cottage Industry to State Enterprise, Colloquium Proceedings.*2(170-180)

Mjøsund, N. H. (2021). A salutogenic mental health model: Flourishing as a metaphor for good mental health. In G. Haugan & M. Eriksson (Eds.), *Health Promotion in health care – Vital theories and research.* Springer. https://doi.org/10.1007/978-3-030-63135-2_5

Montague, A. E., Varcin, K. J., Simmons, M. B., & Parker, A. G. (2015, April–June). Putting technology into youth mental health practice: Young people's perspectives. *SAGE Open, 5*(2)1–10.

Mulvale, A., Miatello, A., Hackett, C., & Mulvale, G. (2016). Applying experience-based co-design with vulnerable populations: Lessons from a systematic review of methods to involve patients, families and service providers in child and youth mental health service improvement. *Patient Experience Journal, 3*(1). https://pxjournal.org/journal/vol3/iss1/15

Mulvale, G., Mall, S., Miatello, A., Murray-Leung, L., Rogerson, K., & Sassi, R. (2019). Co-designing services for youth with mental health issues: Novel elicitation approaches. *International Journal of Qualitative Methods*, *18*, 1–13. https://doi.org/10.1177/1609406918816244

Nakarada-Kordic, I., Hayes, N., Reay, S. D., Corbet, C., & Chan, A. (2017). Co-designing for mental health: Creative methods to engage young people experiencing psychosis. *Design for Health*, *1*(2), 229–244. https://doi.org/10.1080/24735132.2017.1386954

Orygen: The National Centre of Excellence in Youth Mental Health. (2019). *Co-designing with young people: The fundamentals*.

Pinfold, V., Szymczynska, P., Hamilton, S., Peacocke, R., Dean, S., Clewett, N., Manthorpe, J., & Larson, J. (2015). Co-production in mental health research: Reflections from the people study. *Mental Health Review Journal*, *20*(4), 220–231. https://doi.org/10.1108/MHRJ-09-2015-0028

Productivity Commission. (2020). *Mental health* (Report no. 95). Productivity Commission.

Realpe, A., Elahi, F., Bucci, S., Birchwood, M., Vlaev, I., Taylor, D., & Thompson, A. (2019). Co-designing a virtual world with young people to deliver social cognition therapy in early psychosis. *Early Intervention in Psychiatry*, *14*(1), 37–43. https://doi.org/10.1111/eip.12804

Sanders, E. B.-N., & Stappers, P. J. (2008). Co-creation and the new landscapes of design. *CoDesign*, *4*(1), 5–18. https://doi.org/10.1080/15710880701875068

Scholten, H., & Granic, I. (2019). User of the principles of design thinking to address limitations of digital mental health interventions for youth: Viewpoint. *Journal of Medical Internet Research*, *21*(1), 1–14.

Seligman, M. (2011). *Flourish*. Nicholas Brealey Publishing.

Shipley, B., & Stubley, W. (2018). *After the ATAR II: Understanding how Gen Z Make decisions about their future*. Year13.

Slattery, P., Saeri, A. K., & Bragge, P. (2020). Research co-design in health: A rapid overview of reviews. *Health Research Policy and Systems*, *18*(17). https://doi.org/10.1186/s12961-020-0528-9

Szebeko, D., & Tan, L. (2010). Co-designing for society. *Australasian Medical Journal*, *3*(9), 580–590.

Valenti, E., Banks, C., Calcedo-Barba, A., Bensimon, C., M., Hoffmann, K., Pelto-Piri, V., Jurin, T., Mendoza, O. M., Mundt, A. P., Rugkåsa, J., Tubini, J., & Priebe, S. (2015). Informal coercion in psychiatry: A focus group study of attitudes and experiences of mental health professionals in ten countries. *Social Psychiatry and Psychiatric Epidemiology*, *50*, 1297–1308. doi:10.1007/s00127-015-1032-3

Wallace, N., David, A., & Gwilt, I. (2021, June 21). Wellbeing through participation: Creativity and co-design as processes of "welldoing". *Non-Traditional Research Outcomes*, *35*. Retrieved July 7, 2023, from https://ualresearchonline.arts.ac.uk/id/eprint/17864/1/Wellbeing%20through%20participation.pdf

Westerhof, G. J., & Keyes, C. L. M. (2010). Mental illness and mental health: The two continua model across the lifespan. *Journal of Adult Development*, *17*(2), 110–119. https://doi.org/10.1007/s10804-009-9082-y

World Health Organization (WHO). (1946, June 19–22). *Preamble to the constitution of the world health organization as adopted by the international health conference*. WHO.

World Health Organization. (2022, June 17). *Mental health*. https://www.who.int/news-room/fact-sheets/detail/mental-health-strengthening-our-response

4   Spaces of co-design in mental health, neurology and neuroscience

Leigh-Anne Hepburn, Chris L. Smith, Donald McNeill and Jason A. Dibbs

Introduction

Co-design and associated terms, such as co-creation, experience-based co-design, participatory co-design and co-production, are practices of collaborative engagement that enable those connected to a particular context (e.g. users, stakeholders, consumers, partners) to contribute to, and become part of, a design process by sharing their experiential knowledge (Trischler et al., 2018; Sanders & Stappers, 2008). Through the building of collective knowledge, insights are generated that can contribute to socially and contextually relevant impacts. The role of co-design in supporting the development, implementation and evaluation of mental health services, programmes and technologies is well established, with recognition of the potential for co-design to support shared decision-making (Larkin et al., 2015; Martin et al., 2017; Mulvale et al., 2019; Kealy-Bateman et al., 2021; Tindall et al., 2021; Orlowski et al., 2018; Hagen et al., 2012).

By contrast, few studies have explored beyond services, programmes and technologies to consider how co-design might better support the design of physical and interaction spaces within mental health service facilities. Attempts to address the role of spatial design in mental health include the edited book, *The Handbook of Mental Health and Space* (McGrath & Reavey, 2018), which identifies, broadly, spatial design concerns in mental health settings; and the paper, 'Psychosocially Supportive Design' (McLaughlan, 2018), assessing the relationship between the psychosocial and built environment in hospital design. However, there is still a gap in understanding the potential of co-design in physical and interaction space design. The following case study addresses this gap, drawing insights from research with a specific mental health setting.

The Brain and Mind Centre (BMC) is a multidisciplinary centre at the University of Sydney that integrates cutting-edge research with diverse mental health, neurology and neuroscience specialist clinics, laboratories and research infrastructures. Operating at the intersection of academia and private and public health and care service provision, the BMC is uniquely positioned to deliver translational research that directly impacts practice. In this way, the BMC offers a unique site for collaboration across mental health, neurology and neuroscience, with engagement across a diverse group of stakeholders, including mental health clinicians, scientists, researchers, patients, patient advocates and administrators.

The collaborative model of care offered by BMC is integrated, seeking to offer efficient and effective person-centred services. Integrated care (Lee & Porter, 2013) and multidisciplinary approaches are recognised for their ability to move from fragmented, small-scale or localised approaches toward integrating disciplines, sectors and stakeholders, including people with lived experience (Holmes et al., 2020). Despite increased awareness of the importance of integrated multi-disciplinary service provision for mental health (Colizzi et al., 2020), few studies have

DOI: 10.4324/9781003318262-6

explored the design of multidisciplinary facilities that integrate academic research and health and care provision. Fewer still have considered the role of co-design within such contexts.

This chapter first considers the application of co-design in physical and interaction health spaces, explicitly considering the dichotomy between generative and participatory approaches and the demands of a field that relies heavily on evidence-based practice. The chapter then introduces research undertaken at the BMC as part of a process of institutional campus redesign that considered the physical relocation of diverse mental health, neurology and neuroscience specialist clinics, laboratories and research infrastructure. Two conceptual spaces of co-design were uncovered based on the multi-disciplinary perspectives of mental health clinicians, scientists, researchers, patient advocates and administrators. The first space is that of intentional co-design and is informed by learning from a workshop facilitated by the research team. The second space is that of emergent co-design, identified as occurring generatively through existing service provision within the BMC. In discussing the two examples, the chapter considers how co-design can support understanding the perspectives of diverse stakeholders involved in integrated care, particularly those based within a research-intensive multidisciplinary centre. In doing so, the chapter seeks to inform the generation of collaborative spatial design knowledge that can inform current thinking across other contexts of mental health, neurology and neuroscience.

Co-design in health spaces

Evidence-based medicine (EBM) rose to dominate medical research methodologies in the late 1990s (Hooker, 1997) and occupies a privileged position in medical research today. It is unsurprising, then, that questions concerning the evidence-based design of medical services and their spaces have begun to surface in recent years. The field of evidence-based design (EBD) generates knowledge to complement the professional expertise of designers and architects regarding the effect, use and perception of healthcare spaces, with corresponding implications for socialisation, collaboration, productivity and the delivery of care (Berry et al., 2004; Martin & Guerin, 2006). Evidence-based design can be understood as processes whereby design recommendations are derived from, or are 'produced by, research on the relationship between the physical environment and objective outcomes' (Devlin, 2014, p. 17). In the medical setting, just as a clinical diagnosis will often defer to evidence-based research in the hope of improving patient outcomes, according to evidence-based design methodology, spatial design is seen as another 'component of an arsenal to improve not only the quality of the patient experience but also the success and reputation of the physician's practice' (Devlin, 2014, p. xi). Yet, whilst evidence-based medicine – deferring to and valorising comparative clinical studies, meta-analyses and randomized trials – has developed into a paradigm of healthcare over the past three decades, exactly what constitutes the evidence basis for design and, more specifically, spatial design in healthcare settings remains an emerging and highly contested epistemological field (Collins, 2014; Kaji-O'Grady & Smith, 2019).

In recent years, the literature has shifted focus from EBD towards a more nuanced consideration of design that, while still addressing the application of design in a generic sense, has expanded to include co-design and experience-based co-design (EBCD). Retaining the need to understand better the 'myriad relationships' between the many stakeholders involved (Ulrich et al., 2010), co-design also values experience as evidence. As described earlier, co-design is an increasingly significant and prevalent methodology, understood as a process of collaborative design, whereby those involved are 'creating things jointly with others' (Stark et al., 2021; Bjögvinsson et al., 2012; Karasti, 2014). With a historical lineage that traces back to countercultural movements of the late-1960s and a prevalence in the evolution of information technologies, co-design is often considered synonymous with participatory design: motivated by and concerned with questions of 'how collaborative design processes can be driven by the participation of the people who will be affected by' those systems (Simonsen & Robertson, 2013). However, while in participatory design, users take on an active role in contributing to outcomes of the design process – generally, through specifically defined activities, and feedback loops – co-design can also be thought of as co-production, whereby designers and users work together towards 'joint ownership and decision-making over both the process and outcome' (Stark et al., 2021; Manzini, 2015).

In the mental health arena, La Borde, the psychiatric clinic of Jean Oury and Félix Guattari took this to the extreme with the interchanging of the roles of clinicians and patients and simultaneously the restructuring of the architectural organisation of offices and wards. Here the spatial co-design was seen as an opportunity to 'throw an entirely new light on "problems of organisation"' (Guattari, 1984, p. 16). In this way, co-design is favoured for its emphasis on researching and designing user-centric health systems and service delivery. With a focus on meaningful and impactful care, co-design has been particularly active in-patient engagement, involving the community to address health-based challenges or condition-specific care. However, despite examples of good practice and the recognition of value created (Palmer et al., 2019), the application of co-design is often limited to project work that targets incremental quality improvements (Donetto, et al., 2014), creating a missed opportunity for fundamental and generative innovation.

A foundational feature of co-design is its generative capability, which strongly focusses on creativity within the design process. Creativity and the generation of new ideas can be understood as drivers of innovation through which development and change can be realised. Generative approaches encourage participants to be creative and open, exploring both the explicitly stated needs (what people understand as a particular challenge and why) as well as revealing latent needs and experiences – those which are tacit, difficult to articulate and may not yet even be understood as a challenge within people's conscious minds (Sanders & Stappers, 2008; Sleeswijk et al., 2005). In a healthcare setting, generative techniques have been used across four key stages: pre-design – understanding and capturing lived experiences; generative – supporting participants to think beyond the current, reimagining future scenarios and generating ideas; evaluation – reflecting on design experiences; and post-design – developing use-case and practice-based data (Bird et al., 2021; Noorbergen et al., 2021).

Despite the burgeoning role of co-design in health contexts, having the generative approach recognised and valued as a valid method of knowledge creation and data capture can still be challenging. Health research is foregrounded by specific constructions of scientific rigour and measurable outcomes, predominantly quantitative methods aligned with randomised control trials. In the last decade, practices of co-design or co-production in mental health have increasingly explored notions of evidence or experiential bases for the refinement of their processes (Larkin et al., 2015; Martin et al., 2017; Mulvale et al., 2019; Bateman et al., 2021; Tindall et al., 2021). Yet, the potential for co-design in the spaces where these services and programmes are delivered, and the nature of the evidence or experiential basis for co-designing these spaces, require further investigation, because what constitutes evidence in disciplines such as design and architecture is complex.

Whereas science and medicine have long histories of developing (largely statistical) measures for the (largely quantifiable) outcomes, design and architecture have historically been informed by qualitative features resistant to statistical measures. The term EBM was coined in 1991 by Gordon Guyatt whilst leading a group tasked with writing user guides for the *Journal of the American Medical Association.* However, as Paul Glasziou writes, 'the ideas behind it have been evolving for centuries,' with its vocabulary 'invented and developed by statisticians and epidemiologists' (Glasziou, 2011, p. xi). In the hierarchy introduced by EBM, randomised trials are determined to offer 'stronger evidential support than observational studies,' whilst it is claimed that comparative clinical studies, including observational studies, 'offer stronger evidential support than "mechanistic" reasoning' and 'expert clinical judgement' (Howick, 2011, p. xii).

If we consider co-design in the light of this hierarchy, several issues become apparent. For instance, by its very nature, co-design is generally poorly suited for producing the kind of evidence prioritised by EBM. The first-person, phenomenological, embodied moment-to-moment experience of a space is not quantifiable and cannot be captured by cross-sectional questionnaires or by intra-individual longitudinal questionnaires related to theoretically defined psychological constructs of mental health (e.g. Myin-Germeys et al., 2018). An evidence basis for co-design is more complex and tied to notions such as nuance, sense, feeling and aesthetics. Such things are no less logical but are seldom supported by theoretical constructs and are tied less to 'expert clinical judgement' (Howick, 2011, p. xiii) than what might be called 'expert critical judgement'.

One could argue that the evidence base for EBM is similarly complex and should be recognised as such. However, EBM is prevalent despite the paradoxes that it often leads to, including the fact 'that many of the treatments in whose effectiveness we have the most confidence … have never been supported by randomized trials of any description' (Howick, 2011, p. xiii). Some well-known examples include 'external defibrillation to start a stopped heart, tracheostomy to open a blocked air passage, and the Heimlich manoeuvre to dislodge airway obstructions' (Howick, 2011, p. xiii). At the point of co-design, the very question of expert clinical judgment and expert critical judgment come to a head. When experience itself is valued, what makes the experience of a patient, an outpatient or a carer any less valuable than that of a clinician or an architect of the space all might occupy? While it is simple to suggest that 'It is important to understand the perspectives of service-users, carers, and staff, and to bring these groups together to "co-design" potential improvements' (Larkin et al., 2015, p. 1464), in the mental health arena, the longstanding structures that both organisationally and spatially demarcate authority and clinical expertise make the uses of co-design both compelling and complex. Tentative steps have, however, already been taken. As Michael Larkin et al. write,

> the use of EBCD in mental health services is still relatively novel, and we are only aware of two other NHS services that have implemented EBCD in acute mental health care and one that has used it in community services for young people.
>
> (Larkin et al., 2015, p. 1465)

The novelty is even greater regarding spatial rather than services or systems design.

Brain, mind and Mallett Street

Recognising the dichotomy between generative approaches of co-design and the demands of a field that traditionally relies heavily on scientific evidence-based practice, the next section reports on a case study that seeks to highlight both the complexity of, and the opportunities for, co-design in this field. Drawing from a series of exploratory workshops and interviews that engaged health professionals, researchers, scientists and administrators, data was captured and analysed thematically to understand better the current knowledge and use of physical and interaction space within a dedicated building.

The Brain and Mind Centre (BMC) at the University of Sydney is a multidisciplinary initiative that aims to foster collaboration between diverse research disciplines and health and care service providers in the production of translational research and research-informed practice in mental health, neurology and neuroscience. The BMC comprises clinics and laboratories working across areas including autism, cannabinoid therapeutics, child behavioural science, child and youth mental health, dementia, gambling addiction, healthy brain ageing, motor neurone disease, multiple sclerosis, neuroimmunology, Parkinson's disease and psychology. Situated in the Sydney Local Health District and close to Camperdown Health, Education and Research Precinct, the BMC occupies a conceptual space (the intersection between service providers and academia) and physical space, a collection of post-industrial, multi-storey buildings within which various clinics and laboratories are housed. An opportunity arose for the BMC to expand its clinics and laboratories into new spaces. As part of a relocation programme, the BMC engaged The Sydney School of Architecture, Design and Planning (ADP) on a project entitled *Brain, Mind and Mallett Street* to collaboratively explore and re-imagine new spatial futures for mental health, neurology and neuroscience with BMC's diverse range of stakeholders.

The research collaboration commenced with a co-design workshop, bringing together 20 clinicians, researchers, scientists and administrators from the BMC. The workshop aimed to understand the complex nature and scope of the BMC's myriad activities and adopted a participatory focus group format to encourage participants to share and engage with their knowledge and experiences in a group setting (DiCiccio-Bloom et al., 2006). The workshop comprised two activities. In the first workshop activity, participants were asked to map the existing BMC specialisms, services and stakeholders, including patients, families and carers; clinicians and public and private care providers; scientists and lab support technicians; academics and researchers. The broad scope of the BMC's activities – from pre-clinical to post-clinical translation – was considered an asset of the BMC by workshop attendees, as was the BMC's focus on thought leadership, research excellence and prioritisation of early-career research opportunities. However, the broad scope and fragmentation of the BMC's various teams, both on and off-site, were seen to raise challenges for collaboration. Workshop participants discussed the need for improved visibility and awareness across the teams of the BMC, increased opportunities for informal engagement and collaboration and the impact of physical and social barriers created by the 'maze-like' buildings housing BMC's facilities.

In the second workshop activity, participants were asked about their spatial desires and preferences, working in small groups to map these onto a design template. Participants talked about their desire for spaces that can encourage and enable continuous engagement across the natural course of human life. For spaces that involved patients and research participants, this included notions of safety, comfort and trust combined with cutting-edge excellence; the need for a welcoming and understanding approach to way-finding that is more than simply a reception area; for community spaces that responded to and offered value to user groups; and for spaces that offer walk-through stories of education, awareness and understanding. Elements such as signage and waiting areas were also highlighted as important. For staff, research and clinician-orientated spaces were important. The notion of values-based shared spaces increased visibility at individual and team levels, and a desire for a community or living-laboratory model of engagement with the BMC was identified as the translation point between community, hospital and university.

Following completion of the first workshop, the next research activity involved individual and group interviews with BMC stakeholders, including clinicians, researchers, scientists, administrators and patient and client advocates. Recruitment took place via an email invitation, and stakeholders self-elected to participate in a semi-structured one-hour interview with

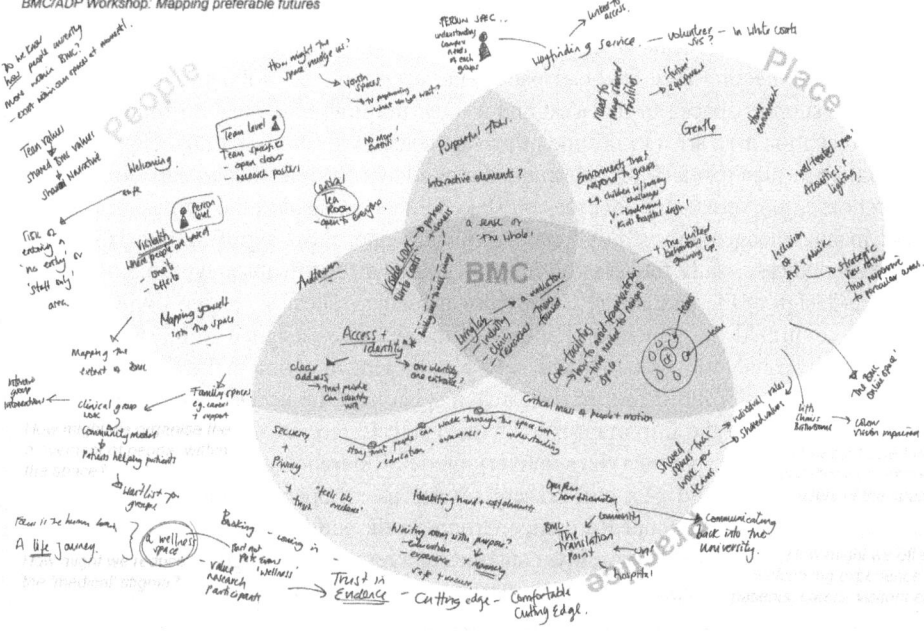

Figure 4.1 'Mapping Preferable Futures' co-design workshop activity, December 2020. Photograph by the authors

the Sydney School of Architecture, Design and Planning research team members. Preference was given to those interviews that could be conducted *in situ*, in the interviewee's workspace at the BMC. However, the ongoing effects of the COVID-19 pandemic meant allowances were made for stakeholders working remotely. In these instances, interviews were conducted online via Zoom. Twenty-two interviews were completed, representing BMC's diverse clinical and research areas: gambling treatment, youth mental health, psychology, geriatrics, sleep and circadian biology, neurology, neuroimaging, multiple sclerosis clinical trials, laboratory services, as well as members of the BMC administration and executive.

Youth mental health care provision at the BMC coalesces around the formal service delivery partnership between the University of Sydney and headspace: the National Youth Mental Health Foundation. The headspace Camperdown facility is co-located with the Sydney Local Health District Early Intervention in Psychosis Service, headspace Early Intervention Team (Nash, 2021) and the Youth Mental Health and Technology research group in the Youth Mental Health Building of the BMC. It provides youth services, including mental and sexual health and drug and alcohol support, to twelve- to twenty-five-year-olds.

The Youth Mental Health Building was purpose-designed by BVN architects in 2010 and consists of four storeys entered via a light-filled atrium with an open staircase, a large reception area on level one, various consulting suites, research laboratories and administrative support spaces. According to the architects, the design 'focussed on flexibility' and 'evolved from discussions about zoning from public spaces to more private areas' (R. Cotrona, personal communication, February 16, 2021). In fact, visitors' journeys to access headspace's services are characterised by the oscillation between private and public spatial zoning, commencing with the private Church Street security entry, immediately followed by the more public atrium and staircase, serving not only headspace's staff and visitors, but also BMC stakeholders accessing other levels of the building. On level one, a small bridge separates the headspace reception area and waiting room from the stair landing and shared kitchen area, which serves as an auxiliary waiting room and meeting area for headspace. The reception area is flanked on either side by administrative support spaces to the west and a large multipurpose meeting room to the east. Behind the reception area are a multitude of private consulting rooms, storage cupboards and a large central open-plan research office arranged around a horseshoe-shaped corridor.

The first case study presented focusses on stakeholders engaged in the co-design workshop, including management, administrative staff, clinicians and, most significantly, patient advocates. The second case study focusses on insights gained through subsequent interviews about emergent co-design at the headspace Camperdown facility. These interviews with headspace stakeholders confirmed the general suitability of the purpose-designed Youth Mental Health Building for delivering youth mental health services, drawing attention to the qualities of certain areas, such as the flexibility of the shared kitchen space and the access to natural light there. Interviewees referred to the important role of the Youth Reference Group or Youth Advisory Group (YAG) in the headspace services delivery model. Reference groups, consisting of youth mental health advocates and past and present service users, operate from the national level, i.e. the headspace Youth National Reference Group, to the individual centre level. The headspace Camperdown YAG meets monthly, constituting a regular and ongoing feedback loop for improving services and the spaces in which those services are delivered.

Co-design in spaces of mental health

As the research progressed, two conceptual spaces of co-design emerged, each characterised by distinct modes and processes. The collaboration between the Sydney School of Architecture, Design and Planning researchers and BMC stakeholders in the initial workshop was intentional, formalised and explicitly structured, while processes of co-design uncovered at headspace Camperdown were emergent, often informal and latent. The following two subsections elaborate on the distinctions and characteristics of each space.

Intentional co-design

Design intent draws from the discipline's traditional goal or solution-orientated nature: design that addresses a particular challenge or identified need (Galle, 1999). In co-design, however, notions of intent are laden with tension and can manifest in many forms. As an approach that seeks to be inherently democratised and empowering, co-design is framed as *power-with* rather than *power-over* (Zamenopoulos et al., 2019), focusing on equitable decision-making. However, whilst this empowerment may be realised in co-design, the original intent behind the proposed co-design is often unacknowledged.

The initial workshop was proposed as a research method to capture experiential data from multidisciplinary stakeholders that could inform the spatial expansion and relocation of BMC services and facilities. This intent was explicit from the start and informed the planning process, with the additional inclusion of the BMC as a strategic project partner. Drawing on the research team's expertise, a decision was made to deliver this event as a co-design workshop, recognising the potential collaborative value offered by engaged and generative practices. This design and delivery of co-design activities in the workshop suggested a further form of intent – this time disciplinary, with activities designed and facilitated by a professional designer.

The exploratory workshop sought better to understand and visualise both physical spaces – the spaces used and occupied by BMC – and social spaces – the day-to-day interactions, collaborations and activities occurring within BMC. As a methodological approach, co-design workshops offer what Muller and Druin (2012, p. 1132) describe as a third space that supports and enables 'negotiation, shared construction, and collective discovery'. In the intentional framing of the workshop activities, co-design supported the sharing of lived experiences whilst also providing a structure that enabled an articulation of the landscape or 'current state' of BMC operations. Through this 'third space' of the workshop, participants arrived at an understanding of the current spatial reality of the BMC and its future aspirations for its expansion.

The intentional co-design in this context, while structured and formalised in the design and delivery of activities, also aligned with the generative approach of established co-design frameworks, for example, the online EBCD toolkit distributed by the King's Fund Charity. In this way, the participatory approach provided a scaffold that could support the engagement of participants with little to no design expertise and, importantly, valued alternative forms of expertise (Donetto et al., 2014). As discussed, the understanding and valuing of evidence differs significantly across disciplines. However, in the space of intentional co-design, this research sought not to gather participants' expert clinical experiences but rather to foreground their expert critical experiences, moving beyond their specific health roles towards a more generic consideration of how they occupy and use space within the BMC.

Co-design, in this example, supported understanding and learning across diverse stakeholders, building a stronger awareness of the interconnected services and research groups housed within the BMC's buildings. In making explicit and sharing participants' experiences, including challenges and opportunities within the current state, new models of future integration were considered. The emerging data offers significant value for spatial design in mental health contexts, whereby those who occupy such spaces can contribute in an engaged and valued manner.

Emergent co-design

Spaces of emergent co-design are responsive to evolving everyday environments (Papoutsi et al., 2021). They differ from intentional co-design in that the context inherently drives them, often emerging without explicit intent and frequently undertaken without the engagement of professional design expertise. In distinguishing between intentional and emergent co-design, Papoutsi et al. (2021, p. 290) suggest that the former is akin to a 'bounded episodic activity,' while the latter offers a mechanism for managing unpredictability and change.

In the experiences shared by headspace stakeholders in interviews, rich and dynamic processes of emergent co-design were identified, illustrating the responsive changes to everyday practices discussed previously. While the co-design activity described by participants did not identify with, nor adhere to, a particular design framework, nor was there any prior engagement of a design professional, the experiences were strongly aligned with underpinning co-design principles, for example, equity, engagement and lived experience.

One result of this co-design initiative at headspace Camperdown has been the move to modify the atmosphere of consulting spaces. Interview participants suggested that the 'rooms were considered too clinical in the past' and that clinical spaces were 'off-putting' to young people seeking mental health support. Through the engagement with YAG, headspace employees have been involved in the co-design of not only clinical spaces but also the reception and waiting area. Through these processes, 'little things' were identified as significant to the atmosphere created in these spaces (interviewee). 'Fidget bowls', containing fidget spinners and other sensory and fidget toys, and a preponderance of indoor plants have been distributed throughout the waiting area and consulting rooms, attempting to address what Nash et al. (2021) describe as 'new models of care featuring low stigmatising youth-friendly services to improve access' (Nash et al., 2021, p. 1637).

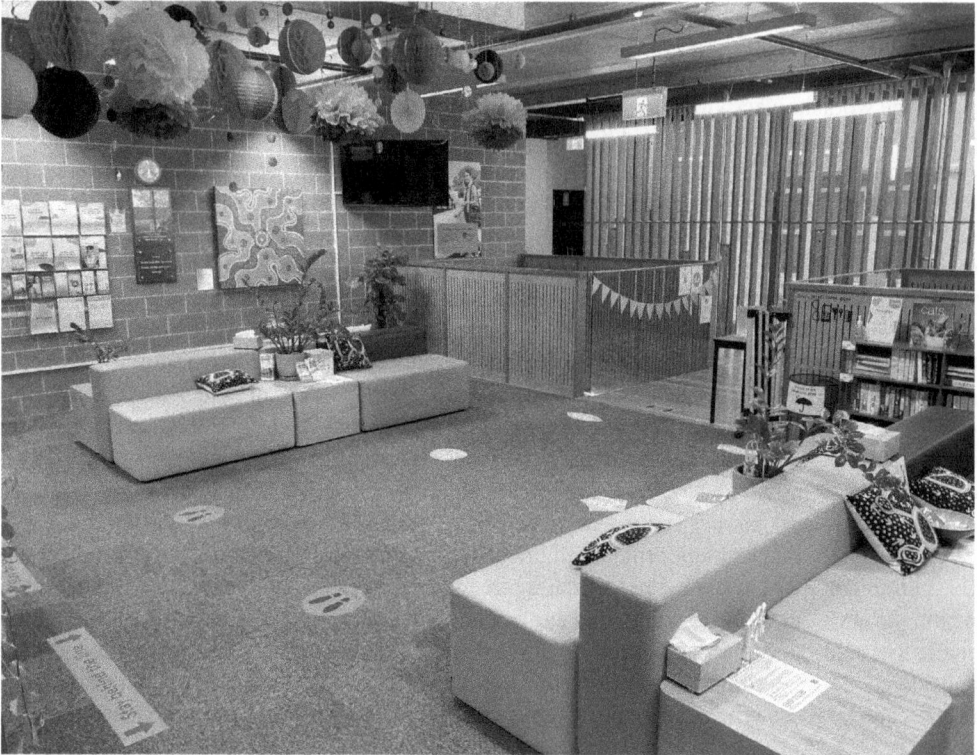

Figure 4.2 Waiting area at headspace, Camperdown. Photograph by the authors

Emergent processes of co-design at headspace Camperdown recognise the power of visual and auditory signifiers to help to engender feelings of inclusivity and alleviate stigma. For example, one interviewee mentioned that in the waiting room, youth-orientated, contemporary music is played at a low volume, Australian Aboriginal artworks feature on the walls, and the rainbow flag is affixed to a windowpane. Participants acknowledged that home may not always be a safe space for headspace clients and, as such, one of the foremost spatial ambitions of headspace Camperdown was to 'create a place where [clients] can come to be free' (interviewee). The shared kitchen area was also described as an important site of emergent co-design: in addition to a refrigerator, food re-heating and tea and coffee facilities, a long table with chairs as well as small round tables and chairs by the east-facing floor-to-ceiling windows were installed, and an informally designed drop-in area – 'headspace youth zone' – was created, replete with lounges, a coffee table, indoor plants and programmable fairy lighting.

Additionally, informal and emergent co-design at headspace Camperdown sought to engage multiple stakeholders equitably, with little distinction between clients and service providers. One example described by participants referred to the personalisation of physical spaces. An interviewee also discussed how clients would sometimes ask clinicians if they could make changes to a room – i.e. move furniture – while some clinicians would bring in their furniture and personal objects.

The informal or emergent co-design reflected in these experiences provides examples of integrated care in practice as realised within one mental health service. While the generative elements described in the experiences were not initiated or led by design per se, they were

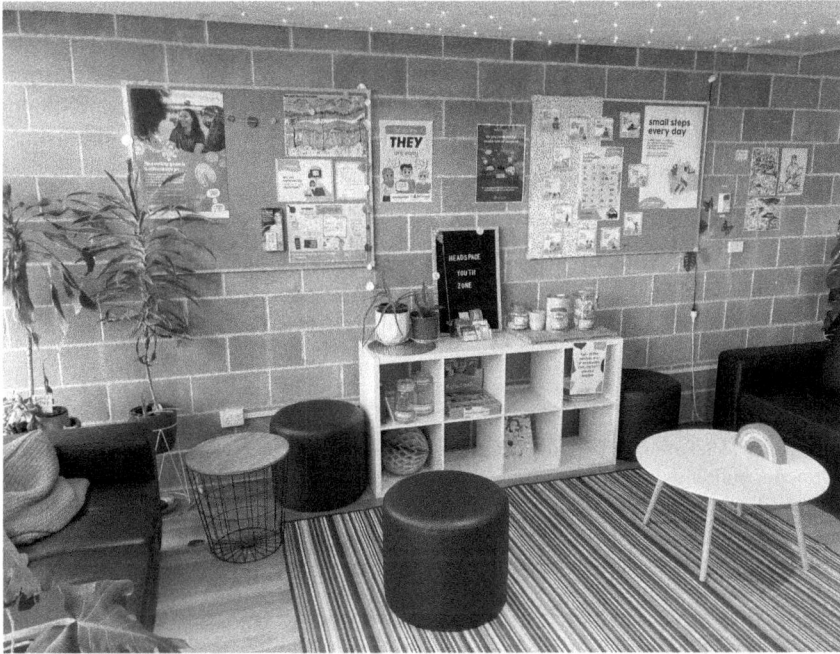

Figure 4.3 Headspace Youth Zone. Photograph by the authors

suggestive of inherent creative practices. Similarly, they demonstrate a values-led approach that seeks to respect stakeholder contributions and insights equitably. In making these experiences explicit, it is possible to apply learnings to inform current thinking across other contexts of mental health, neurology and neuroscience.

Conclusion

The *Brain, Mind and Mallett Street* research collaboration between ADP and BMC set out to investigate and deploy co-design in expanding BMC's services and facilities. The activities of this research collaboration – the workshops and interviews – questioned the status of knowledge in processes of co-design in mental health, neurology and neuroscience settings. These activities identified the significance of expert critical judgement rather than expert clinical judgement in understanding spatial design in these settings. Through these activities, two conceptual spaces of co-design were identified: the first constituting an intentional and formal collaboration between ADP researchers and BMC stakeholders; the second, the emergent and, at times, informal practices of headspace Camperdown. These respectively illustrate the different modes by which co-design can generate spatial understandings: that is, spatial knowledge that is experience-based, derived from expert critical judgement and characterised by nuance, emotions and aesthetics.

Emergent processes of co-design, already entrenched in the headspace youth mental health centre, focus on the co-design of interior spaces, including consultation rooms, the reception area and waiting room and the shared kitchen. These processes are non-hierarchical, dynamic and informed equitably by the experiences, observations and expert critical judgement of the various users and stakeholders of headspace Camperdown, including the youth mental health advocates and past and present service users comprising the YAG.

Identifying these two conceptual spaces of co-design described in the experiences of BMC stakeholders creates an opportunity to understand better and leverage the knowledge and experience of those interacting in the space. Intentional and emergent co-design offer learnings that can inform future collaboration in integrated and multidisciplinary contexts and, importantly, can contribute to collaborative spatial design knowledge for integrated care in mental health, neurology and neuroscience.

Acknowledgements

The authors wish to acknowledge the valuable contributions of all research participants and extend their thanks to the project partner, The Brain and Mind Centre.

References

Berry, L. L., Parker, D., Coile, R. C., Hamilton, D. K., O Neill, D. D., & Sadler, B. L. (2004). The business case for better buildings. *Frontiers of Health Services Management, 21*, 3–24.

Bird, M., McGillion, M., Chambers, E. M., Dix, J., Fajardo, C. J., Gilmour, M., Levesque, K., Lim, A., Mierdel, S., Ouellette, C., & Polanski, A. N. (2021). A generative co-design framework for healthcare innovation: Development and application of an end-user engagement framework. *Research Involvement and Engagement, 7*, 1–12.

Bjögvinsson, E., Ehn, P., & Hillgren, P. A. (2012). Design things and design thinking: Contemporary participatory design challenges. *Design Issues, 28*(3), 101–116.

Colizzi, M., Lasalvia, A., & Ruggeri, M. (2020). Prevention and early intervention in youth mental health: Is it time for a multidisciplinary and trans-diagnostic model for care? *International Journal of Mental Health Systems, 14*(1), 1–14.

Collins, E. (2014). *Architects and research-based knowledge: A literature review*. RIBA.

Devlin, A. S. (2014). *Transforming the doctor's office: Principles from evidence-based design*. Routledge.

DiCicco-Bloom, B., & Crabtree, B. F. (2006). The qualitative research interview. *Medical Education, 40*(4), 314–321.

Donetto, S., Tsianakas, V., & Robert, G. (2014). *Using experience-based co-design (EBCD) to improve the quality of healthcare: Mapping where we are now and establishing future directions* (pp. 5–7). King's College London.

Galle, P. (1999). Design as intentional action: A conceptual analysis. *Design Studies, 20*(1), 57–81.

Glasziou, P. (2011). Foreward. In J. H. Howick (Ed.), *The philosophy of evidence-based medicine* (pp. xi–xii). John Wiley & Sons.

Guattari, F. (1984). *Molecular revolution: Psychiatry and politics*. Puffin Books.

Hagen, P., Collin, P., Metcalf, A., Nicholas, M., Rahilly, K., & Swainston, N. (2012). *Participatory design of evidence-based online youth mental health promotion, intervention and treatment*. http://pandora.nla.gov.au/pan/141862/20160405-1343/www.youngandwellcrc.org.au/wp-content/uploads/2014/03/Young_and_Well_CRC_IM_PD_Guide.pdf

Holmes, E. A., O'Connor, R. C., Perry, V. H., Tracey, I., Wessely, S., Arseneault, L., Ballard, C., Christensen, H., Silver, R. C., Everall, I., & Ford, T. (2020). Multidisciplinary research priorities for the COVID-19 pandemic: A call for action for mental health science. *The Lancet Psychiatry, 7*(6), 547–560.

Hooker, R. C. (1997). The rise and rise of evidence-based medicine. *The Lancet, 349*(9061), 1329–1330.

Howick, J. H. (2011). *The philosophy of evidence-based medicine*. John Wiley & Sons.

Kaji-O'Grady, S., & Smith, C. L. (2019). *LabOratory: Speaking of science and its architecture*. MIT Press.

Karasti, H. (2014, October). Infrastructuring in participatory design. In V. D'Andrea, H. Winschiers-Theophilus (eds.) *Proceedings of the 13th participatory design conference*. Research Paperseries (Vol. 1, pp. 141–150).

Kealy-Bateman, K.-B. W., Ouliaris, C., Viglione, L., Wetton, R., & Bullen, P. (2021). Use of a quality improvement strategy to introduce co-design of the mental health discharge plan in rural and remote New South Wales. *Australian Journal of Rural Health*, *29*(4), 596–600.

Larkin, M., Boden, Z. V., & Newton, E. (2015). On the brink of genuinely collaborative care: Experience-based co-design in mental health. *Qualitative Health Research*, *25*(11), 1463–1476.

Lee, T., & Porter, M. (2013). *The strategy that will fix healthcare*. Harvard Business Review.

Manzini, E. (2015). *Design, when everybody designs: An introduction to design for social innovation*. MIT Press.

Martin, C. S., & Guerin, D. A. (2006). Using research to inform design solutions. *Journal of Facilities Management*, *4*(3), 167–180.

Martin, K., Stevens, A., & Arbour, S. (2017). The process of developing a co-design and co-delivery initiative for mental health programming. *Journal of Psychosocial Rehabilitation and Mental Health*, *4*(2), 247–251.

McGrath, L., & Reavey, P. (Eds.). (2018). *The handbook of mental health and space: Community and clinical applications*. Routledge.

McLaughlan, R. (2018). Psychosocially supportive design: The case for greater attention to social space within the pediatric hospital. *HERD: Health Environments Research & Design Journal*, *11*(2), 151–162.

Muller, M. J., & Druin, A. (2012). Participatory design: The third space in human–computer interaction (1125–1153). In J. Jacko (Ed.), *Human computer interaction handbook: Fundamentals, evolving technologies, and emerging applications*[MS1] . CRC Press.

Mulvale, G., Moll, S., Miatello, A., Murray-Leung, L., Rogerson, K., & Sassi, R. B. (2019). Co-designing services for youth with mental health issues: Novel elicitation approaches. *International Journal of Qualitative Methods*, *18*. doi:10.1177/1609406918816244

Myin-Germeys, I., Kasanova, Z., Vaessen, T., Vachon, H., Kirtley, O., Viechtbauer, W., & Reininghaus, U. (2018). Experience sampling methodology in mental health research: New insights and technical developments. *World Psychiatry*, *17*(2), 123–132.

Nash, L., Isobel, S., Thomas, M., Nguyen, T., & van Der Pol, R. (2021). Clinician stakeholder experiences of a new youth mental health model in Australia: A qualitative study. *Early Intervention in Psychiatry*, *15*(6), 1637–1643.

Noorbergen, T. J., Adam, M. T., Roxburgh, M., & Teubner, T. (2021). Co-design in mHealth systems development: Insights from a systematic literature review. *AIS Transactions on Human-Computer Interaction*, *13*(2), 175–205.

Orlowski, S., Matthews, B., Lawn, S., Jones, G., Bidargaddi, N., & Venning, A. (2018). Designing for practice: Understanding technology use in rural community-based youth mental health contexts. *CoDesign*, *15*(2), 163–184.

Palmer, V. J., Weavell, W., Callander, R., Piper, D., Richard, L., Maher, L., Boyd, H., Herrman, H., Furler, J., Gunn, J., & Iedema, R. (2019). The participatory zeitgeist: An explanatory theoretical model of change in an era of coproduction and co-design in healthcare improvement. *Medical Humanities*, *45*(3), 247–257.

Papoutsi, C., Wherton, J., Shaw, S., Morrison, C., & Greenhalgh, T. (2021). Putting the social back into sociotechnical: Case studies of codesign in digital health. *Journal of the American Medical Informatics Association JAMIA*, *28*(2), 284–293.

Sanders, E. B. N., & Stappers, P. J. (2008). Cocreation and the new landscapes of design. *Co-Design*, *4*(1), 5–18.

Simonsen, J., & Robertson, T. (Eds.). (2013). *Routledge international handbook of participatory design* (Vol. 711). Routledge.

Sleeswijk Visser, F., Stappers, P. J.van der Lugt, R. & Sanders, E. B. N. (2005). *Sanders*Contexmapping. Contexmapping: Experiences from practice EBN. *CoDesign*, *1*(2), 119–149.

Stark, E., Ali, D., Ayre, A., Schneider, N., Parveen, S., Marais, K., & Pender, R. (2021). Coproduction with autistic adults: Reflections from the authentistic research collective. *Autism in Adulthood*, *3*(2), 195–203.

Tindall, R. M., Ferris, M., Townsend, M., Boschert, G., & Moylan, S. (2021). A first-hand experience of co-design in mental health service design: Opportunities, challenges, and lessons. *International Journal of Mental Health Nursing*, *30*(6), 1693–1702.

Trischler, J., Pervan, S. J., Kelly, S. J., & Scott, D. R. (2018). The value of co-design: The effect of customer involvement in service design teams. *Journal of Service Research*, *21*(1), 75–100.

Ulrich, R. S., Berry, L. L., Quan, X., & Parish, J. T. (2010). A conceptual framework for the domain of evidence-based design. *HERD: Health Environments Research & Design Journal*, *4*(1), 95–114.

Zamenopoulos, T., Lam, B., Alexiou, K., Kelemen, M., De Sousa, S., Moffat, S., & Phillips, M. (2019). Types, obstacles and sources of empowerment in co-design: The role of shared material objects and processes. *CoDesign*, *17*(2), 139–158.

5 Co-design of eHealth in the context of severe mental illness

Tessa Dekkers, Nienke Beerlage-de Jong, Stephanie Schouten, Tahnee Heirbaut, Saskia Kelders, Jeroen Deenik and Hanneke Kip

People with severe mental illness and eHealth

Approximately 1% of the world's population lives with severe mental illnesses (SMI), such as schizophrenia (20 million) or bipolar disorder (46 million) (GBD 2017 Disease and Injury Incidence and Prevalence Collaborators, 2018). SMI has a major impact on a person's daily life and is often associated with severe limitations in social and societal functioning. These range from difficulties in finding and retaining employment, housing, relationships, finances and physical health (Firth et al., 2019). To navigate these challenges in daily living, many people with SMI require long-term, complex care from multiple caregivers (Delespaul, 2013).

Care and support needs of people with SMI vary over time, fluctuating with the severity of the illness and the presence of its symptoms. Therefore, treatment must be adapted frequently. During acute stages (e.g. a developing psychotic crisis, attempted suicide) people with SMI require immediate medical assistance through psychiatric emergency services. For people with SMI whose behaviour has led or may lead to a criminal offence, care may also include forensic mental health treatment, focused on preventing criminal recidivism next to treatment of the mental illness (Mullen, 2000). Still, chronic illness can often be managed through medication and support in self-care and daily activities from their general practitioner, psychiatric nurse or informal caregivers (Oud et al., 2009). However, due to shortages in healthcare staff and resources, it is not always possible to deliver optimal care.

Therefore, the person with SMI also has a crucial role in self-managing their illness. Self-management refers to 'the individual's ability to manage the symptoms, treatment, physical and psychosocial consequences, as well as the lifestyle changes inherent to living with a chronic condition' (van Gemert-Pijnen et al., 2018, p. 340). For people with SMI, this may include gaining knowledge about their illness and treatment, having the skills to correctly self-administer medication, knowing how to cope with persistent symptoms or being able to recognise early signs of relapse (Mueser et al., 2002). Equipped with such skills, people with SMI have greater control over their own care.

eHealth, i.e. the use of technology to support health, wellbeing and healthcare (van Gemert-Pijnen et al., 2018), can improve treatment and help people with SMI's self-management. eHealth technologies, such as mobile apps, online modules, wearables or virtual reality (VR) have specific advantages. They can be used by people with SMI in their own time and at their own pace, are scalable and easy to implement since they can be accessed by many people without requiring time from healthcare staff (van Gemert-Pijnen et al., 2018). Furthermore, eHealth can be used to improve the quality of treatment by offering new ways to treat patients, for example, by skills-training in realistic environments in VR. Finally, persuasive eHealth technology can engage people, for example, by including virtual rewards or sending reminders. This can improve adherence to interventions (Kelders et al., 2012; Ludden et al., 2015) and is specifically

DOI: 10.4324/9781003318262-7

relevant to people with SMI in forensic treatment who show generally low treatment motivation (Deenik et al., 2019; Drieschner & Boomsma, 2008).

Despite these potential benefits, eHealth has not yet been broadly adopted in mental healthcare. A large project in Dutch forensic mental healthcare investigated benefits and barriers of 12 different types of technology (e.g. VR, mobile apps, web-based modules, robotics) (Kip et al., 2018). The (in)accessibility of current eHealth was considered a major barrier. Healthcare professionals were concerned that some forensic psychiatric patients did not have the necessary technological and cognitive skills to use eHealth. This concern may be warranted as many existing eHealth interventions rely heavily on users' cognitive and adaptive skills. For example, often-used internet-based interventions are very text-heavy, include written assignments focused on goal-setting and require much intrinsic motivation to complete (Kip et al., 2020). While this project focused specifically on forensic mental health care, people with SMI from both forensic and non-forensic populations may experience deficits in these areas, including shorter attention spans, limited working memory and language skills or difficulties in generalising and applying new knowledge to daily life (Rehm & Shield, 2019; VanDerNagel et al., 2017). This shows that there is a need to design eHealth interventions that better fit the preferences and abilities of people with SMI.

The importance of co-design

One way to develop eHealth interventions that fit people with SMI's preferences and abilities is through co-design. Co-design is characterised by *active involvement* of *non-designers* throughout the design process in a collective creative partnership established through *design activities* (Sanders & Stappers, 2008; Vandekerckhove et al., 2020). Here, the term *non-designers* refers to individuals without a professional background in design, which may include end-users (e.g. people with SMI, friends and family) and other stakeholders (e.g. healthcare professionals and management) (Sanders et al., 2010). *Active involvement* means that these people have influence in the design process beyond the mere usage of a final product. Their role may range from testing, to informant, to co-design partner (DeSmet et al., 2016). Co-design particularly values the latter, which means that co-design research is conducted with end-users and stakeholders as active partners instead of as passive research subjects (Orlowski et al., 2015). *Design activities* are embedded in focus groups or workshops that facilitate collective creativity by allowing all parties to share their experiences and knowledge through acts of making (e.g. a foam mock-up), telling (e.g. sharing experiences) or acting (e.g. role play) (Sanders et al., 2010).

Many benefits of co-design have been proposed and tested, ranging from improving effectiveness of interventions to empowering patients (Frauenberger et al., 2015). For example, the co-design process can improve user experience and usability of eHealth through a better fit with users' needs (Frauenberger et al., 2015; Kip et al., 2019; Orlowski et al., 2015; Visser et al., 2005). eHealth interventions are expected to benefit from such improvements in multiple ways, including increased effectiveness (Orlowski et al., 2015), adherence (Killikelly et al., 2017; Zhang & Ying, 2019) and long-term use.

Involvement in co-design may also provide people with SMI with a method to (re)gain ownership and a sense of power (Frauenberger et al., 2015; Orlowski et al., 2015). This is important, as stereotypical beliefs of people with SMI as dangerous, uncooperative, frightening and lacking self-control and intelligence persist and lead to stigmatisation in the general population, among healthcare professionals and by people with SMI themselves (i.e. self-stigma) (Abiri et al., 2016; Penn & Martin, 1998). Such stigmatic beliefs contribute to an overly pessimistic outlook on the ability of people with SMI to make changes in their health (self-)management and might result in loss of self-esteem, avoidance and increased symptom severity (Abiri et al., 2016; Boyd et al., 2014; Deenik et al., 2019). Finally, some people with SMI have had experiences during their treatment that seriously impede autonomy, including seclusion, restraint, involuntary admission and forced medication (Daya et al., 2020), forcing them to adopt a compliant and passive patient role (Byrne & Wykes, 2020). Together with stigmatisation, this can result in a hierarchical treatment context where opinions of people with SMI are at risk of being disregarded and undervalued. We believe that co-design may help disrupt this hierarchy by showing the importance and value of their perspective.

Until now, co-design has been used sparingly in designing eHealth collaboratively with people with SMI. Examples of studies that have applied co-design include co-design with young adults with schizophrenia to design a smartphone application supporting early phase schizophrenia care (Terp et al., 2016); co-design with people with bipolar disorder to design a mobile self-management app (Switsers et al., 2018); and co-design with teenagers who experienced psychosis to design an educational website (Nakarada-Kordic et al., 2017). All studies were considered successful and endorse the pragmatic and empowering benefits of co-design described above: co-design enabled active engagement of patients and made them feel 'lucky, important, and valuable, not as patients, but as experts of their experience' (Terp et al., 2016); it highlighted the diversity in patients' preferences for eHealth so that the fit of the app could be improved (Switsers et al., 2018); and it dispelled misconceptions about people with mental illness (Nakarada-Kordic et al., 2017).

However, conducting and managing co-design projects in the context of SMI can be challenging. It involves navigating an often highly hierarchical environment. It also requires flexibility to adapt to possibly rapidly fluctuating symptoms, moods or limited cognitive skills of people with SMI. These challenges can all impede design research in healthcare (Groeneveld et al., 2018). A good fit between person, technology and context is essential to any product, but identifying the specific needs of people with SMI is especially important as existing eHealth design conventions may not work for them due to their social, cognitive, physical, psychological and sensory impairments (Kip et al., 2019; Merter & Hasırcı, 2018; Rotondi et al., 2017). In this chapter, we provide recommendations for design researchers to constructively engage in co-design projects in this context. The recommendations are based on earlier work describing best practices for involving people with SMI in co-design and are illustrated with multiple co-design projects from practice.

Best practices for co-design with people with SMI

To determine best practices, we conducted a qualitative multi-method approach incorporating a scoping review of existing literature, a survey and interviews with patients and experts by experience (for full details see Schouten et al., 2022). The identified literature focused on co-design projects with people with SMI. We reviewed each paper for recommendations regarding co-design. In the online survey, 25 researchers participated who had conducted co-design with vulnerable populations. The survey invited respondents to identify challenges faced in co-design and offer recommendations to overcome them. Finally, group interviews were conducted with six current SMI patients and people with lived experience of SMI who had participated in a co-design process. The interviews focused on opinions and preferences regarding participation, activities, communication and continued involvement.

All three sources were combined to identify 23 best-practices for managing co-design projects endorsed by literature, design-researchers and people with SMI (see Box 5.1). Best-practices related to four overarching aspects of co-design, namely: (1) activities to carry out prior to a co-design project; (2) fruitful collaboration within the co-design team; (3) accommodating skills and abilities of SMI participants; and (4) mitigating challenges of power and hierarchy.

Box 5.1 Best-practices for co-design involving people with severe mental illness (adapted from Schouten et al., 2022)

Plan and structure of co-design study

1   Combine multiple methods (e.g. focus groups, interviews and design workshops) to gain different types of data and completeness of information.
2   Set up a flexible study design to allow for an iterative and adaptive development approach.
3   Determine the recruitment strategy in collaboration with stakeholders (e.g. vulnerable members, care organisations, care supervisors, people with lived experience).
4   Secure the availability of sufficient resources (i.e. time, budget, materials and participants) in the early preparation phase of the study.
5   Provide and coordinate a clear structure between and within study activities (e.g. setting regular meetings).
6   Reflect with an open and critical mindset on the chosen methods, tools and materials.

Create and maintain a participatory team

7   Collaborate with multiple stakeholders, including patients, to incorporate all relevant perspectives in the design, development and delivery process.
8   Ensure voluntary and informed participation by briefing participants on study goals and set-up, through clear but brief session introductions and informative flyers.
9   Contact team members and participants in between sessions to send reminders and updates, secure participation and provide them with support for their role as contributor.
10   Stimulate a collaborative work relationship between team members and participants through icebreaker activities.
11   Provide transparency in design decisions by showing (concept) designs and explaining decision rationale.

Accommodate vulnerable participants

12   Use concrete tools (e.g. scenarios, personas and prototypes) that account for the cognitive abilities (e.g. abstract reasoning and decreased attention span) of the SMI participants.
13   Adapt the order of research activities in a bespoke manner during data collection, according to the state and preference of the SMI participants.
14   Prior to the study, determine with participants how to solve practical barriers that might affect participation to improve (repeated) attendance.
15   Offer intrinsically valuable incentives (e.g. money, coupons, personal goals) to participants.
16   Employ researchers skilled in conducting qualitative research (e.g. asking effective probing questions) to guarantee the quality of data.
17   Put measures in place that minimise the risk of harm or distress for vulnerable participants, such as having psychologists in attendance and offering ample opportunities for breaks.

Strive for power balance

18   Approach participants with lived experience as experts and equal partners to minimise the sense of power imbalance.

19 Stimulate equal dialogue and interaction by encouraging reserved members to provide input.
20 Conduct formal evaluations (e.g. brief interviews, exit questionnaires) with vulnerable participants to reflect on both the designs and the co-design process.
21 Create an informal and relaxed physical environment (e.g. through music, decorations and by providing refreshments) during data collection sessions.
22 Enhance accessibility for participation by offering remote research methods to vulnerable participants.
23 Provide skills training on digital literacy and research methods to promote equal participation.

Case studies

Some of these recommendations are relevant to any co-design project, in- and outside the scope of SMI. For example, an iterative study design (#2) is key to co-design in healthcare generally, as is collaboration with multiple stakeholders early and throughout the project (#7) (Melles et al., 2021). The importance of securing time, resources and funding (#4) is often stressed in co-design as well as the need to identify and offer ways to make participation in co-design intrinsically meaningful (#15) (Pirinen, 2016). Finally, minimising existing power imbalances in healthcare systems (#18) is critical to successful co-design (Lindblom et al., 2021; O'Brien et al., 2021; Pirinen, 2016).

Other best practices are more specific to the SMI setting, such as the need to adapt to abilities in abstract reasoning and reduced attention span (#12) and to minimise the risk of harm or distress (#17). The next section illustrates these recommendations for co-design with people with SMI through four concrete case studies. The case studies (SCIPP, LeaveHelp, Forward with VR, WELLBE) are all part of several eHealth projects conducted by researchers from the University of Twente between 2018 and 2022. They all directly involved people with SMI in the design process in some way, though the extent and nature of their involvement varied. For example, LeaveHelp involved people with SMI as informants for feedback on early prototypes through usability tests, while SCIPP involved people with SMI in multiple design workshops as active co-creators.

Self-control intervention app (SCIPP) for people with severe mental illness

The eHealth intervention

Self-control refers to the ability to prevent or override unwanted thoughts or behaviours (Muraven et al., 1999; Tangney et al., 2004). Training self-control is relevant to people with SMI as self-control has a positive impact on problems they may struggle with, including aggression, emotion regulation and physical activity (Tangney et al., 2004). The SCIPP project was initiated to explore the perspectives of people with SMI on self-control training (SCT) to ultimately design a usable, engaging and effective SCT mobile app.

Co-design activities

The SCIPP project consisted of three generative design workshops and one-on-one usability tests conducted with people currently in treatment for their SMI as well as people with lived experience of SMI and who were employed at the time as experience expert.[1] All participants were supplied with a booklet of co-design exercises to create awareness of when and how they use self-control in their daily life (Visser et al., 2005). The first workshop focused on experiences with, and attitudes towards, self-control. Experiences were elicited through two activities: 2D-collaging during which participants created a collage to represent self-control and a moderated group discussion. During the second workshop, mock-ups of elements of the app were discussed. For example, participants discussed ways in which the app could track progress (e.g. using a dashboard, a timeline, a visual etc.). After this workshop, a professional design company developed three paper prototypes based on desired qualities and drawings made by participants. In the final workshop, participants explored these prototypes. The session closed with a general group interview, asking patients for their views regarding (elements of) the prototypes and the extent to which they found them appealing, usable and intuitive. Afterwards, a functioning high-fidelity prototype of the app was developed and tested. Three new participants with SMI were recruited to navigate through the app using structured scenarios (e.g. set up an account and navigate to the daily self-control challenge) and to provide recommendations for improvement.

Co-design recommendations

It is important to address existing power imbalances and approach people with lived experience as equal partners with equal rights (#18). For example, in the SCIPP project, this meant that people who participated were able to use their phones during design workshops, even if phone use is normally prohibited for them. Another way that equality was fostered was by transparently showing and crediting contributions. In the SCIPP project, design workshops were conducted sequentially, with each workshop incorporating knowledge gained in previous workshops. For example, in workshop 1, patients stated that self-control is trained together with other people who can support them. For the second workshop, we prepared several mock-ups illustrating how social support could be embedded in the app. Ultimately, a virtual coach who encouraged users to share their successes with close others was included in the app. As this direction emerged collaboratively, everyone was credited as a co-designer in the 'about us' page of the SCIPP app. In the exit interviews, we discovered that this experience of equality was part of the intrinsic motivation of patients to participate (#15). Patients shared that they valued seeing that their contributions mattered and that this would motivate them to participate in co-design again.

Leave app (*VerlofHulp* app) for patients in forensic care

The eHealth intervention

At a given moment in their treatment, forensic psychiatric inpatients go on (unescorted) leave. This is an exciting moment, both for the patient and the healthcare provider, as patients will have to deal with difficult situations in the world outside the institution by themselves. The Leave app (Dutch: *VerlofHulp* app) supports patients during their leave by self-monitoring leave goals, such as activities (e.g. work or family visits), skills (e.g. social or coping skills), problem behaviours (e.g. focused on alcohol use or sexually transgressive behaviour) and thoughts and feelings, providing tailored advice for patients on leave. The goal of the Leave app project was to investigate the acceptability of the app's content and design and how the app could be further improved.

Co-design activities

As part of the iterative design process and to check whether the language used in the app was suitable for the target group of forensic patients – a group that often has mild intellectual disabilities – the texts in the app were submitted to two healthcare professionals experienced in treating patients with intellectual disabilities. Based on their advice, the language was simplified, shortened and formulated in a more direct manner. After a first version of the app was developed, usability tests were conducted with forensic patients.

In the usability tests, a Think Aloud protocol combined with interviews was used. Patients performed three tasks in the app (e.g. completing a diary) while expressing their thoughts about the process and afterwards answered questions regarding the perceived benefits and points of improvement of the app. During the usability tests, the researchers specifically paid attention to the findability of buttons and functions in the app, the ease of navigation through the app, as well as the comprehensibility of the texts.

Co-design recommendations

The usability tests identified many issues with the app. Patients found that it included too much text and had problems navigating the app. As one participant put it: "I am in a mental maze right now" (Dutch: "*Ik zit in een mentaal doolhof*", personal translation by first author). As indicated earlier, this can be due to a misfit between the design and content of the app and the level of abstract reasoning and attention span of the user. Typical usability tests of medical devices last one to two hours and may take up to four, covering multiple tasks (Wiklund et al., 2010). To account for the general shorter attention spans of this target group (#12) in the Leave App project, the time was limited to a maximum of 45 minutes and a maximum of three tasks. The tasks within the usability test were made as concrete as possible and were embedded in real-life scenarios. These scenarios were short, clear and specific so that participants could easily imagine that they were the person in the generic situation outlined in the scenario, reducing the need for abstract reasoning. This was also helpful in allowing the researchers to observe first hand where errors arose.

Virtual reality project: forward with VR

The eHealth intervention

To treat patients with SMI and aggressive or sexual delinquent behaviour, both therapist and patient need a clear idea of what triggers this behaviour. This is challenging, as many patients have difficulties with reflecting on, and talking about, their behaviour in a treatment room, which is very different from the context in which their delinquent behaviour occurs. VR offers opportunities to observe and practice behaviour in immersive scenarios that feel realistic. In the 'Forward with VR' (Dutch: *VooRuit met VR*) project, a co-design development process was initiated to identify the needs and wishes of patients and therapists regarding a VR-application. This resulted in the 'Triggers & Helpers' VR intervention. In this interactive VR application, therapist and patient build personalised VR-scenarios to gain more insight into challenging situations and provide personalised opportunities to safely practice coping skills to prevent delinquent behaviour.

Co-design activities

Triggers & Helpers was designed by means of an extensive, multi-method development process (Kip et al., 2019), structured by means of the CeHRes Roadmap – an interdisciplinary framework for the development, implementation and evaluation of eHealth interventions (van Gemert-Pijnen et al., 2011). Specifically relevant to the co-design was the multidisciplinary project team that included a coordinator, researchers, a policy advisor, patients and therapists. The team was responsible for the coordination and decision-making within the project. Decisions were made based on data that were collected from participants (other than the project team) via multiple methods. These included focus groups on potential applications of VR, semi-structured interviews on points of improvement of current care, idea generation with video-based scenarios, evaluation of potential VR applications, low-fidelity prototyping and a second round of interviews to investigate whether the VR application was in line with previously defined values. Based on this process and the resulting prototype, multiple versions of the VR application were developed by the VR developer and tested with therapists and patients via usability tests. After multiple iterations, a final version of the VR application was released in 2022 and is now commercially available and used by multiple treatment centres. Based on experiences of therapists and patients, ongoing improvements and additions will be made to continue to ensure the most optimal user experience for therapists and patients.

Co-design recommendations

The project that led to the intervention took several years and was coordinated by a multidisciplinary project team (#7). To use the team most effectively, patients and therapists were involved both as *participants* in separate data collection activities as well as *decision-makers* based on the collected data. This ensured involvement of end-users in determining the problem at hand, in mapping contextual factors and in setting-up the project, i.e. before data collection started. Another benefit of the multidisciplinary team was the ability to reflect on the suitability of co-design activities with this target group from multiple perspectives (#6).

The necessity of accounting for the capabilities of people with SMI in setting up research methods (#12) was stressed in this project. For example, the first round of interviews took about an hour and contained relatively abstract questions, which appeared to be challenging for participating patients. In line with recommendation #6 on reflecting critically on the methods, this experience was used to shape the next methods, e.g. by ensuring a shorter time span and by using concrete examples. These findings were also shared with the research community by means of an open-access paper, in which the importance of sharing these lessons learnt was emphasized (Kip et al., 2019).

Web-based positive psychology app (WELLBE) for patients with bipolar disorder

The eHealth intervention

Mood monitoring is an important element in the treatment of bipolar disorder (BD). The prospective Life Chart Method (Denicoff et al., 1997) helps people with BD to monitor their mood on a daily basis, which facilitates early recognition and intervention in relapse (Denicoff et al., 2002; Gershon & Eidelman, 2015). However, people with BD can experience daily monitoring as taxing and confrontational (Saunders et al., 2017). The WELLBE project was conducted to develop a digital version of the Life Chart Method informed by patients and healthcare professionals and to investigate the opinions and preferences of people with BD relating to positive psychology interventions (PPI's) more generally (Geerling et al., 2021, 2022)

Co-design activities

Three two-hour focus group meetings were held with patients with BD and mental health professionals treating patients with BD. The first focus group explored experiences with positive psychology, monitoring and technology. Participants wrote down their experiences, needs and requirements of a PPI app on Post-its. Agreements and disagreements about preferences were summarised and checked with participants for validation and comments. Based on the outcomes, an illustrative example of a positive psychology exercise on gratefulness was developed. During the next focus group, participants evaluated the content, wording and design of this prototype and discussed possible other positive psychology interventions. Based on these findings, a functioning app-prototype was developed, containing several short positive psychology interventions. Nineteen patients and healthcare professionals (a mix of people who had or had not previously participated in the focus groups) participated in the pilot test to gain a broad mix of opinions. They used the app as they went about their daily activities. While using the prototype, they posted remarks and evaluations, which were discussed in a final moderated discussion during the third focus group.

Co-design recommendations

People with SMI can come into co-design projects with distressing and traumatic experiences (Tindall et al., 2021). Therefore, an important recommendation for co-design in the SMI context is to minimise risk of harm and distress (#17). In the WELLBE project, harm and distress was minimised in several ways. First, the lead researcher explicitly took on a dual role of monitoring both the co-design process and wellbeing of participants therein. In addition, all recruitment material was written in clear, understandable language and stressed that participants could stop participation at any time, also allowing participants to advocate for their own wellbeing. Prior to the final workshop, one person with SMI was no longer able (and willing) to participate. The lead researcher debriefed this participant personally and ensured that they still received their small gift for participation (in line with recommendation #15 on incentives). Because the workshops were set up with flexible exercises that could work with any number of participants (#2), the project could still continue as planned.

Conclusion

Taking a co-design approach to eHealth development has the potential to create technology that closely fits the unique capabilities and characteristics of people with SMI. This may improve the use and effectiveness of eHealth, resulting in patients with an increased capacity to cope with the daily impact of their (chronic) mental illness. Still, to reach these goals, design-researchers should critically reflect on the extent to which co-design is accessible as a method and take steps to make the method as inclusive as possible for people with SMI. In this chapter, we have discussed best practices in four case studies that illustrate how to adapt co-design planning, management and activities.

We found that working with people with SMI forces design researchers to fully understand their target group and their strengths and weaknesses as well as the primary aims of each stage of the co-design process. If the participants' attention span only allows for a short usability test, it must be focused on the core functionalities of the design. If the benefit of a technology can only be discussed through a simple, concrete storyboard, it must be made very clear what this benefit is. While the current chapter focused primarily on the co-design of mobile apps, it can be conjectured that this increased clarity of focus can also benefit co-design projects conducted in other settings.

We have also discussed that co-design may empower people with SMI, disrupting (self) stigmatisation and hierarchy in the mental healthcare system. In recent years, many authors have called for a mental healthcare system that is better informed by, and more attuned to, people with lived experience (Byrne & Wykes, 2020; Daya et al., 2020; Tindall et al., 2021). The case studies demonstrate that considerate co-design that fits with people with SMI is not only possible but also very valuable in this regard. It results in better-fitting products, services and systems. But even more important is the culture shift that occurs when designers, researchers, clinicians, people with SMI and their caregivers are brought together to be truly empathic to each other's experiences.

Note

1 Dutch: *ervaringsdeskundige*, a care professional who provides care informed by their own experiential knowledge following one to two years of vocational or college education.

References

Abiri, S., Oakley, L. D., Hitchcock, M. E., & Hall, A. (2016). Stigma related avoidance in people living with Severe Mental Illness (SMI): Findings of an integrative review. *Community Mental Health Journal, 52*(3), 251–261. https://doi.org/10.1007/s10597-015-9957-2

Boyd, J. E., Adler, E. P., Otilingam, P. G., & Peters, T. (2014). Internalized Stigma of Mental Illness (ISMI) scale: A multinational review. *Comprehensive Psychiatry, 55*(1), 221–231. https://doi.org/10.1016/j.comppsych.2013.06.005

Byrne, L., & Wykes, T. (2020). A role for lived experience mental health leadership in the age of Covid-19. *Journal of Mental Health, 29*(3), 243–246. https://doi.org/10.1080/09638237.2020.1766002

Daya, I., Hamilton, B., & Roper, C. (2020). Authentic engagement: A conceptual model for welcoming diverse and challenging consumer and survivor views in mental health research, policy, and practice. *International Journal of Mental Health Nursing, 29*(2), 299–311. https://doi.org/10.1111/inm.12653

Deenik, J., Tenback, D. E., Tak, E. C. P. M., Blanson Henkemans, O. A., Rosenbaum, S., Hendriksen, I. J. M., & van Harten, P. N. (2019). Implementation barriers and facilitators of an integrated multidisciplinary lifestyle enhancing treatment for inpatients with severe mental illness: The MULTI study IV. *BMC Health Services Research, 19*(1), 740. https://doi.org/10.1186/s12913-019-4608-x

Delespaul, P. (2013). Consensus over de definitie van mensen met een ernstige psychische aandoening (EPA) en hun aantal in Nederland [Consensus on the definition of people with a serious mental illness (SMI) and their numbers in the Netherlands]. *Tijdschrift Voor Psychiatrie, 55*(6), 427–438.

Denicoff, K. D., Ali, S. O., Sollinger, A. B., Smith-Jackson, E. E., Leverich, G. S., & Post, R. M. (2002). Utility of the daily prospective National Institute of Mental Health Life-Chart Method (NIMH-LCM-p) ratings in clinical trials of bipolar disorder. *Depression and Anxiety, 15*(1), 1–9. https://doi.org/10.1002/da.1078

Denicoff, K. D., Smith-Jackson, E. E., Disney, E. R., Suddath, R. L., Leverich, G. S., & Post, R. M. (1997). Preliminary evidence of the reliability and validity of the prospective Life-Chart Methodology (LCM-p). *Journal of Psychiatric Research, 31*(5), 593–603. https://doi.org/10.1016/S0022-3956(96)00027-1

DeSmet, A., Thompson, D., Baranowski, T., Palmeira, A., Verloigne, M., & De Bourdeaudhuij, I. (2016). Is participatory design associated with the effectiveness of serious digital games for healthy lifestyle promotion? A meta-analysis. *Journal of Medical Internet Research, 18*(4). https://doi.org/10.2196/jmir.4444

Drieschner, K. H., & Boomsma, A. (2008). The treatment motivation scales for forensic outpatient treatment (TMS-F). *Assessment, 15*(2), 224–241. https://doi.org/10.1177/1073191107311650

Firth, J., Siddiqi, N., Koyanagi, A., Siskind, D., Rosenbaum, S., Galletly, C., Allan, S., Caneo, C., Carney, R., Carvalho, A. F., Chatterton, M. L., Correll, C. U., Curtis, J., Gaughran, F., Heald, A., Hoare, E., Jackson, S. E., Kisely, S., Lovell, K., … Stubbs, B. (2019). The Lancet Psychiatry Commission: A blueprint for protecting physical health in people with mental illness. *The Lancet Psychiatry, 6*(8), 675–712. https://doi.org/10.1016/S2215-0366(19)30132-4

Frauenberger, C., Good, J., Fitzpatrick, G., & Iversen, O. S. (2015). In pursuit of rigour and accountability in participatory design. *International Journal of Human-Computer Studies, 74*, 93–106. https://doi.org/10.1016/j.ijhcs.2014.09.004

GBD 2017 Disease and Injury Incidence and Prevalence Collaborators. (2018). Global, regional, and national incidence, prevalence, and years lived with disability for 354 diseases and injuries for 195 countries and territories, 1990–2017: A systematic analysis for the global burden of disease study 2017. *The Lancet, 392*(10159), 1789–1858. https://doi.org/10.1016/S0140-6736(18)32279-7

Geerling, B., Kelders, S. M., Kupka, R. W., Stevens, A. W. M. M., & Bohlmeijer, E. T. (2021). How to make online mood-monitoring in bipolar patients a success? A qualitative exploration of requirements. *International Journal of Bipolar Disorders*, *9*(1), 39. https://doi.org/10.1186/s40345-021-00244-2

Geerling, B., Kelders, S. M., Stevens, A. W. M. M., Kupka, R. W., & Bohlmeijer, E. T. (2022). A web-based positive psychology app for patients with bipolar disorder: Development study. *JMIR Formative Research*, *6*(9), e39476. https://doi.org/10.2196/39476

Gershon, A., & Eidelman, P. (2015). Inter-episode affective intensity and instability: Predictors of depression and functional impairment in bipolar disorder. *Journal of Behavior Therapy and Experimental Psychiatry*, *46*, 14–18. https://doi.org/10.1016/j.jbtep.2014.07.005

Groeneveld, B., Dekkers, T., Boon, B., & D'Olivo, P. (2018). Challenges for design researchers in healthcare. *Design for Health*, *2*(2), 305–326. https://doi.org/10.1080/24735132.2018.1541699

Kelders, S. M., Kok, R. N., Ossebaard, H. C., & Van Gemert-Pijnen, J. E. W. C. (2012). Persuasive system design does matter: A systematic review of adherence to web-based interventions. *Journal of Medical Internet Research*, *14*(6), 1–24. https://doi.org/10.2196/jmir.2104

Killikelly, C., He, Z., Reeder, C., & Wykes, T. (2017). Improving adherence to web-based and mobile technologies for people with psychosis: Systematic review of new potential predictors of adherence. *JMIR MHealth and UHealth*, *5*(7), e94. https://doi.org/10.2196/mhealth.7088

Kip, H., Bouman, Y. H. A., Kelders, S. M., & van Gemert-Pijnen, L. J. E. W. C. (2018). eHealth in treatment of offenders in forensic mental health: A review of the current state. *Frontiers in Psychiatry*, *9*. https://doi.org/10.3389/fpsyt.2018.00042

Kip, H., Kelders, S. M., Bouman, Y. H. A., & Van Gemert-Pijnen, L. J. E. W. C. (2019). The importance of systematically reporting and reflecting on eHealth development: Participatory development process of a virtual reality application for forensic mental health care. *Journal of Medical Internet Research*, *21*(8). https://doi.org/10.2196/12972

Kip, H., Sieverink, F., van Gemert-Pijnen, L. J. E. W. C., Bouman, Y. H. A., & Kelders, S. M. (2020). Integrating people, context, and technology in the implementation of a web-based intervention in forensic mental health care: Mixed-methods study. *Journal of Medical Internet Research*, *22*(5), 1–24. https://doi.org/10.2196/16906

Lindblom, S., Flink, M., Elf, M., Laska, A. C., von Koch, L., & Ytterberg, C. (2021). The manifestation of participation within a co-design process involving patients, significant others and health-care professionals. *Health Expectations*, *24*(3), 905–916. https://doi.org/10.1111/hex.13233

Ludden, G. D., van Rompay, T. J., Kelders, S. M., & van Gemert-Pijnen, J. E. (2015). How to increase reach and adherence of web-based interventions: A design research viewpoint. *Journal of Medical Internet Research*, *17*(7), e172. https://doi.org/10.2196/jmir.4201

Melles, M., Albayrak, A., & Goossens, R. (2021). Innovating health care: Key characteristics of human-centered design. *International Journal for Quality in Health Care*, *33*(Suppl. 1), 37–44. https://doi.org/10.1093/intqhc/mzaa127

Merter, S., & Hasırcı, D. (2018). A participatory product design process with children with autism spectrum disorder. *CoDesign*, *14*(3), 170–187. https://doi.org/10.1080/15710882.2016.1263669

Mueser, K. T., Corrigan, P. W., Hilton, D. W., Tanzman, B., Schaub, A., Gingerich, S., Essock, S. M., Tarrier, N., Morey, B., Vogel-Scibilia, S., & Herz, M. I. (2002). Illness management and recovery: A review of the research. *Psychiatric Services*, *53*(10), 1272–1284. https://doi.org/10.1176/appi.ps.53.10.1272

Mullen, P. E. (2000). Forensic mental health. *British Journal of Psychiatry*, *176*(4), 307–311. https://doi.org/10.1192/bjp.176.4.307

Muraven, M., Baumeister, R. F., & Tice, D. M. (1999). Longitudinal improvement of self-regulation through practice: Building self-control strength through repeated exercise. *The Journal of Social Psychology*, *139*(4), 446–457. https://doi.org/10.1080/00224549909598404

Nakarada-Kordic, I., Hayes, N., Reay, S. D., Corbet, C., & Chan, A. (2017). Co-designing for mental health: Creative methods to engage young people experiencing psychosis. *Design for Health*, *1*(2), 229–244. https://doi.org/10.1080/24735132.2017.1386954

O'Brien, J., Fossey, E., & Palmer, V. J. (2021). A scoping review of the use of co-design methods with culturally and linguistically diverse communities to improve or adapt mental health services. *Health and Social Care in the Community*, *29*(1), 1–17. https://doi.org/10.1111/hsc.13105

Orlowski, S. K., Lawn, S., Venning, A., Winsall, M., Jones, G. M., Wyld, K., Damarell, R. A., Antezana, G., Schrader, G., Smith, D., Collin, P., & Bidargaddi, N. (2015). Participatory research as one piece of the puzzle: A systematic review of consumer involvement in design of technology-based youth mental health and well-being interventions. *JMIR Human Factors, 2*(2), e12. https://doi.org/10.2196/humanfactors.4361

Oud, M. J., Schuling, J., Slooff, C. J., Groenier, K. H., Dekker, J. H., & Meyboom-De Jong, B. (2009). Care for patients with severe mental illness: The general practitioner's role perspective. *BMC Family Practice, 10*, 1–8. https://doi.org/10.1186/1471-2296-10-29

Penn, D. L., & Martin, J. (1998). The stigma of severe mental illness: Some potential solutions for a recalcitrant problem. *Psychiatric Quarterly, 69*(3), 235–247. https://doi.org/10.1023/A:1022153327316

Pirinen, A. (2016). The barriers and enablers of co-design for services. *International Journal of Design, 10*(3), 27–42. http://www.ijdesign.org/index.php/IJDesign/article/view/2575

Rehm, J., & Shield, K. D. (2019). Global burden of disease and the impact of mental and addictive disorders. *Current Psychiatry Reports, 21*(2), 10. https://doi.org/10.1007/s11920-019-0997-0

Rotondi, A. J., Spring, M. R., Hanusa, B. H., Eack, S. M., & Haas, G. L. (2017). Designing eHealth applications to reduce cognitive effort for persons with severe mental illness: Page complexity, navigation simplicity, and comprehensibility. *JMIR Human Factors, 4*(1), e1. https://doi.org/10.2196/humanfactors.6221

Sanders, E. B.-N., Brandt, E., & Binder, T. (2010). A framework for organizing the tools and techniques of participatory design. *ACM International Conference Proceeding Series*, 195–198. https://doi.org/10.1145/1900441.1900476

Sanders, E. B.-N., & Stappers, P. J. (2008). Co-creation and the new landscapes of design. *CoDesign, 4*(1), 5–18. https://doi.org/10.1080/15710880701875068

Saunders, K. E. A., Bilderbeck, A. C., Panchal, P., Atkinson, L. Z., Geddes, J. R., & Goodwin, G. M. (2017). Experiences of remote mood and activity monitoring in bipolar disorder: A qualitative study. *European Psychiatry, 41*(1), 115–121. https://doi.org/10.1016/j.eurpsy.2016.11.005

Schouten, S. E., Kip, H., Dekkers, T., Deenik, J., Beerlage-de Jong, N., Ludden, G. D. S., & Kelders, S. M. (2022). Best-practices for co-design processes involving people with severe mental illness for eMental health interventions: A qualitative multi-method approach. *Design for Health, 6*(3), 316–344. https://doi.org/10.1080/24735132.2022.2145814

Switsers, L., Dauwe, A., Vanhoudt, A., Van Dyck, H., Lombaerts, K., & Oldenburg, J. F. E. (2018). Users' perspectives on mHealth self-management of bipolar disorder: Qualitative focus group study. *JMIR MHealth and UHealth, 6*(5). https://doi.org/10.2196/mhealth.9529

Tangney, J. P., Baumeister, R. F., & Boone, A. L. (2004). High self-control predicts good adjustment, less pathology, better grades, and interpersonal success. *Journal of Personality, 72*(2), 271–324. https://doi.org/10.1111/j.0022-3506.2004.00263.x

Terp, M., Laursen, B. S., Jørgensen, R., Mainz, J., & Bjørnes, C. D. (2016). A room for design: Through participatory design young adults with schizophrenia become strong collaborators. *International Journal of Mental Health Nursing, 25*(6), 496–506. https://doi.org/10.1111/inm.12231

Tindall, R. M., Ferris, M., Townsend, M., Boschert, G., & Moylan, S. (2021). A first-hand experience of co-design in mental health service design: Opportunities, challenges, and lessons. *International Journal of Mental Health Nursing, 30*(6), 1693–1702. https://doi.org/10.1111/inm.12925

Vandekerckhove, P., De Mul, M., Bramer, W. M., & de Bont, A. A. (2020). Generative participatory design methodology to develop electronic health interventions: Systematic literature review. *Journal of Medical Internet Research, 22*(4), 1–18. https://doi.org/10.2196/13780

VanDerNagel, J. E. L., Kiewik, M., Didden, R., Korzilius, H. P. L. M., van Dijk, M., van der Palen, J., Buitelaar, J. K., & de Jong, C. A. J. (2017). Substance use in individuals with mild to borderline intellectual disability: An exploration of rates and risks in the Netherlands. *Advances in Neurodevelopmental Disorders, 1*(4), 283–293. https://doi.org/10.1007/s41252-017-0035-3

van Gemert-Pijnen, L. J. E. W. C., Kelders, S. M., Kip, H., & Sanderman, R. (Eds.). (2018). *eHealth research, theory and development*. Routledge. https://doi.org/10.4324/9781315385907

van Gemert-Pijnen, L. J. E. W. C., Kip, H., Kelders, S. M., & Sanderman, R. (2018). Introducing ehealth. In S. M. Kelders, H. Kip, & R. Sanderman (Eds.), *eHealth research, theory and development* (pp. 3–26). Routledge.

van Gemert-Pijnen, L. J. E. W. C., Nijland, N., van Limburg, M., Ossebaard, H. C., Kelders, S. M., Eysenbach, G., & Seydel, E. R. (2011). A holistic framework to improve the uptake and impact of eHealth technologies. *Journal of Medical Internet Research*, *13*(4), e111. https://doi.org/10.2196/jmir.1672

Visser, F. S., Stappers, P. J., van der Lugt, R., & Sanders, E. B.-N. (2005). Contextmapping: Experiences from practice. *CoDesign*, *1*(2), 119–149. https://doi.org/10.1080/15710880500135987

Wiklund, M. E., Kendler, J., & Strochlic, A. Y. (2010). *Usability testing of medical devices*. CRC Press. https://doi.org/10.1201/b10458

Zhang, M. W. B., & Ying, J. (2019). Incorporating participatory action research in attention bias modification interventions for addictive disorders: Perspectives. *International Journal of Environmental Research and Public Health*, *16*(5). https://doi.org/10.3390/ijerph16050822

6 Guidelines for facilitation

Articulating tacit knowledge on co-designing within mental health

Erika Renedo Illarregi

Introduction

This chapter presents a framework for facilitating co-design within mental health care contexts. It has been developed by reflecting on two projects – the *Co-design for Wellbeing* case study and the *Design at Psychosis Therapy Project* (*Design at PTP*) – and is illustrated through participant interview data alongside extracts from the author's reflective diary.

Most co-designers have learnt facilitating through practice, often intuitively, and the tacit skills involved are rarely taught formally nor discussed in design research. Escalante et al. (2017) also point out that research on the transformative impact of co-design processes on design researchers themselves is lacking. Furthermore, when conducting co-design work within a mental health context, designers may be required to adopt the role of a listener or support person, engaging in co-design through reciprocity (Kenning and Bennett, this book). To call attention to these unspoken dimensions of facilitators' experiences, this chapter draws on the personal insights of the author's role and experience as a facilitator.

The reflection is structured in three parts: the first part proposes the metaphorical concepts of *weaving and layered participation*, the second introduces the notion of *nurturing mattering* and the third discusses *facilitation attitudes, emotions and ethics*. Weaving and layered participation have been developed to encourage meaningful and ethical engagement (Renedo Illarregi, 2022, p. 272). The *weaving* metaphor was chosen to express how one *thread* of engagement may weave the next, while *layered* participation refers to participants being able to engage at different levels simultaneously. *Mattering* refers to the extent to which we make a difference in the world around us (Elliott et al., 2010). Perceiving that we are noticed by, and are important to, others is known as the experience of mattering to others (Rosenberg, 1985). Within weaved or layered participation, a sense of mattering is intrinsically developing as everyone is encouraged to contribute one way or the other. This sense can be nurtured further by using certain strategies that help raise awareness of each person's contribution to the design, to each other and the world. These strategies are discussed and illustrated with examples in the section *nurturing mattering*. Finally, within a participatory situation where mattering is nurtured, certain *attitudes and emotions* emerge, which in turn are favourable to weaving layered participation, closing the circle. In the following, two case studies are discussed to illuminate this cycle. The chapter concludes with a discussion on these concepts in relation to the literature.

Methods

The two case studies presented here were part of a PhD project by the author that explored the experiences of co-design participants facing mental health problems (Renedo Illarregi, 2022).

DOI: 10.4324/9781003318262-8

The research followed the ethical guidelines of collaborators Islington Mind and *Psychosis Therapy Project* and was approved by the Human Research Ethics Committee (HREC) of The Open University.

Design at PTP

Design at PTP was part of the service for people with psychosis (Psychosis Therapy, 2021), which was held at Islington Mind, London. Participants were recruited from those attending the charity's drop-in service by informing them about the project. Nealy, David, Anthony, Nestor, Amara, Baris, Ellaria, Uriel and Jack participated in this research. Names were pseudonymised, unless otherwise preferred by participants – like in the case of Anthony. More on the ethics around privacy versus participants' willingness for recognition can be found in Renedo (Illarregi, 2022, p. 319). During the spring of 2019, weekly design workshops were delivered in the drop-in space for six months, loosely structured in three stages: understanding design, finding and mapping situations and creating design(s). The first stage aimed to help participants familiarise with each other and with design. It consisted of activities chosen ad hoc for the project, such as bringing meaningful objects and discussing their design process in relation to a historical timeline; or prototyping design solutions to respond to each other's improvised design problems. Unlike boundary objects (Star & Griesemer, 1989), which mediate among stakeholders through belonging to diverse, intersecting social worlds, these were personal to each individual and helped participants express themselves before the group could comment on how they related to the timeline. Prototyping was used in a collaborative context (Peter et al., 2013) with the additional requirement that they were addressing design briefs devised by other group members. In the second stage, a version of cultural probes (Gaver et al., 1999) was used to explore participants' common interests and curiosities and to inform the development of a design brief, or purpose. The brief emerged following collective work of organising the responses thematically (Figure 6.1). As a result, 'stewardship' and 'taking care of humanity' were proposed as purposes for the collective design project. Finally, brainstorming activities were organised to generate ideas. Three different aims (to heal, to wonder and to connect) and three different target groups (spiritual creatives, the wisening population and nature) were distilled from the themes that emerged during the cultural probes. Participants chose to pair these randomly to create three brainstorming sessions: 'To help Nature heal'; 'To help spiritual creatives wonder'; and 'To help the wisening population connect'. The final outcome was a board game, which was showcased alongside other participants' work in an exhibition at the Islington Mind charity. Most of the activities in the workshops were designed or redesigned by me while getting to know the participants, and they were informed by, and the result of, intuitive processes which I aim to articulate through the conceptual framework described in this chapter. A detailed description of all workshops and activities can be found in Renedo Illarregi (2022, p. 136).

Co-design for Wellbeing

The *Co-design for Wellbeing* project (Renedo-Illarregi et al., 2020) was delivered through eight structured weekly sessions at Islington Mind. Four participants – Damian, Bea, Liam and Raymond – engaged throughout the project (names pseudonymised except Raymond).

The idea was to explore a design project that could be easily implemented across health and care contexts. The project began with a process of identifying matters of concern around the subject of wellbeing. There was less emphasis on coordination towards a unifying goal, aiming instead at the mutual enhancement of different ideas. Participants shared and explored issues

- No expectations
- Flexibility
- Curiosity
- Humour
- Navigating conflict

- Making space for lateral discussions
- Appreciation, affirmation, and acknowledgement
- Equalizing contributions
- Bridging
- Reframing experiences
- Communicating impact
- Your own sense of mattering

- Interlacing designing with other activities
- Adding activities to respond to disengagement
- Sharing your own research challenges
- Designing through use
- Emergent briefs
- The use of physical space and materials
- From week to week
- Navigating uncertainty
- The use of randomness and serendipity

contributing   bettering   intentioning

connecting   thinking

Facilitation attitudes and emotions
Nurturing mattering
Weaving and layered participation

less intentional

more intentional

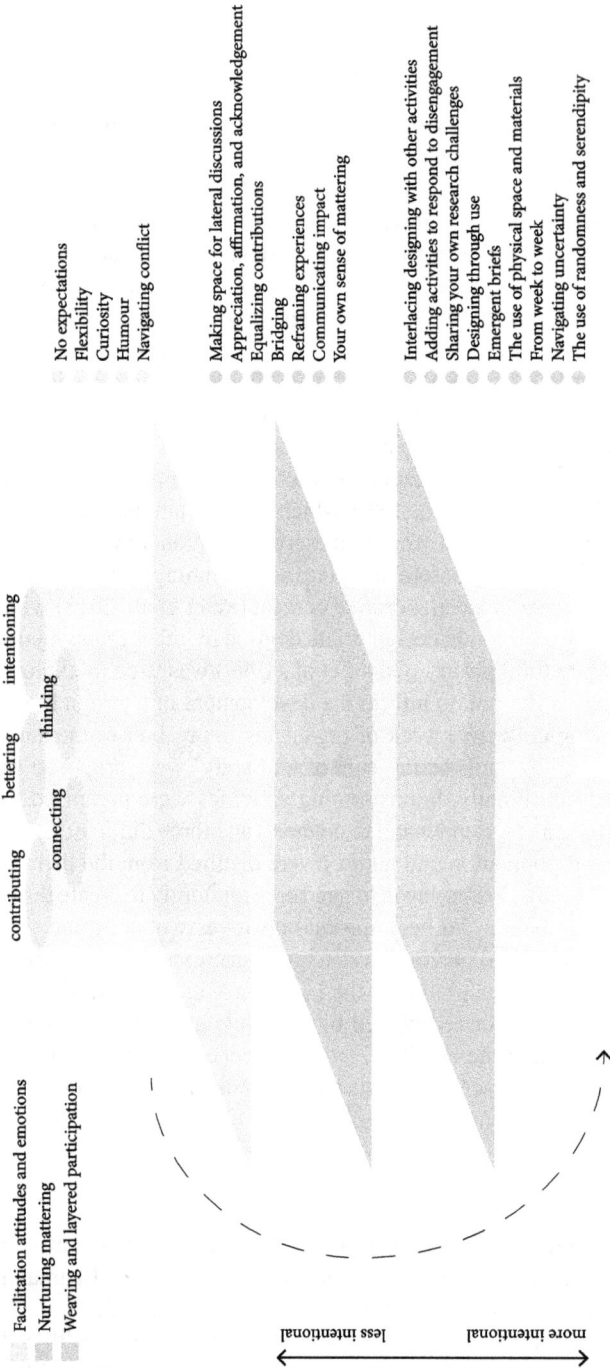

Figure 6.1 Conceptual illustration of co-design framework

anonymously to articulate design challenges that aimed to support wellbeing. This was followed by a process of brainstorming ideas and developing prototypes, which generally focused on wellbeing. The project was guided by a process called 5 Is, which guided participants through five stages: Identify, Ideate, Invent, Initiate and Implement (Renedo-Illarregi et al., 2020). More details can be found in Renedo-Illarregi (2022, p. 113; Renedo-Illarregi et al., 2020).

Reflective analysis

Both projects were analysed separately through different methodologies (Renedo-Illarregi, 2022). Interpretative phenomenological analysis (IPA) (Smith et al., 2009) and mixed methods were used for *Design at PTP*, which combined wellbeing questionnaires (Stewart-Brown et al., 2011) *with semi-structured interview data*. IPA was used to look at participants' experiences inductively, and mixed methods to look at whether the project had an impact on their wellbeing. Case study analysis (Yin, 2018) was used for *Co-design for Wellbeing*. The findings from these analytical processes – mixed methods, IPA and case study – are reported in Renedo-Illarregi (2022) and their detailed discussion is beyond the scope of the present chapter. Here I build on these findings through abductive analysis (Tavory & Timmermans, 2014), further reflecting on the data across both projects to elaborate guidelines for facilitation and propose a framework (Figure 6.1). To signify the subjective nature of the reflection, the chapter is written in the first person.

Figure 6.1 portrays the interconnectedness of the notions discussed throughout the chapter. Each level or subsection of the framework is represented by a different colour. The vertical axis represents how much control or intention the facilitator might have over the situations that unfold. For example, as facilitator, I had most control over weaving and layering participation (lower part of graph), but nurturing mattering was not always experienced as intentional. I had even less control over how my attitudes could affect participants or how our collective emotional landscape would unfold over time (top of graph). *Situated examples* pertaining to each subsection are shown on the right-hand side. Concepts referring to experiences of participants are represented by the cylinders that reach across all levels as they interact with, and emerge from, these.

Findings 1: weaving and layered participation

Reflecting on and contrasting both case studies revealed that participant engagement was encouraged differently in each. The metaphors of weaving (in the *Design at Psychosis Therapy Project*), or layered participation (in the *Design for Wellbeing* project), portray the different dynamics.

Weaving participation

During *Design at PTP*, I came to understand the way I was encouraging participation as *weaving*. I began interacting with some clients in the charity's drop-in area, talking about the project and recruiting participants. Some began with the first activity, bringing meaningful objects, which raised the intrigue of others. One participant's contribution engaged another and vice versa. The weaving metaphor is useful because one thread of participation, e.g. Anthony bringing his objects, would pull another thread, e.g. another participant being curious and joining.

I felt myself in the middle of an ecosystem, pulling threads and weaving them into the design project, which in turn would continue forming the ecosystem. I was reading from and into what was brought and using it to pull more threads, constantly rearranging the situation. What some-one brought was used to raise interest from another, whose questions were used to motivate yet another, and so on. Often, I would comment on what one participant shared one day with another who missed that session, weaving their engagement back into the process.

Anthony used a religious analogy to describe this *weaving* role. He called it the 'coordinating force or mind'.

> The story is, (…) in Mecca [there] is a big square based around an old black meteorite, is set into the wall inside (…) and when they were setting it into the wall (…) the chiefs argued about who [should] pick up this holy [meteorite] (…) and Mohamed (…) put it in the mid-dle of the rug (…) they all stood around the carpet he said right, now all of you lift the carpet together (…) so the idea is that you needed a coordinating force, a coordinating mind (…) you were the coordinating element in bringing the co-designed elements together (…) you are the Mohamed in this situation …
>
> (Anthony, 2nd interview)

Layered participation

The *Co-design for Wellbeing* case, rather than weaving together contributions, focused on ena-bling various *layers* of engagement. Each individual could come up with their own design or help others. A set of pre-planned activities aimed to help participants move along the process, enabling engagement at various layers. What these layers entail may differ depending on partici-pants and the project. I came to understand my role as facilitating layering when I noticed that one participant might immerse imaginatively into the activities, while another would engage somewhat peripherally, not directly 'doing' the activities. While one of the participants' imagi-nation developed in tangents hard to follow, another would respond that '*nothing came to mind*', pushing me to craft, or improvise, new layers to support different kinds of engagement.

Situated examples of weaving and layered participation

The examples below illustrate the variety of strategies that can be used to weave or layer participation.

Interlacing designing with other activities

My PhD project was embedded within existing mental health services, which favoured engage-ment. For example, Bea regularly attended the art room where the co-design project was going to happen, enabling her to be at the design sessions informally. Anthony's previous engagement with craft helped the project, which motivated him to join new activities too.

> (…) it [the design project] gave me direction and inspiration…
>
> (Anthony, 1st interview)

> the creative writing and the poetry groups sort of are as a follow on from the design group
>
> (Anthony, 3rd interview)

Adding activities to respond to disengagement

Activities can be added or adapted to engage participants who seem to drift apart. The reflective diary illustrates these insights.

I couldn't keep defining and defining especially because (…) some of the participants are more vocal than others (…), so there needs to be, in every session, more or less a bit of action, even if (…) I think [it is] unrelated to the project as a whole, and so that everyone has got the chance to be active in different ways

(Reflective diary, 20.03.19)

Splitting an activity into different tasks may help. For instance, in the *Co-design for Wellbeing* project, I used the metaphor of a tree to discuss how issues interconnect with one another. If I saw someone who was disengaging from the discussion, I might ask for their help to cut the cardboard to make the tree. At other times, the very tools needed for an activity (e.g. boxes) could be made by participants, adding layers of engagement.

Sharing your own research challenges

Sharing one's doubts and welcoming participants' input may motivate their involvement as researchers, as reflected in my diary and the interviews:

I am even trying to figure out a framework to sort of gather information (…) Uriel said OK so you have come two levels up abstraction (…) to then figure out (…) how is populated (…)

(Reflective diary, 24.04.19)

the game! it was from my experience because I said a game like Trivial Pursuits we have lots of questions that is exactly where it came from… my experience! ouh… we have discovered something!

(Amara, 2nd interview)

Sometimes I would be asked questions that corresponded with those of the research (how will this project help me?). By replying that *we* were going to try to find out together, I invited participants to reflect.

Designing through use

This was particularly prominent in *Co-design at PTP* during the development of the board game, which took form by pretend playing. In improvising our play without the product, it progressively formed while encouraging engagement.

'what colour is your soul?' and she said 'well it is lilac, and it is also the green, but is also changing '(…) [I say] 'ok that is perfect (…) you get five lilac points' (laughs) (…) Anthony was saying (…) 'maybe we should have a master', and then I said to him (laughing)' no we don't like masters… the master idea, right Amara?' (…) Amara was like 'yes! no everyone is equal', (…) we could think about facilitator? (…)

(Reflective diary, 12.6.19)

Emergent briefs

Emergent briefs are as much a consequence of weaving participation as an enabler. Inputs are constantly being reconfigured toward common goals. In *Design at PTP*, the brief emerged from our interactions, threading together a wide range of views and ideas, ultimately endorsing everyone's contribution. We put all the cultural probe responses together, looking for common themes (Figure 6.2). Based on this, a participant suggested stewardship as the collective purpose.

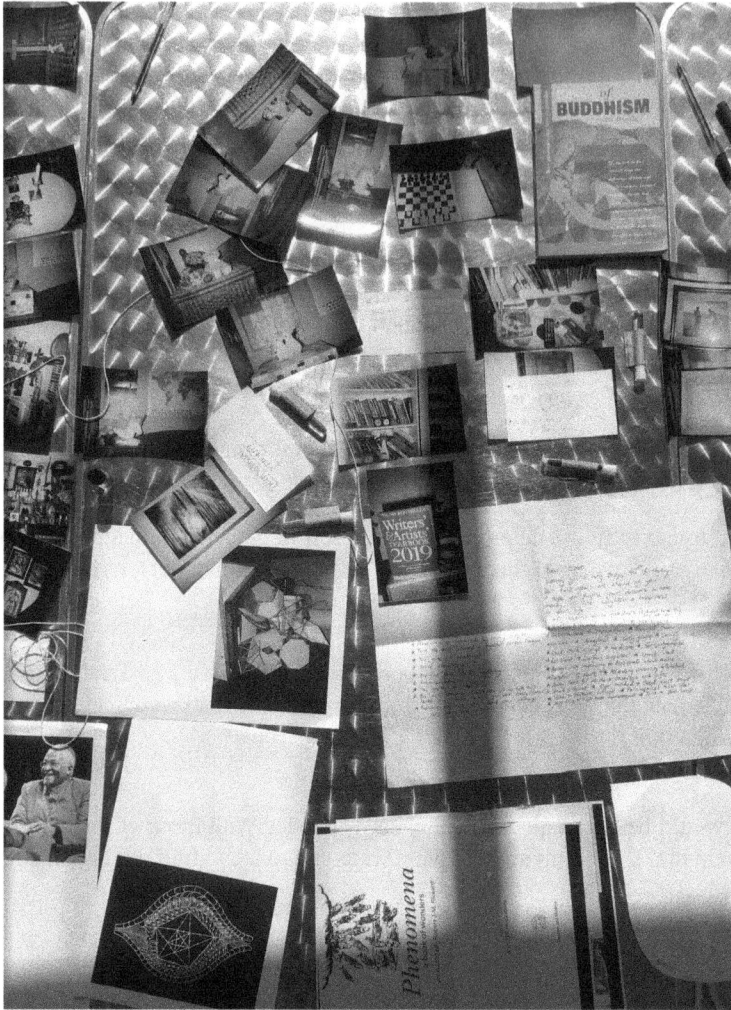

Figure 6.2 Various responses to the cultural probes

> (…) I quite enjoyed us all contributing bits and pieces and sort of (…) finding (…) common themes I didn't think (…) many common things would come up but apparently they did
>
> (Anthony, 1st interview)

> (…) Uriel [mentioned] that stewardship, so like taking care of the world, was what all the religious and spirituality [within cultural probes] have in common, and that could be the function of our design (…)
>
> (Reflective diary, 22.5.19)

The use of physical space and materials

Toward the end of *Co-design at PTP*, different elements of the game needed to be designed. I began to use the physical space to encourage engagement and decision-making by distributing materials and writing design questions across the table, which participants would encounter

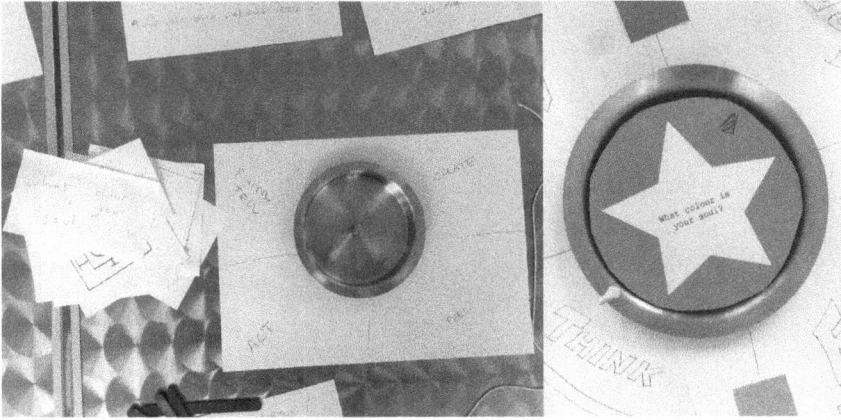

Figure 6.3 (left) Participant wrote a question for a card, which was prototyped for the next session. (right) In the following week, another participant thought the card itself could be the spinner too and drew a pointer

upon taking a seat. This way, they were encouraged to engage with the different aspects of the design and discuss them, too.

From week to week

Comments or ideas were implemented into the design process from the previous week. Weekly insights helped to inform the following sessions, keeping a sense of continuity and acknowledging contributions' value.

> Not much went past you (…) like a throwaway comment you may hear and incorporate it (…) into the following [week], which is good in a way; it shows you what you say has a certain validity
>
> (Anthony, 1st interview)

Toward the end, this week-to-week implementation became more literal (e.g. designing the cards) (Figure 6.3).

Navigating uncertainty

Navigating uncertainty is a key aspect of co-design facilitation, and it may even impact participants' engagement and recovery.

> Design creation I mean is more (…) because my art mostly is abstract but the design wasn't abstract was it?, or maybe it kind of started abstract and then it had to be structured at the end
>
> (Amara, 2nd interview)

As we were co-designing the game, Anthony found it difficult to deal with the fact that the rules were not defined. On one occasion, appointing the concept as 'prototype' and writing it on a sign legitimised it being hazy, I conceptualised this strategy as the 'bracketing of uncertainty'.

> the rules of the game was a bit hazy and (…) fair enough I wrote prototype (…) it was a weight off my mind because it give (…) sense to the fact (…) that the game was unfinished (…) or haven't been figured out totally (…)
>
> (Anthony, 1st interview)

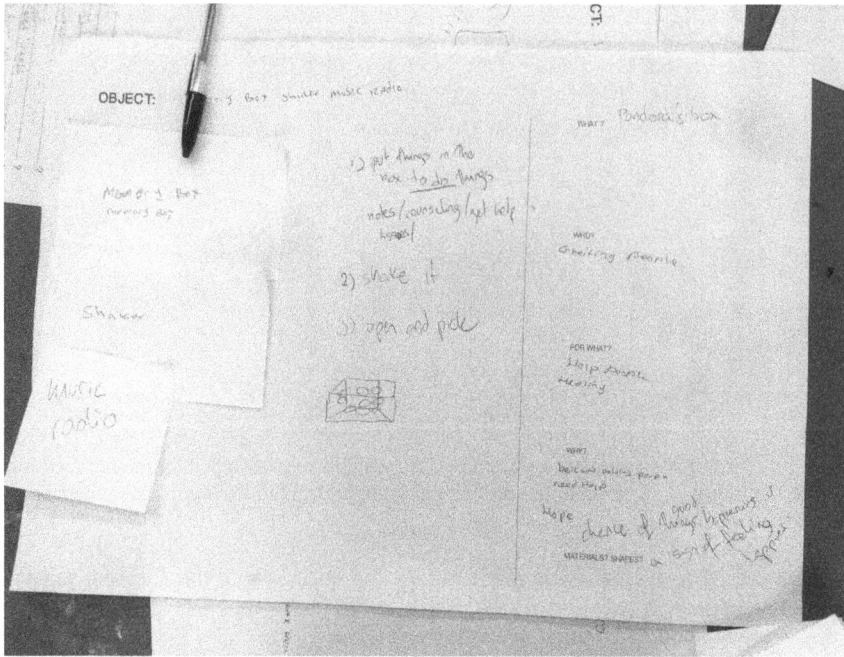

Figure 6.4 Music radio, shaker and memory box are the terms randomly combined to stimulate idea generation in response to designing something for people in grief

The use of randomness and serendipity

In the project, the use of randomness, as having no particular order or following no pattern, and serendipity, understood as good luck discoveries occurring coincidently or by chance, appeared to enable dealing with indecision, mitigating stagnation and stimulating creativity. For example, in the *Co-design for Wellbeing* case, the use of randomness helped to stimulate the creation of ideas (Figure 6.4) by randomly (without looking, by chance) combining three different terms (e.g. music radio, shaker and memory box) and encouraging participants to create a concept from their combination, which responds to the challenge at hand (e.g. designing something for people in grief). On another occasion, in *Design for PTP*, when forming the brief out of cultural probe responses, participants decided to match the three different groups that we could design for and the three different possible purposes of the brief (to wonder, to heal and to connect) using chance to determine the pairs randomly with one another. More details and photographs can be found in Renedo Illarregi (2022, p. 290).

Findings 2: nurturing mattering

When practising weaving or layered participation, participants are not only involved in the design process. The design process emerges because of them. What is designed together matters to participants and potentially people beyond. Hence, practising weaving or layered participation also nurtures mattering. Yet certain additional strategies can nurture it further. In general terms, this involves sharing personal experiences and exploring how those inform design briefs, raising awareness of how design's purpose ultimately involves others. In the two projects, this happened in slightly different ways: in *Design at PTP*, this emerged as 'from personal sharing to societal mattering', and in *Co-design for Wellbeing* as 'from problems that hurt to solutions that matter'.

From personal sharing to societal mattering

In *Design at PTP*, we started with participants' personal contributions, which were woven towards a common goal. Initially, participants brought objects and talked about them, choosing how much of themselves they wanted to share with others, which was intended to make them feel more comfortable with each other. In parallel, short design projects were introduced, helping participants familiarise themselves with the notion of designing for others. Later, through cultural probes, participants began looking at common themes emerging to inform a design brief. These processes merged to create a collective sense of purpose and an understanding of the impact beyond one's immediate sphere.

From problems that hurt to solutions that matter

In *Co-design for Wellbeing*, participants shared issues in an anonymous way, whether drawing on their personal experiences, from imagination, or people they knew. How these individual challenges related to other issues was explored, revealing their complexity. Each individual challenge was used to inform group brainstorming sessions, transforming them into collective matters of concern. Later, each participant was encouraged to develop one idea further individually. Hence, individual problems ultimately informed solutions that mattered to others.

Situated examples of nurturing mattering

In the following, processes from both projects are elaborated, which promote mattering.

Making space for lateral discussions

To nurture mattering, it was important to create space, where possible, for stories that may go off on a tangent. Participants should feel comfortable talking about their interests, which may be unexpected. One of the particularities of design is that, with some imagination, these lateral discussions can be threaded back to the main process in one way or another. It may also mean taking note of these suggestions for revisiting later when there is time.

Appreciation, affirmation and acknowledgement

Continuous acknowledgement or appreciation of contributions is key, as reported in the interviews.

> Very little challenge, you appreciate it and you encourage.
>
> (Nealy, 2nd interview)

> helps the world and it helps each person in the group (…) as well, yes because I think the attention you gave to each (…) of us (…) that is very important (…) you know affirming us (…) bringing, acknowledging the positive and or acknowledging us in some way.
>
> (Amara, 2nd interview)

Equalising contributions

It is also important to acknowledge different contributions equally to counter a natural bias for valuing certain kinds of tasks over others. This can be challenged through continuous reflection, considering everyone irreplaceable. This may also involve reassurance. In the reflective diary, I recall:

'I feel like I am not contributing very much' [said Nestor]... and I said why... how you feel?... why is that? (...) they [participants] kind of create this (...) hierarchy (...) themselves so (...) how do you change that (...) make sure that everyone feels that the value of the participation is equal or (...)

(Reflective diary, 19.06.19)

Amara said (...) I am not doing much again...[discredit her contribution] [yet] at some point she said again 'oh no! yes, the idea of the game was mine (...) There is something happening here, about not being willing to take (...) a serious stake or (...) acknowledgement of oneself as part of a collective and I think I need to take an active role (...) [in] addressing it.

(Reflective diary, 19.06.19)

In *Design at PTP*, participants often downplayed their own input, although in the interviews most participants acknowledged their contribution. In a collective situation, it is possible that feelings of inferiority may manifest. Querying skewed perceptions and acknowledging them can help, as does giving attention to those who participate less intensely to emphasise to them and others what the value of their unique contribution is. An external perspective can sometimes help, too. In *Co-design for Wellbeing,* with the projects being individual, participants had no trouble in acknowledging their role. However, where participants support others rather than creating their ideas, this should equally be acknowledged. Equalising contributions also involves being aware of earlier associations, as therapeutic and learning environments may often imply certain power dynamics. To challenge this, I tended to stay away from using educational or therapeutic concepts, such as project outcomes or recovery.

Bridging

I use the concept of bridging to refer to the process of encouraging reflection on how a personal problem connects with a group of people who may have the same issue (user group). Bridging nurtures mattering by building a notion that designing involves serving others in some way. In *Design at PTP*, I asked participants to think about groups of people they would like to design for. Amara and Nealy both wrote about a person they knew. Asking questions about other people in similar situations promoted awareness of design serving a collective, which is empowering.

Reframing experiences

Experiences are reframed throughout the process of design, for instance from being conceptualised as personal symptoms or beliefs to stories that matter in another capacity, as input for the design process. In *Co-design for Wellbeing*, issues were turned into challenges. In *Design at PTP*, experiences, such as unusual beliefs and psychosis, were shared in a new light in relation to the design process. Through reframing, these experiences become part of a purposeful activity where they function as insights that inform designs and where they are perceived as empowering, rather than being seen as disempowering symptoms.

Communicating impact

Keeping participants informed about the development and impact of the research, e.g. how the design outcome is tested elsewhere, research publications, is important to nurture mattering.

By keeping participants informed about how my thinking evolved and the feedback I received, participants engaged critically with the research.

Your own sense of mattering

Feeling that my presence was welcomed and appreciated was also important, as nurturing mattering is often reciprocal. In *Design at PTP*, I felt welcomed and comfortable. A particularly funny and touching passage from Anthony's interview illustrates this:

> I don't, wouldn't change you, you are practically perfect in every way, like Mary Poppins, the Mary Poppins of the design project.
>
> (Anthony, 1st interview)

I also felt welcomed at the *Co-design for Wellbeing* project. However, at the time, the charity was going through a retendering process, which meant that most staff members were busier than usual. I sometimes felt that I was taking resources (e.g. people's time) that were needed elsewhere. Although I do not believe this affected the project, it highlighted the importance of the facilitator's sense of mattering.

Findings 3: facilitating attitudes, emotions and ethics

Below, I discuss the way we bring ourselves into the practice. Some attitudes were intentionally brought into the process, but others, such as humour, emerged spontaneously, challenging assumptions around how we can or cannot express ourselves in response to unusual experiences or strange situations.

Attitudes and emotions

No expectations

Unlike many other projects, this project did not have an initial design agenda or brief. Having no expectations for outcomes did not mean that I did not encourage participants to engage. Nealy describes the nuances of this encouragement in her interview.

> You were so friendly, so close, one of us, you behaved like one of us, that affected us also very important (…) very little invention, you told us again and again is good thought, good thing to do it, and that helped us. (…) You would just explain [the] project, and you didn't care much [if] we wouldn't interact that much.
>
> (Nealy, 2nd interview)

Flexibility

Flexibility is an implicit part of weaving and layered participation. Sometimes it is built into the activities. For instance, in both projects, I suggested various ways to conduct research, which participants could choose. At other times, flexibility reflected the response to the situation at hand, for instance when I changed an activity that I had planned for that day to another which seemed to respond better to the context.

Curiosity

Curiosity about each other's ideas and about the world was encouraged. A particularly important insight from *Design at PTP* was that we seemed to share an inclination toward one another, which is a particular kind of curiosity, with no pressure in terms of sense-making, which made understanding in intellectual terms secondary.

> so... insight from today is that it doesn't really matter if we understand each other or not as long as we are sharing the space, (...) it is fine if we don't understand, we are not sure if we are interpreting things in a similar way, it is ok to be like that, (...) because we orient ourself towards one another nevertheless.
>
> (Reflective diary, 17.4.19)

Humour

The use of humour was remarked on by participants, who remembered times of laughter, the use of banter, or described the project as fun. This occurred spontaneously and was not considered when planning the workshops.

> there was a good bit of banter and sometimes there were jokes and they were specific.
>
> (Anthony, 1st interview)

> (...) thinking all together as a group playing games and laughing, yes, it was change I mean, we laugh a lot, yes.
>
> (Nealy, 1st interview)

The use of humour was also helped with communicating more challenging experiences. For example, in one of the brainstorming sessions at *Design at PTP*, we were talking about insects and how an appreciation toward their role might benefit the world when Anthony mentioned the 'adopt an ant' campaign (Figure 6.5). We all burst into laughter, and he continued to tell us about his psychotic episode, where an ant led his way home. The story was shared in humorous terms, in reference to the design situation. However, it was significant in that it led to sharing unusual experiences which challenged stigma. At the same time, humour could also be offensive. Experience and time spent with participants helped navigate such delicate boundaries. The power of using humour in the design process came from it not being the focus of attention, but a side effect, emerging from our co-designing.

> Banter was also appreciated by participants. (...) Nealy said how can I lose weight? and (...) I wrote have Ramadan all year long (...) and you could read it upside down (...) she thought was funny (...) there seemed good banter (...)
>
> (Anthony, 1st interview)

> I got confidence and I had lots of fun, I have lots of fun, with lots of laughter ... banter, I discovered that I can do banter, (laughs)
>
> (Amara, 1st interview)

Navigating conflict

One strategy when navigating disagreements, is to bring attention to how these conflicting views relate to the design situation. Alternatively, participants' individual attention could be temporarily diverted to different tasks, and brought back together later, de-escalating tension without repressing the discussions content.

My emotional landscape

Facilitators' emotions are a generally neglected dimension within co-design, despite their impact. Designers have not always worked in emotionally challenging contexts, and it is

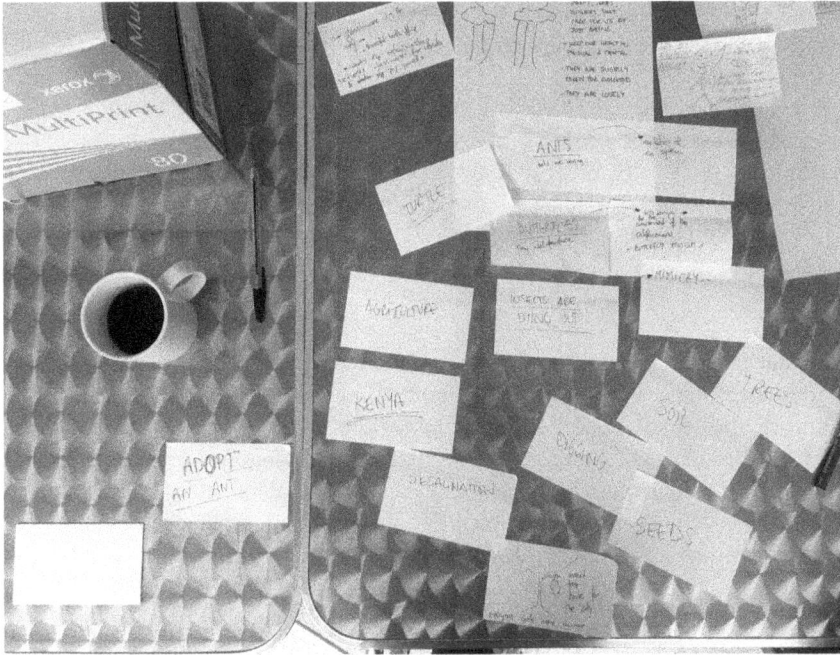

Figure 6.5 Anthony's 'Adopt an ant' idea written in a post it note, responding to 'how to help nature heal' brainstorming

not in the tradition to discuss these personal aspects. Within mental health, on the other hand, spaces are held for practitioners to discuss emotions. Throughout the project, I had the opportunity to discuss my experiences with a therapist, exploring how the project affected me, and reflecting on how my beliefs and background could affect participants. By reporting this aspect of the project, I aim to open a discussion and advocate for creating these spaces for facilitators, to prevent harm and support personal growth. In my reflective journal, I recorded insights on my emotional landscape. The experience was enriching and transformational. The verbatim fragments below illustrate the richness of this journey (Renedo-Illarregi, 2022):

> Amara was like well (…) we are kind of making it up now… and like she was so happy about saying that… (…) I mean I felt so blessed, I felt really good (…)
> (Reflective diary, 12.06.19)

> They [participants] affect you… I mean I dreamt with …I think it was Anthony making like … a kind of white (…) lamp which was an Angel, so like you move the lamp [which] gets kind of stabbed by wood (…) like a stab that makes the wings light up (…)
> (Reflective diary, 10.07.19)

> I felt a bit nervous because I thought like they may get bored wasn't sure what to say, how to say it, I wanted to see what it emerged naturally, so it was very interesting in that sense
> (Reflective diary, 27.02.19)

That was the last session. I think I will be quite sad when this ends actually, very sad (…) Anthony is funny (…) [he] said you know I would like to know if you managed (…) I am crying now actually. (…) there is a lot happening in (…) those interactions (…) where you are making something out of a lot of living experiences (…) somehow you go there you don't know what you are doing you kind of get things here get thing there (…) So much serendipity on the design process I have never seen so much I think, I don't know if it is because people are more vulnerable to ... to just what is happening there (…)

(Reflective diary, 10.07.19)

Ethical encounters

An ethical dimension is embedded in the whole of this chapter, reflecting a deep commitment to working with one another with utmost respect and care during the projects. Having mental health support for participants and someone to discuss any ethical issues was important. Notwithstanding, formal ethical procedures and guidelines are considered insufficient in preparing researchers for the complexity of the field and they are but one aspect of research ethics (Guillemin & Gillam, 2004). In practice, some issues often remain partly unresolved. Some such moments – termed *ethical encounters* – are illustrated below. These are encounters with situations that were ethically meaningful in some way and open interesting questions (Renedo-Illarregi, 2022).

Ethical encounter 1

Uriel begun engaging in the project informally, but he did not seem keen on paperwork. I talked to the ethics committee and supervisors about the consent form and agreed I should explain the importance of this procedure. He finally read through the information sheet and completed the consent form. I noticed that in the section 'I have understood...' he had ticked 'no'. When I asked him if we could go over it again, he refused, simply stating that not he, nor anyone, can ever be sure of understanding anything. It struck me that he was right. I found myself in a difficult situation with the ethical form, yet it was clear that he understood the research, the likelihood of it being published, and that he was simply challenging the form philosophically. Paradoxically, by ticking 'no', he demonstrated a deeper understanding of the complexities behind such process. I then had to make a judgement and considered his form valid.

Ethical encounter 2

Uriel had agreed to be interviewed after the project. However, in the summer the project ended, he had surgery, and he emailed his therapist and me saying we could visit him at his home. At the time, I thought perhaps it was not appropriate to visit him for an interview considering he was possibly recovering and that interviewing in the charity was preferable. When he recovered, I tried to schedule the interview a couple more times, but he said he was tired. At that point, I thought it best to stop asking. Uriel died a few months later, which was very hard to hear. I revisited my decisions and doubts arose due to his death. Was being tired a way to communicate he was not interested in the interview? Or was he really just tired, and I lost the opportunity to honour his voice when he offered to visit at home?

Ethical encounter 3

When writing the thesis, I had moments when I had to consider participants' ability to recognise themselves or others from the group. With such small samples, participants may be able to recognise each other from the contents of data fragments when they read the thesis. It is important to reflect on this to ensure participants' ongoing relationships are not compromised. In this project, I did not have to omit any data relevant to the research questions. However, I remained vigilant to any sensitive fragments and that researchers need to be aware of, and consider, the possibility of coming across ethical dilemmas in relation to privacy of participants versus transparency of findings.

Discussion

The discussion draws together the individual findings under the three main themes to highlight their importance as guidance and tools for co-designing in a mental health context. Furthermore, those situated examples, which in one way or other align with earlier work, have been briefly highlighted in relation to the literature.

Weaving and layered participation

In co-design, there are different ways in which participants may interact and work together (Zamenopoulos & Alexiou, 2018). The concepts of weaving and layered participation have been introduced and developed as an empathic approach to co-design that aids facilitators in crafting ways of encouraging engagement that prioritises participants' experiences and wellbeing. Weaving participation aligns with the work of Sawyer and DeZutter (2009) who, in the context of theatre, report that collaborative emergence is more likely to be found when: (1) the activity has an unpredictable outcome; (2) there is moment-to-moment contingency; (3) the interactional effect of any given action can be changed by the subsequent actions of other participants; and (4) the process is collaborative, with each participant contributing equally.

The two projects discussed exemplified different applications of these concepts: the *Co-design for Wellbeing* project focused on cooperation in which participants find synergies across their different interests but work independently on their respective goals. Still, other forms of co-design emerged and were encouraged when it was considered favourable (e.g. when participants preferred to adopt a supporting role). This research refers to such engagement as *layered*, which aligns with the work of Kanstrup and Bertelsen (2018) who point to the designers' obligation to legitimise a mixture of investments in participation, including peripheral and low participation. In contrast, *Co-design at PTP* was collaborative, working toward a common goal. This goal was emergent, and the outcome – the board game – was reflective of the process itself. It became a physical manifestation of how we – the participants – related to one another and in due course might help people connect in ways that we, as a group, also did.

In conclusion, the role of the designer in the context of the co-design process is to weave or layer engagement and experiences and, by doing so, not to control emergent processes, but to coordinate them to nurture mattering.

Some of the examples I describe under weaving and layered participation can be discussed in relation to earlier work, such as designing through use, emergent briefs, navigating uncertainty and randomness and serendipity.

Designing through use may be said to align with (Schleicher et al., 2010) description of embodied storming, which differs from bodystorming in that it requires us to act first, as physical actors in a situation, and not conceiving designers as distanced from things. Embodied storming deploys the strengths of humans acting together. In that particular moment, we were really playing first, and the boardgame was taking shape as a result.

Emergent briefs contributes toward the discussion of emergence in co-design (Alexiou, 2010) and, more specifically, what the author describes as a bottom-up definition of emergence, used to indicate that solutions are not obtained through direct modelling of the desired outcome ('top-down' modelling), but they are formulated as an aggregate effect of distributed processes carried by a number of individual entities (agents) that interact with each other. Furthermore, in this case not even the problem was set out before the project. Hence, the name 'emergent briefs' aims to remark on this quality that the brief, and not only the design, is created through people's interactions and not a priori, which is a far more common co-design practice. When we facilitate, we might want to be aware on how bottom-up or top-down our approach might be in deciding what we are doing. In this context, cultural probes were not used to find out anything specific and instead were explored openly. In this sense, it aligns with the original use of cultural probes which, as Gaver et al. (2004) describe, were playful and subjective, not as rational as it has often been used thereafter.

The subject of *uncertainty* has been extensively explored in design literature (see, for instance, Akama et al., 2018; Ball et al., 2010; Ball & Christensen, 2009; Cash & Kreye, 2018; Christensen, Bo Thomas & Ball, 2017; Dilnot, 1998). Akama et al. (2018), for instance, reveal how uncertainty can be engaged as a generative 'technology' for understanding, researching and intervening in the world, drawing on key themes in creative methodologies, such as making, essaying, inhabiting and attuning. Within mental health, uncertainty is also a key concept, as it may be difficult to deal with, making it a key aspect to reflect on in facilitation. Although a detailed discussion on the role of uncertainty is beyond the scope of the present chapter, the principles described in this situated action align with earlier theory around *co-design and mental health* (Renedo-Illarregi, 2018).

The use of randomness and serendipity within co-design as a way to spark creativity is in line with Verbeeck's (2006) hypothesis that the early design process is in need of the unexpected, rather than of iron logic. Their research investigated how the use of randomness as a generative principle could present the designer with a creative design environment (Verbeeck, 2006).

Nurturing mattering

This concept contributes to our understanding of how facilitation may be intertwined with the participants' sense of mattering. It partially contrast Arnstein's ladder of participation (Arnstein, 1969), in that it questions hierarchical paradigms of power and acknowledges mattering in its multiplicity of forms. This is not to say that hierarchies of power do not exist, but that Arnstein's framing of these inequalities carries within it the very seeds through which they re-emerge.

Arnstein (1969) envisioned different rungs labelled Manipulation and Therapy, Informing Consultation and Placation, and Partnership, Delegated Power and Citizen control, out of which only the last three demonstrate citizen power or influence in decision-making. Reviewing Arnstein's ladder in the context of user involvement in health, Tritter and McCallum (2006) remark that the model does not acknowledge the fact that some users may not wish to be involved. This challenges the assumption that disempowered communities are those who are not participating. Furthermore, assuming power as everyone's goal devalues other purposes.

Ramírez Galleguillos and Coşkun (2020) have reviewed 46 papers to distil how participatory design projects have been developed in practice with underprivileged or disadvantaged individuals. Nurturing mattering articulates a variety of strategies that concur with their findings of how to raise higher levels of involvement, such as (1) cultural immersion to understand the group of participants before starting (Winschiers-Theophilus et al., 2012); (2) including the participants as research partners (Xu & Maitland, 2019); and (3) adapting the process to how the participants are doing, thinking, feeling (Kanstrup & Bertelsen, 2016).

Nurturing mattering is trying to transcend the notion that participants are unprivileged per se, without losing sight that there might be serious consequences for being in their situation. In this case, a sincere appreciation of the profoundly enlightening experiences that participants might have had enabled this. They had lived something I did not, they could understand something I could not. This approach does not mean forsaking vulnerability, but it tries to transcend the hierarchy that such awareness already projects into our interactions. As limiting as psychosis could be, as serious as its consequences may be, nurturing mattering is a commitment to try to avoid abiding by those binaries 'needed and needy' or 'powerful and powerless'. Rather than focusing on finding ways of enabling people to engage in projects that seek to improve *their* lives, as Ramírez Galleguillos and Coşkun (2020) termed it in summarizing the participatory designer's role, I tried to wonder whose lives might need improving – or healing – to begin with. Nurturing mattering is trying to move beyond the notion that some people matter more than others because of what they are or do. It considers every human being as mattering no matter what.

Attitudes, emotions and ethics

Flexibility, curiosity and humour, are notions that are familiar to designers, and attitudes discussed in this chapter generally align with those promoted within co-design.

Humour was often mentioned by participants. It appears that participants were referring to the ways in which they could laugh about their own or other experiences in appreciative and respectful ways. The finding aligns with (Gelkopf, 2011), who reviews and discusses the use of humour and laughter in treating people with serious mental illness. There is a good understanding of the range of effects, which humour and laughter can have on perceptions, attitudes, judgements and emotions, and how they can potentially benefit a person's physical and psychological state (Gelkopf, 2011). As in individual therapy, humour within a group context may enable and facilitate the development of a sense of proportion and may help overcome exaggerated seriousness that often serves as a defence against ambiguity (Gelkopf, 2011). The presentation of one's life in a humorous manner may often help patients accept certain difficult situations in a more existential way, accepting life's absurdities and quandaries (Gelkopf, 2011). Conversely, humorous stimuli may lead to different affective responses, ranging from very pleasant to very unpleasant ones, depending on the person (Levine & Abelson, 1959), because historically people with mental health problems have often been ridiculed (Foucault, 1973). This warrants facilitators to carefully navigate this issue, perhaps by not making it intentional but letting it emerge spontaneously as part of the co-design process. In fact, unlike humour or laughter-based interventions (Gelkopf, 2011), which might target it directly, within our project, humour was not the aim, but a side effect, which emerged spontaneously from the collective undertaking of designing together.

In terms of my own attitude and emotions, I found special resonance with Akama and Light's concept of readying ourselves for contingent participatory design and the need for attunement (Akama & Light, 2018). They argue that readiness, on the micro-scale, helps us respond to small moments of intersubjective nuance and to feel a way through; and at a macro scale, to be dexterous and willing to work on turbulent, shifting sands. Indeed, notions described earlier such as flexibility, appreciation align with such concept of attunement.

Research on the impact of design research projects on the wellbeing of researchers is lacking (Escalante et al., 2017) and, by emphasising on my own journey, I seek to encourage such discussion. The ethical principles implicit in such projects resonate with principles described by previous practitioners (Kelly, 2018): free and informed participation, balancing participation with minimising the risk of harm, maximising the benefits of the experience and outcomes of participation and supporting fair and appropriate empowerment. This chapter articulates how to embody such values in practice.

The involvement of participants can also sometimes unintentionally lead to a disregard for ethical principles, such as tokenistic participation or not giving equal opportunity to participate (Losada et al, this book). Hence, by reflecting on what we do, often intuitively, the framework aims to prevent such problems. In addition, examples of moments which raised important ethical questions were described. As Kelly (2018) proposes, our research community has an important role to play by providing examples of ethical stories for practitioners to learn from. The *ethical encounters* align with Guillemin and Gillam's (2004) definition of 'ethically important moments', which are moments which do not necessarily involve ethical dilemmas, points 'where the approach taken or the decision made has important ethical ramifications' (p. 265). The ethical encounters also illuminate the participant's understanding what is good, what is bad and everything in between, encouraging the cultivation of what Dewey (1932) termed a 'reflective' morality, a form of negotiated, open-ended, imaginative inquiry undertaken in response to contextual concerns (Dixon, 2020).

References

Akama, Y., & Light, A. (2018). Practices of readiness: Punctuation, poise and the contingencies of participatory design. In *PDC '18: Proceedings of the 15th participatory design conference: Full papers* (pp. 1–12). https://doi.org/10.1145/3210586.3210594

Akama, Y., Pink, S., & Sumartojo, S. (2018). *Uncertainty and possibility: New approaches to future making in design anthropology.*

Alexiou, K. (2010). Coordination and emergence in design. *CoDesign, 6*(2), 75–97. https://doi.org/10.1080/15710882.2010.493942

Arnstein, S. R. (1969). A ladder of citizen participation. *Journal of the American Planning Association, 35*(4), 216–224. https://doi.org/10.1080/01944366908977225

Ball, L. J., & Christensen, B. T. (2009). Analogical reasoning and mental simulation in design: Two strategies linked to uncertainty resolution. *Design Studies, 30*(2), 169–186. https://doi.org/10.1016/j.destud.2008.12.005

Ball, L. J., Onarheim, B., & Christensen, B. T. (2010). Design requirements, epistemic uncertainty and solution development strategies in software design. *Design Studies, 31*(6), 567–589. https://doi.org/10.1016/j.destud.2010.09.003

Cash, P., & Kreye, M. (2018). Exploring uncertainty perception as a driver of design activity. *Design Studies, 54*, 50–79. https://doi.org/10.1016/j.destud.2017.10.004

Christensen, B. T., & Ball, L. J. (2017). Fluctuating epistemic uncertainty in a design team as a metacognitive driver for creative cognitive processes. *CoDesign.* https://doi.org/10.1080/15710882.2017.1402060

Dewey, J. (1932). *Theory of the moral life.* Rinehart and Winston.

Dilnot, C. (1998). The science of uncertainty: The potential contribution of design to knowledge. In *Proceedings of the Ohio conference.* https://www.academia.edu/447813/The_Science_of_Uncertainty_the_Potential_Contribution_of_Design_to_Knowledge?auto=download

Dixon, B. S. (2020). *Dewey and design: A pragmatist perspective for design research.* Springer International Publishing AG.

Elliott, G., Kao, S., & Grant, A.-M. (2010). Mattering: Empirical validation of a social-psychological concept. *Http://Dx.Doi.Org/10.1080/13576500444000119, 3*(4), 339–354. https://doi.org/10.1080/13576500444000119

Escalante, M. A. L., Tsekleves, E., Bingley, A., & Gradinar, A. (2017). 'Ageing Playfully': a story of forgetting and remembering. *Https://Doi.Org/10.1080/24735132.2017.1295529, 1*(1), 134–145. https://doi.org/10.1080/24735132.2017.1295529

Foucault, M. (1973). *Madness and civilization : A history of insanity in the age of reason / Michel Foucault* (R. Howard, Trans.). Vintage Books.

Gaver, B., Dunne, T., & Pacenti, E. (1999). Design: Cultural probes. *Interactions*, *6*(1), 21–29. https://doi .org/10.1145/291224.291235

Gaver, W. W., Boucher, A., Pennington, S., & Walker, B. (2004). Cultural probes and the value of uncertainty. *Interactions*, *11*(5), 53. https://doi.org/10.1145/1015530.1015555

Gelkopf, M. (2011). The use of humor in serious mental illness: A review. *Evidence-Based Complementary and Alternative Medicine : ECAM*, *2011*, 342837. https://doi.org/10.1093/ecam/nep106

Guillemin, M., & Gillam, L. (2004). Ethics, reflexivity, and "Ethically important moments" in research. *Qualitative Inquiry*, *10*(2), 261–280. https://doi.org/10.1177/1077800403262360

Kanstrup, A. M., & Bertelsen, P. (2016). Bringing new voices to design of exercise technology: Participatory design with vulnerable young adults. *ACM International Conference Proceeding Series*, *1*, 121–130. https://doi.org/10.1145/2940299.2940305

Kanstrup, A. M., & Bertelsen, P. (2018). Participatory rhythms: Balancing participatory tempi and investments in design with vulnerable users. In *Proceedings of the 15th participatory design conference on short papers, situated actions, workshops and tutorial - PDC '18* (pp. 1–5). https://doi.org/10.1145 /3210604.3210631

Kelly, J. (2018). Towards ethical principles for participatory design practice. *CoDesign*, *15*(4), 329–344. https://doi.org/10.1080/15710882.2018.1502324

Levine, J., & Abelson, R. (1959). Humor as a disturbing stimulus. *The Journal of General Psychology*, *60*(2), 191–200. https://doi.org/10.1080/00221309.1959.9710220

Peter, A., Lotz, N., Mcdonnell, J., & Lloyd, P. (2013). *The effect of prototyping material on verbal and non-verbal behaviours in collaborative design tasks*. 5th International Congress of International Association of Societies of Design Research, pp. 2382–2393. http://oro.open.ac.uk/38801/1/IASDR2013_Paper _Final_corrected_3-7-2013.pdf

Psychosis Therapy Project. (2021). *Psychosis therapy project*. https://psychosistherapyproject.com/author /psychosistherapyproject/

Ramírez Galleguillos, L. M., & Coşkun, A. (2020). How Do I matter? A review of the participatory design practice with less Priv-ileged participants. In *Proceedings of the 16th participatory design Con-Ference 2020 - Participation(s) otherwise - Vol 1 (PDC '20: Vol. 1)* (p. 1). https://doi.org/10.1145 /3385010.3385018

Renedo-Illarregi, E. (2018). What are the effects of co-designing on participants' mental health and does uncertainty play a role in this change process? In *Proceedings of the 5th international conference on Design4Health*.

Renedo Illarregi, E. (2022). *Co-design as healing : Exploring the experiences of participants facing mental health problems* (Degree Granting Institution Open University, Ed.). The Open University.

Renedo-Illarregi, E., Alexiou, K., & Zamenopoulos, T. (2020). Co-design for wellbeing with mental health participants: From identifying a problem to creating prototypes. In *Proceedings of the 6th international conference on Design4Health* (pp. 23–30).

Rosenberg, M. (1985). Self-concept and psychological well-being in adolescence. In R. Leahy (Ed.), *The development of the self* (pp. 205–246). Academic Press.

Sawyer, R. K., & DeZutter, S. (2009). Distributed creativity: How collective creations emerge from collaboration. *Psychology of Aesthetics, Creativity, and the Arts*, *3*(2), 81–92. https://doi.org/10.1037 /a0013282

Schleicher, D., Jones, P., & Kachur Niedzielski, O. (2010). Bodystorming as embodied designing. *Interactions*, *17*(6), 47–51. https://doi.org/10.1145/1865245.1865256

Smith, J. A., Flowers, P., & Larkin, M. (2009). *Interpretative phenomenological analysis: Theory, method and research*. Sage Publications. https://books.google.co.uk/books?id=WZ2Dqb42exQC

Star, S. L., & Griesemer, J. R. (1989). Institutional ecology, "translations" and boundary objects: Amateurs and professionals in Berkeley's museum of vertebrate zoology, 1907-39. *Social Studies of Science*, *19*(3), 387–420. http://www.jstor.org/stable/285080

Stewart-Brown, S., Platt, S., Tennant, A., Maheswaran, H., Parkinson, J., Weich, S., Tennant, R., Taggart, F., & Clarke, A. (2011). The Warwick-Edinburgh Mental Well-Being Scale (WEMWBS): A valid and reliable tool for measuring mental well-being in diverse populations and projects. *Journal of Epidemiology & Community Health, 65*(Suppl. 2), A38–A39. https://doi.org/10.1136/jech.2011.143586.86

Tavory, I., & Timmermans, S. (2014). *Abductive analysis: Theorizing qualitative research.* https://doi.org/10.7208/chiacgo/9780226180311.001.0001

Tritter, J. Q., & McCallum, A. (2006). The snakes and ladders of user involvement: Moving beyond Arnstein. *Health Policy, 76*(2), 156–168. https://doi.org/10.1016/j.healthpol.2005.05.008

Verbeeck, K. (2006). *Randomness as a generative principle in art and architecture.* Massachusetts Institute of Technology.

Winschiers-Theophilus, H., Bidwell, N. J., & Blake, E. (2012). Altering participation through interactions and reflections in design. *CoDesign, 8*(2–3), 163–182. https://doi.org/10.1080/15710882.2012.672580

Xu, Y., & Maitland, C. (2019, January 4). *Participatory data collection and management in low-resource contexts: A field trial with urban refugees.* ACM International Conference Proceeding Series. https://doi.org/10.1145/3287098.3287104

Yin, R. K. (2018). *Case study research and applications : Design and methods* (6th ed.). Sage.

Zamenopoulos, T., & Alexiou, K. (2018). Co-design as collaborative research. *Connected communities foundation series.* University of Bristol/ AHRC Connected Communities Programme.

7 Psychosocial design and engagement at *The Big Anxiety* festivals

Gail Kenning and Jill Bennett

Introduction

In Australia as elsewhere, the mental health system has been criticised for failing to provide the range of supports needed to address mental health and wellbeing across a diverse population. A recent national inquiry highlighted a 'disproportionate focus on clinical services', a corresponding lack of community-based supports, and a general failure to respond to changing needs in a system that is 'insufficiently people-focused' (Productivity Commission, 2020). Government reports have also noted that a lack of 'trauma-informed' service provision has left service-users, particularly First Nations Australians, alienated from or retraumatised by the health service (Prevention and Response to Violence Abuse and Neglect Government Relations (PARVAN), 2023). Here we highlight some benefits of non-clinical approaches to trauma that respond to lived experience operating outside the biomedical model of healthcare in social and cultural venues within communities.

The projects were co-designed by the authors as part of *The Big Anxiety* – a research-based mental health arts festival – with lived experience contributions being central in the design process. Within the healthcare system, co-design has been widely adopted as a means of re-designing services with input from service-users (Dawda & Knight, 2019). But the extent and scope of service-user engagement is often limited by the 'top-down' nature of the mental health system, which has traditionally marginalised lived experience (Bennett et al., 2022, 2023). By contrast, a psychosocial design paradigm is characterised by bottom-up, emergent and responsive practices that derive *from* lived experience and adhere to trauma-informed principles of care (Bennett et al., 2022, 2023; Levenson, 2017). At the core of such an approach is creating a 'potential space' where participants develop trust to enable them to engage in new experiences that can bring about change (Winnicott, 2005 [1971]). The first project, a *Long Table* event, was staged as part of a community-based workshop programme in the regional town of Warwick, Queensland, Australia, to address the trauma and youth suicide which disproportionately affects the Indigenous population. The second, *We're just gonna call it all BPD* – developed with service users – was premiered in *Spaces Between People*, a gallery exhibition as part of *The Big Anxiety* festival in Naarm, Melbourne, Australia.

Our conceptualisation of the psychosocial in relation to design and engagement is informed by psychosocial studies, a field of research and practice situating the psychology of embodied, lived experience within a social nexus (Bennett et al., 2022 p. 93). As such, it draws on concepts developed in psychoanalysis and psychotherapy to envisage psychodynamic relationships and the way in which these are facilitated and examined in a given setting. Using psychosocial design, we develop a contained space that can 'hold' shifting relationships between participants (Bennett, 2022a). The generative processes that occur in this 'contained' space actuate embodied feelings and emotions that are not yet formed in language but may emerge through

DOI: 10.4324/9781003318262-9

a process of discovery as individual or shared understandings in the present or later on. In this space, there is an intent to dissolve the hierarchies apparent in many co-design processes that prioritise systems and services requiring consumers and stakeholders to 'fit in'. We use trauma-informed care (TIC) principles that attend to how discomfort, distress and the unfamiliar may be experienced because of a trauma history (Levenson, 2017). It entails a focus on safety, trust, choice, collaboration and empowerment with the goal of minimising the likelihood of 'repeating dysfunctional dynamics' and creating the potential for supportive or flourishing experiences (Bennett et al., 2023; Levenson, 2017).

Psychosocial design

Psychosocial design practices engaging with mental health and trauma require designers to attune to the ways in which people interact with the physical, institutional and social structures of existing systems as well as to trauma histories and negative experiences within systems (Bennett et al., 2022; Bennett et al., 2023). In this sense, it addresses the ongoing politics of co-engagement with regard to who gets 'a seat at the table', who gets 'to have a say' and, more importantly, who is considered worthy of being listened to (Bødker & Kyng, 2018, p. 43). The primary and enduring focus is on psychosocial outcomes, or improving mental health for individuals and the community, rather than on outputs such as an artwork, exhibition or event per se. This extends to the psychosocial engagement offered to viewers of artworks that are not simply *about* mental health but advance cultural, social and philosophical questions about individual and collective mental health.

This psychosocial paradigm, discussed more fully in Bennett et al. (2023), attends to the material affordances of space, place and social context – and the psychosocial dimensions of those affordances in terms of who is enabled to participate (Gibson, 1979). It entails creating the aforementioned potential space as a 'container' or facilitating space in which to build trust and shared understanding. Bennett et al. (2022a, p. 109) frame this as follows:

> If a psychosocial understanding of affordances emphasizes the social nature of the environment, and the environmental nature of our social relations, its application in design attends not only to the optimal facilitating environment but to the internalized, pre-reflective capacities which enable the actor to make sense of – and act on – an affordance in the first place.

In the design of projects such as *The Big Anxiety f*estival or *Spaces Between People* exhibition (discussed here), which privilege socio-cultural/psychosocial, rather than bio-medical understandings of trauma, arts-based practices are used to engage with intersubjective experience or with feelings, affect and emotions, generating rich experiential engagements that can in turn prove therapeutic (Hustvedt & Bennett, 2022). These art experiences realise and enact sense-based connections that, within a psychosocial design context, can support the processing of trauma within a safe container or holding space (Bennett, 2022b; Bennett et al., 2022).

Design in this lived experience-oriented context addresses the barriers to engagement (negatively experienced affordances) by designing-in options for action. In design terms, this focus on the psychosocial extends beyond what Cruickshank (2014) identifies as a paradigm shift towards 'openness'. While Cruickshank (2014) positions the designer as an active participant or facilitator, allowing lived experience to become central, for him the designer retains a degree of orchestration throughout. Within psychosocial design, however, we seek to activate a "container-contained" relationship whereby participants are supported to engage with their own internal process using creative resources (Auger, 2013; Bennett et al., 2023; Bion, 1993 [1970]); Dunne & Raby, 2013; Lyckvi et al., 2018; Norman, 2016; Rieger et al., 2018).

Psychosocial design and engagements can be challenging both for designers well-versed in co-design, participatory approaches and action research methodologies as well as for health professionals enmeshed in the complex systems and relational structures of the mental health services. The relational foundation of the psychosocial calls for a 'letting go', or at least a delay in the application of diagnostic approaches, trained-in responses and standardised problem/solution processes – thereby allowing fully agentic participants to emerge and potential to be realised. Psychosocial approaches resist designed-in 'interventions' (which Vogelpoel and Gattenhof (2012) suggest is a heavily laden clinical term in itself); they are active and purposeful in holding a space for action to emerge that is not curated, orchestrated or choreographed.

The Big Anxiety

The Big Anxiety (TBA)[1] art and mental health festival was founded in 2017 in Sydney and is now a multi-city festival with a research hub, the Big Anxiety Research Centre (BARC),[2] at the University of New South Wales (UNSW), Sydney. Initially taking place in metropolitan cities, the festival programme has now expanded to regional communities. The design and delivery team comprises trauma specialists and arts-based researchers who have evolved a distinctive practice of event design informed by psychosocial practice, combined with the use of creative resources (Bennett et al, 2022; Bennett et al., 2023). TBA programme for Warwick initially consisted of a longer-term exhibition and a two-day forum focusing on addressing experiences of trauma, loss and suicidality. The programme content and outcomes are addressed more fully elsewhere, but here we will focus on how psychosocial design responds to situations as they emerge. Warwick had experienced high levels of youth suicide, and just weeks before *The Big Anxiety* event, the community had been deeply impacted by the death of a 16-year-old First Nations man who had reached out to services for support (Bennett et al., 2023). The festival design team and members of the community felt compelled to address this loss, which had intensified grief and anger and, more specifically, the feeling that these emotions were not being publicly acknowledged (Bennett et al., 2023). In discussion with the community, we determined to add an additional event to the programme – a *Long Table* discussion – to occur on the night before the two-day intensive forum. Significantly, this late change prompted some nervousness from institutional partners. However, it was clear from discussions with the community lead that the heightened level of emotion needed to be met with empathy rather than ignored or side-stepped. First Nations community partners expressed the view that the programme could offer a glimmer of hope and that opening up a space for discussion would be a welcome first step (Bennett et al., 2023).

The *Long Table* is an arts-based psychosocial engagement focused on the elaboration of lived experience and designed to facilitate dialogue by bringing together people with common interests in a non-hierarchical format that allows for marginalised voices to be heard. In this instance, it served as a vehicle for listening to the community and for designing a trauma-informed approach attuned to epistemic injustice and the institutional silencing of those whose knowledge is marginalised within systems of power (Moran & Bennett, 2022). It epitomises the aims of psychosocial design in facilitating a considered space for agentic participants to flourish. The *Long Table* was originally conceived by artist, activist, writer, director and performer Lois Weaver, inspired by Marleen Gorris' film *Antonia's Line*, in which the protagonist hosts a diverse array of characters at her ever-expanding table (Weaver & Hunter Petree, 2022). It is a stylised, hybrid performance-installation-roundtable-discussion-dinner-party and has occurred in a range of experimental open public forums with topics including women's prisons, Brexit and queer theatre (Weaver & Hunter Petree, 2022). It has been developed within TBA as a method for non-hierarchical, lived experience-led discussion of mental health and trauma. The format promotes difficult conversations but moves away from the conventional panel approach with experts behind a table in front of a listening audience (Weaver & Hunter Petree, 2022, p. 113).

The table is designed to seat 12 people and usually commences with six of twelve seats filled by people willing to seed discussion, with anyone in the room able to join or leave the table at any time, but there is no pressure to speak. People are invited to share their thoughts one at a time, but not in a turn-taking format, addressing the table as a whole (as at a dinner table) rather than responding to specific individuals. The published etiquette for a *Long Table event* states: 'There can be silence—There might be awkwardness—There could always be laughter—There is an end but no conclusion' (Shaw et al., n.d). The unmoderated discussion may be wide-reaching with emotions, such as grief and anger surfacing at any time. There is no intention to control or achieve specific outcomes or reach a consensus. The *Long Table* thus serves as a vehicle for creating a holding space for attentive listening (Bennett et al., 2022, 2023; Winnicott, 1965). Here, we provide insights into the dynamics of the space.

The *Long Table* in Warwick

The creative team for the overall programme of events (primarily Jill Bennett and Marianne Wobcke) worked closely with a key member of the community to extend invitations to the *Long Table* to people with lived experience of suicide. While some accepted the invitation beforehand, many chose to decide on the day whether they would attend. To support a sense of safety and comfort, food and drinks were supplied, and information was given about self-care. This included reiterating that participants were free to make decisions about what they needed at any time during the event, which might mean taking time away from the *Long Table* room. Recognising that additional support is often needed in contexts where trauma or histories of oppression are present, a Bowen therapist was available in the room to help people de-compress. This type of therapy is particularly appropriate and can be used in group situations because it is a clothed, non-invasive, invitation to the body to relax to gentle, rolling movements (Personal Communication: Heather Graham, 9 December 2022). Skilled trauma counsellors were also present and available on request.

On the evening, 30+ people were in attendance, including the organising team and a camera crew. First Nations midwife, artist and trauma worker Marianne Wobcke acted as host, supported by Mandandanji artist Aaron Blades, at the table. On entering the room, many participants took seats in the back rows, some suggesting 'they were not here to take part and they just wanted to watch and listen'. Wobcke introduced the concept of the *Long Table* to participants, identifying its connection to First Nations practices:

> The *Long Table* is not about control or achieving a specific outcome but rather about holding a space of deep listening – resonating with the Aboriginal practice of Dadirri.
>
> (The *Long Table*, Warwick unpublished recordings 6–8 April 2022)

The topic for conversation was introduced as the impact of suicide on the community and individuals within a First Nations approach to grief and dying, Wobcke continued:

> When someone we love dies, we wait a long time with the sorrow. We own our grief, and we allow it to heal slowly. We wait for the right time for our ceremonies and meetings. The right people must be present. Careful preparation must be made.
>
> (The *Long Table*, Warwick unpublished recordings 6–8 April 2022)

Wobcke set expectations as follows:

> We express gratitude for the commitment that you have made for yourself to turn up for such an important meet up … the format is a space to hold and respect and express emotions, it is not about control it is about people coming together to safely express themselves.
>
> Sometimes it's messy. Sometimes we don't know what to say. And we have to sit in silence to stumble. All of that we give you our heartfelt permission to do this.
>
> (The *Long Table*, Warwick unpublished
> recordings 6–8 April 2022)

Artist Aaron Blades began by sharing his experiences of being disconnected 'from Country' and his 'mob',[3] and of interactions with the justice system and mental health services. He spoke of the impact of mental health and suicide on his family and how, in reconnecting to his grandmother, he had found a pathway forward. The participants in the *Long Table* ranged in age from late teens to sixties; five men and primarily First Nations women. Many openly identified as having lived experience of mental health challenges, including complex trauma, diagnoses of schizophrenia or borderline personality disorder (BPD). Throughout the two-hour event, many people came to the table. Each talked for between two and fifteen minutes, sharing personal experiences of grief, loss, suicidality, depression and abuse. People disclosed experiences of multiple suicides in families, some very recent occurrences. First Nations women in particular talked about the loss of sons, daughters, nieces and nephews. Every speaker, and many on the sidelines, had been touched in some way by suicide.

As stories unfolded, there was an increasing recognition of similarities in their experiences, emotional histories and struggles. Some talked about being misdiagnosed and being given too little support from general practitioners, hospitals, nurses, doctors and counsellors. They shared frustrations in trying to get help for themselves or family members, but also acknowledged how people had helped. Many people, both speaking and listening, cried, laughed and expressed levels of frustration and anger. Some speakers were too distressed to continue, while others took up their story on their behalf. In general, the group experienced a shared discharge of emotion, which ultimately motivated ongoing discussion.

As the *Long Table* drew to a close, pizza was delivered, and participants were keen to reflect on the conversations while sharing food. Some acknowledged that they had pushed through levels of discomfort to engage; a few people left the room overwhelmed by emotion and then felt motivated to return. People lingered in one-on-one or group conversations. No one was in a rush to leave, and it was almost two hours after the close of the *Long Table* that the last people left. There was an overwhelming sense in the room that more needed to be done, a recognition that formal services were at breaking point and that the community could find a way to help itself. In this sense, the *Long Table* had focused the intent of the community.

The *Long Table* effectively served as an impromptu introduction to the two-day programme of workshops focusing on trauma recovery and wellbeing explored via immersive audio-visual sessions, Forum Theatre exercises and virtual-reality experiences. It reinforced the value of designing a container and safe space for experience, the 'potential space' positively impacting on the subsequent two days (Bennett, 2022a; Winnicott, 2005 [1971]). The process of creating the space enacts a form of experience design where experience is made possible rather than defined, being highly responsive and, where necessary, pivoting to allow events to take whatever shape needed. For such design to be effective and meaningful as well as safe, designers must remain attuned to the emotional valence of the event and to the needs of participants, building in options and flexibility. In this sense, it is grounded in TIC principles, which begin with ensuring trust and safety and enabling self-determined action within a collaborative context.

Participants reported on the impact of the programme in its entirety (reporting via interviews and survey, discussed in detail elsewhere) but noted that the *Long Table* played a particular function:

> The long table was a great beginning, it helped me feel safe and heard. For me it set the stage for the next two days. By the end of the programme, I was floored by the safe space that was created and the hope that was rebirthed in me. I feel like I discovered parts of me that were never allowed to flourish.
>
> *(The Long Table, Warwick unpublished recordings 6–8 April 2022)*

It provided an opportunity to speak and be 'valued, safe and heard'. This sense of safety built trust in the process, a trust that was noted as being absent in engaging with mental health services and systems. For some, this allowed for a greater focus on their personal wellbeing in the subsequent two days. Several spoke of a journey and process of unfolding: 'I feel like I have gone through a journey of self-growth, but mainly self-acceptance.'

The *Long Table* in its open format appears 'light touch', in that the number of decisions made to shape the event are not clearly evident to all; however, the design choices made and the entire process of establishing the event attends assiduously to the whole environment (Bennett et al., 2023). Its open format is under-engineered, creating a container to 'hold' emotions and for unscripted conversations to emerge expressing deep emotion, of grief in particular, but then the feelings of hope, togetherness and optimism that had been eroded in the community through lack of services and support.

Spaces between people

The theme for *The Big Anxiety*, Naarm, was learning from lived experience. As with the engagement at Warwick, establishing a container or holding space for people to engage with issues around mental health was key. *Spaces between People* was an exhibition aimed at creating such a container for the audience to engage with, learn from and share their own stories of lived experience. As part of the arts and mental health festival, its aim was to create an intimate environment in which the external conditions that perpetuate trauma are both illuminated and momentarily displaced as new possibilities for engagement are realised. Again, the concept derives from Winnicott's notion '[i]t is in the space between inner and outer world, which is also the space between people – the transitional space – that intimate relationships and creativity occur' (Winnicott, 1953, p. 92).

The works in the *Spaces between People* exhibition (including *We're Just Gonna Call It all BPD* discussed here) embody this transitional potential space, presenting accounts of difficult internal experiences in relation to external conditions, and generating new forms of intimate connection with these experiences. Rather than simply representing stories of trauma, the aim was to design an exhibition as a container in which stories (mediated through digital technology in this case) could be processed and placed in an environment that invited audiences to sit with the emotions presented. In these approximations of therapeutic listening encounters, emotions can be shared (illuminated and understood) without judgement in a safe space. If the *Long Table* built trust, optimism and connection through the sharing of experience in such a space, *Spaces Between People* used the format of the exhibition to activate a similar space of holding and connection but this time the goal was to open up the potential for participation with an audience who may have resonant lived experiences. Exemplified by *We're Just Gonna Call It all BPD*, the viewer can experience 'sitting with' emotions, along with the participants of different ages and experiences talking about how they develop coping strategies. The gallery space provides an opportunity that is available to all with lived experience, in inviting the viewer to join with a community of peers.

We're just gonna call it all BPD was developed from interviews with people reflecting on the experience of being given a diagnosis of borderline personality disorder (BPD). BPD is one of the most stigmatised of all mental health diagnoses – both in the public imagination and within the health sector itself. As such, it has been criticised as a 'highly contentious and damaging label' with calls for its abolition pointing to the high correlation between childhood abuse or neglect and BPD diagnoses (Warrender et al., 2021). Created by fEEL in association with RMIT and University of Technology Sydney (UTS), the art experience is shaped by a three-channel video installation set up akin to a physical group therapy meeting. The installation presents a revolving array of six people (three on view at any time) talking about their lived experience and the impact of receiving a BPD diagnosis. As one story ends, another begins, the entire loop running for over an hour (Figure 7.1). At any one time, three life-sized characters are seated

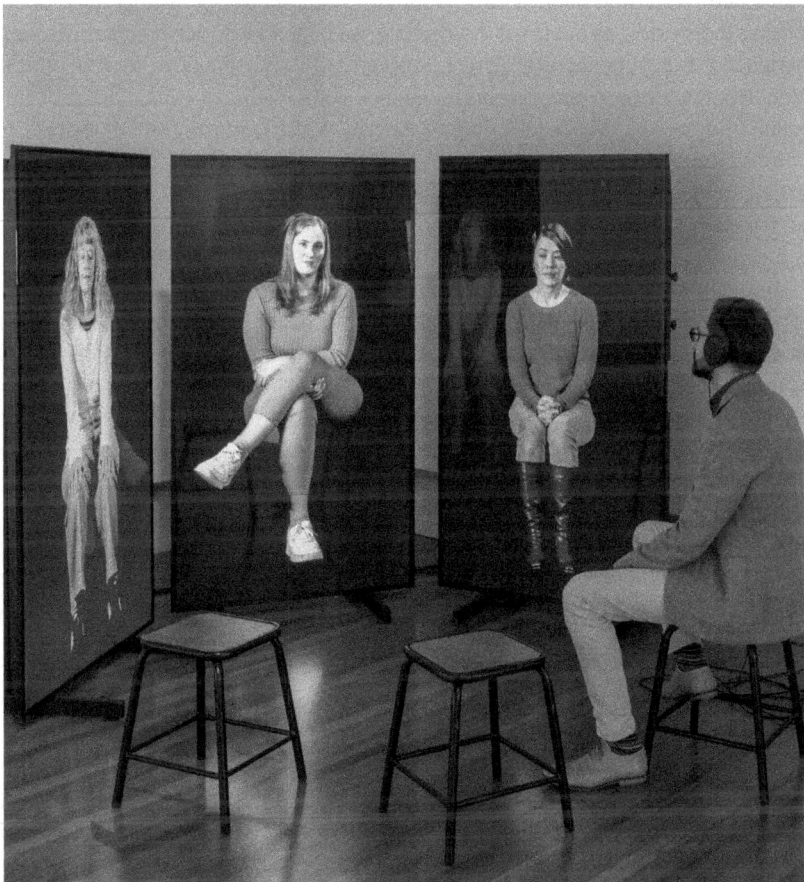

Figure 7.1   We're just gonna *call it all BPD,* a video installation designed to facilitate a close relationship to experience. RMIT Galleries Photo: Tobias Titz

on stools on separate free-standing screens, forming a semi-circle. Three seats, completing the circle are available for the viewers. The central character begins narrating their story as the characters on either side of them listen, sometimes intently, sometimes fidgeting or drifting off. The narrator, for the most part, holds eye-contact with the viewer, at times seemingly scanning the group for acknowledgement.

The spoken words are verbatim scripts produced from the audio recordings of six people of differing age and background – five female, one non-binary – each describing histories of early and persisting trauma and unmet emotional needs. They shed light on the impulse to self-harm and on the struggle to regulate intense emotion in the absence of carers able to recognise and attend to needs. They are often critical of the levels of formal support and diagnosis they received, although in each case they have found connections to sustain them and learnt various techniques to enable 'sitting with' and processing difficult feelings.

A creative team, including the participants, worked verbatim with wide-ranging content from the semi-structured interviews with researchers to create scripts that conveyed both the emotional depth and intensity of the narrative and amplified the agency of participants and their experiences of posttraumatic growth. The design process drew on verbatim theatre approaches that allow meaning to emerge both for the participant in the telling of their stories and for the listening audience (Kenning et al., 2022; National Theatre, 2014). Rather than summarising and condensing the stories, as occurs in journalistic and agenda-driven storytelling, the creative team, experienced in psychosocial practice, worked with recordings to identify not only thematic content but the valence and emotional nuance conveyed in speech. The process allowed for the rhythm and flow of the story-telling to emerge while capturing the embodied feeling of the interactions (Kenning et al., 2022).

The participants suggested that in the telling of their stories it was as if they were talking to a trusted friend or therapist – one who may or may not exist. This inspired the format of the artwork in the gallery setting in re-enacting of the stories with actors collectively sharing within a group therapy style encounter. The format constitutes a holding space for listening without judgement – with the potential benefits of empathetic listening and of hearing others speak about their experiences. This is of particular value in relation to diagnoses such as BPD which can be alienating and lonely.

The interviews revealed the frustrations of how, once participants had received a diagnosis of BPD, all behaviours were put down to the diagnosis rather than being acknowledged as a normal response to adverse life-events that included neglect, sexual abuse and complex trauma. As participant (A) explained:

> I found myself caught up in the Black Saturday bushfires…I ended up with Post Traumatic Stress Disorder … and then I started to develop these symptoms that were, you know, in line with BPD. So, I got labelled with BPD.

The participant explained how this impacted her behaviours and attitudes towards her. She suggested health care staff behaved as if:

> We're going to ignore the PTSD. We're going to ignore all other symptoms that that preceded trauma and we're just going to call it all BPD. And now we're going to treat you as a person with BPD, which means you're an attention seeker.

Another, in the words of a woman who worked in the health system, expressed both understandings and frustrations about the care needed (Participant AN):

It could be absolutely amazing to delve into trauma and to start to process and kind of adapt to some of that. I've got friends that have done it and have had amazing kind of success, but yeah. In the public system they quite blatantly will tell you that they don't deal with [trauma]. I've heard that over and over and over.

The voices of the characters on screen shared strategies they had been given and provided insights into how they learnt to work with overwhelming emotions (Participant L):

I had emotion disproportionate to the event – and I remember saying to the counsellor, 'I hate this', … I said, 'What [else] can I do?' and he said, 'You could sit with it', and I went 'What?', and he said, 'You could sit with this feeling'. I remember being so shocked I forgot to ask him what he meant. And I went home, and I sat in the chair, and I thought 'I'm going to figure out this sitting with it shit and I'm not going to get off this chair until I can figure it out and sit with this feeling that I'm feeling'.

In this telling, the character is restating the very act the viewer is charged with in this space: to simply sit with emotions.

These works and the exhibition room were specifically designed to facilitate a close relationship to experience; an experience-near encounter. In the signage, we alerted people to the terms of this encounter (as opposed to issuing trigger warnings), inviting visitors to engage in active listening, attuning to the internal world of another with 'unconditional positive regard' (Rogers, 1959, p. 195). To this end, we attempted to design a slow, attentive listening experience, in which judgement is withheld in favour of an openness to intersubjective experience. In other words, rather than evaluating the work as good/bad art, the invitation is to engage with a mode of subjectivity. Following this, there was an open invitation to sit and share thoughts and feelings, in a journal provided, as well as a formal survey. The design of the space and content supported a deep connection with subjectivity and with creativity, as expressed by one exhibition audience member who responded in the journal:

How do we survive this world? Through exchanging stories and experiences, we learn that each individual from our communities and societies have their own narratives. Being able to think & imagine a person more than just a number. Being creative with who we are!

(Personnel communication via Gallery
Journal 16 November 2022)

Designing a safe space for mental health

Given the stated shortfall in health services to adequately address trauma, we advocate for mental health being understood and supported in communities in social and cultural contexts. Psychosocial design as a relational process emerges out of psychosocial practices long used in the support of mental health (Bennett et al., 2023). It offers support and opportunities for healing, drawing on trauma-informed principles that place lived experience at the centre and offer the much-needed non-clinical supports being called for.

The central argument of this chapter is that psychosocial design, by attending to the affordances of any given situation or environment, can create a holding space to engage with and learn from lived experience. This bottom-up generative approach allows insights to emerge, in contrast to the often top-down approaches of co-design and care, evident in many healthcare systems and services. The design process uses deep listening practices throughout to build the trust and connection already identified as lacking in interactions with health care systems and to create experiences in which judgement is withheld and individual and collective agency empowered. In Warwick, the *Long Table* created affordances or opportunities for action by constituting a potential space for those who felt disenfranchised by health systems and services and grounding the event in lived experience – positioning people as experts in their own lives was key. Participants in the *Long Table* were given space to talk and be heard and, as such, this ultimately allowed for a focus on long-term *outcomes* (personal growth, supporting mental health at the community level), rather than simply *outputs* (the festival event itself).

We're gonna call it all BPD exemplifies the process of trust-building through a creative collaboration that entailed paying close attention to what was being said, how it was said and to whom – and by collaboratively shaping an artwork that enabled audiences to experience and engage with resonant experiences. This was not just an expressive work but a context for audience engagement and reception. How the audience accessed the work was a direct response to how the participants conceived of their 'ideal listener'. The environment, designed as a group therapy space, allows the audience to engage with trauma histories and complex emotions in ways that feel considered, resourced and supported.

The visitors' experiences that arise out of affective-led, arts-based interactions are fluid and open-ended. As such, designers are effectively creating a potential space, rather than a defined experience. This often means 'standing back' or 'letting go' and creating the space for fully agentic participants and audiences to make use of what is offered. Thus, the projects that we have described focus on building strength in people and communities, creating opportunities for communities to form, and/or on creating projects with communities that can in turn serve as resources.

Acknowledgements

Research for this chapter was supported by an Australian Research Council Laureate Fellowship. Full credits for the works described can be found on the website feel-lab.org. Special thanks to Cynthia Hoffman, Marianne Wobcke and all Warwick Big Anxiety team; BPD research team: Renata Kokanović (lead), Emma Seal, Tamara Borovica (RMIT); Natasha Swingler, Karolina Krysinska, Jess Dee, Linnie M and other anonymous participants. *We're just* gonna *call it all BPD* builds on research from an Australian Research Council [ARC] Linkage project. *Spaces Between People* was designed for Archives of Feeling at RMIT Galleries, commissioned by Andrew Tetzlaff.

Notes

1 thebiganxiety.org
2 https://unsw.to/barc
3 'Country' does not only reference place but is irrevocably linked to Aboriginal cultural practices, law/ lore, language and identity and kinship, known as 'mob' (Holmes, M. C. & Jampijinpa, W., 2013). Law for country: The structure of Warlpiri ecological knowledge and its application to natural resource management and ecosystem stewardship. *Ecology and Society, 18*(3).

References

Auger, J. (2013). Speculative design: Crafting the speculation. *Digital Creativity (Exeter)*, *24*(1), 11–35. https://doi.org/10.1080/14626268.2013.767276

Bennett, J. (2022a). *The big anxiety: Taking care of mental health in times of crisis* (J. Bennett, Ed.). Bloomsbury Academic.

Bennett, J. (2022b). The politics of experience. In J. Bennett (Ed.), *The big anxiety: Taking care of mental health in times of crisis* (pp. 3–13). Bloomsbury Academic.

Bennett, J., Froggett, L., & Muller, L. (2022). Facilitating environments: An arts-based psychosocial design approach. In J. Bennett (Ed.), *The Big Anxiety: Taking care of mental health in times of crisis*, (pp. 117-143). Bloomsbury.

Bennett, J., Kenning, G., Gitau, L., Moran, R., & Wobcke, M. (2023). Transforming trauma through an arts festival: A psychosocial case study. *Social Sciences (Basel)*, *12*(4), 249. https://doi.org/10.3390/socsci12040249

Bion, W. R. (1993 [1970]). *Attention and interpretation*. Maresfield Library.

Bødker, S., & Kyng, M. (2018). Participatory design that matters-facing the big issues. *ACM Transactions on Computer-Human Interaction*, *25*(1), 1–31. https://doi.org/10.1145/3152421

Cruickshank, L. (2014). *Open design and innovation: Facilitating creativity in everyone*. Gower.

Dawda, P., & Knight, A. (2019). *Experience based co design - A toolkit for Australia*.

Dunne, A., & Raby, F. (2013). *Speculative everything: Design, fiction, and social dreaming*. The MIT Press.

Gibson, J. J. (1979). *.The ecological approach to visual perception*. Psychology Press.

Holmes, M. C., & Jampijinpa, W. (2013). Law for country: The structure of Warlpiri ecological knowledge and its application to natural resource management and ecosystem stewardship. *Ecology and Society*, *18*(3).

Hustvedt, S., & Bennett, J. (2022). Why do art therapies work? In J. Bennett (Ed.), *The big anxiety: Taking care of mental health in times of crisis* (pp. 17–27). Bloomsbury Academic.

Kenning, G., Bennett, J., & Kuchelmeister, V. (2022). The Visit: A collaborative confabulation. In J. Bennett (Ed.), *The big anxiety: Taking care of mental health in times of crisis* (pp. 104–115). Bloomsbury Academic.

Levenson, J. (2017). Trauma-informed social work practice. *Social Work*, *62*(2), 105–113. https://doi.org/10.1093/sw/swx001

Lyckvi, S., Roto, V., Buie, E., & Wu, Y. (2018). *The role of design fiction in participatory design processes*. ACM International Conference Proceeding Series.

Moran, R., & Bennett, J. (2022). The Warwick long table on suicide and mental health. *Human rights defender*. https://protect-eu.mimecast.com/s/G4l0Cy6P1clQjAOHZ8Fye?domain=mailchi.mp [accessed 2 February 2024]

National Theatre. (2014). *An introduction to verbatim theatre*. National Theatre. https://www.youtube.com/watch?v=ui3k1wT2yeM

Norman, D. A. (2016). When you come to a fork in the road, take it: The future of design. *The Journal of Design, Economics, and Innovation*, *2*(4), 343–348. https://doi.org/10.1016/j.sheji.2017.07.00

Prevention and Response to Violence Abuse and Neglect Government Relations (PARVAN). (2023). *Integrated trauma informed care framework: My story, my health, my future*. PARVAN.

Productivity Commission. (2020). *Mental health*. Commonwelath of Australia. https://www.pc.gov.au/inquiries/completed/mental-health/report/mental-health-volume1.pdf

Rieger, K. L., Lobchuk, M. M., Duff, M. A., Chernomas, W. M., Campbell-Enns, H. J., Demczuk, L., Nicolas, S., & West, C. H. (2018). Effectiveness of mindfulness-based arts interventions on psychological wellbeing and fatigue in adults with a physical illness: A systematic review protocol. *JBI Database System Rev Implement Rep*, *16*(7), 1476–1484. https://doi.org/10.11124/JBISRIR-2017-003446

Rogers, C. R. (1959). A theory of therapy, personality and interpersonal relationships as developed in the client-centered framework. In S. Koch (Ed.), *Psychology: A study of a science. Study 1, volume 3: Formulations of the person and the social context* (Vol. 3, pp. 184–256). McGraw-Hill.

Shaw, P., Weaver, L., & Mergolin, D. (n.d.). *The long table*. http://www.split-britches.com/long-table?rq=long%20table

Vogelpoel, N., & Gattenhof, S. (2012). Arts-health intersections: A model of practice for consistency in the arts-health sector. *Journal of Applied Arts and Health, 3*(3), 259–274.

Warrender, D., Bain, H., Murray, I., & Kennedy, C. (2021). Perspectives of crisis intervention for people diagnosed with "borderline personality disorder": An integrative review. *Journal of Psychiatric and Mental Health Nursing, 28*(2), 208–236. https://doi.org/10.1111/jpm.12637

Weaver, L., & Hunter Petree, L. (2022). I have a thing about tables. In J. Bennett (Ed.), *The big anxiety: Taking care of mental health in times of crisis* (pp. 112–121). Bloomsbury Academic.

Winnicott, D. W. (1953). Transitional objects and transitional phenomena - A study of the first not-me Possessional. *International Journal of Psycho-Analysis, 34*(2), 89–97.

Winnicott, D. W. (1965). *The maturational processes and the facilitating environment: Studies in the theory of emotional development*. Hogarth and the Institute of Psycho-analysis.

Winnicott, D. W. (2005 [1971]). *Playing and reality*. Routledge.

8 Designing community arts engagement for people with dementia and their informal care partners

Laura Malinin, Jennifer E. Cross, Deana Davalos, Meara Faw, Lindsey Wilhem and Rebecca Lassell

Introduction

'What role might community performing arts programmes play in improving quality of life (QoL) for people with dementia and their informal care partners?" This question underpinned a grass-roots effort in a mid-sized city in the United States where concerned stakeholders from local healthcare organizations, non-profit organisations, government agencies and a nearby research university came together to co-design a new music-enrichment programme for community members who were navigating the challenges of dementia. The community partnership began with the local symphony orchestra and a healthcare provider envisioning a community-based programme to improve the QoL for people with dementia and care partners. They brought together a coalition of stakeholders to develop community activities to provide ways for people with dementia and care partners to engage together in enriching experiences shown to improve their sense of wellbeing. They also sought research partners to document how participation might provide cognitive and physiological benefits for people with dementia. This chapter discusses the informal co-design process that evolved over eight years, specifically focusing on the role of empathy in the human-centred design approach as well as the key concepts of interdisciplinary collaboration and the iterative feedback loop characteristic of design thinking. Through discussion of our co-design processes, we articulate lessons learned and recommendations for best practices.

Psychosocial programming for people with dementia

Dementia encompasses a broad range of disorders, often characterised by progressive neurological degeneration and accompanied by an atypical decline in cognitive, behavioural, emotional, occupational or interpersonal functioning. The population affected by dementia is projected to increase from approximately 57.4 million cases globally in 2019 to 152.8 million cases in 2050 (GBD, 2019; Dementia Forecasting Collaborators, 2022). Pharmaceutical interventions have dominated treatment since the first drug was approved by the Food and Drug Administration in 1993 to target memory and thinking difficulties. However, these treatments have shown limited efficacy and can be accompanied by a range of undesirable side effects. While research into effective treatments for symptoms and causes of dementia continues, increased interest has turned to modifiable risk factors and non-pharmaceutical interventions (Gillis et al., 2021). Research on non-pharmacological interventions shows immense promise for improving QoL, relational connectedness and wellbeing among people with dementia and care partners (Cooper et al., 2012). Psychosocial interventions are particularly promising as they have been found to improve psychological and/or social functioning, interpersonal relationships, wellbeing, cognition and everyday functional abilities (Moniz-Cook et al., 2011). One benefit of psychosocial interventions is that they can be efficacious

DOI: 10.4324/9781003318262-10

across nearly all stages of dementia – from mild to moderate to severe symptoms – unlike cognitive-enhancement–focused interventions that may become too cognitively demanding past certain stages of disease progression (Mabire et al., 2022). Psychosocial interventions are also holistic in that they may involve family members, caregivers and others with whom the person with dementia resides. In this chapter, the term caregiver describes formal caregiver roles (e.g. nursing staff, home health aids), whereas the term care partner refers to the primary informal caregiver (e.g. spouse, adult child). Research into psychosocial interventions consistently highlights positive outcomes for people with dementia and care partners. They are associated with reduced conflict and agitation for people with dementia in residential facilities (Thomas & Sezgin, 2021). Interventions with people with dementia and care partners together improve the subjective sense of burden and depression for care partners (Brotons & Marti, 2003; Wiegelmann et al., 2021) and create a greater sense of connection with people with dementia (Faw et al., 2021a; Wilhelm & Wilhelm, 2020). Additionally, psychosocial interventions in public spaces (e.g. art galleries) reduce perceptions of stigma for people with dementia and care partners (Bienvenu & Hanna, 2017; Lepp et al., 2003). Our own research shows potential for psychosocial interventions to increase the care partners' sense of connection with their community as well as restored dignity for people with dementia and their care partners (Faw et al., 2021a).

Co-designing the programme: a human-centred design thinking approach

The community arts programmes described in this chapter were inspired by a community music programme called *B-Sharp Music Wellness* (Phoenix Symphony, n.d.), which consisted of small groups of musicians who provided performances for people with dementia. While this programme was perceived as valuable to the community and people with dementia (Walton & Bartleet, 2021), comprehensive impact assessments were lacking. The new community music programme in Fort Collins, Colorado, also called *B Sharp,* was jointly designed and implemented by a steering committee of members from the local symphony orchestra, community partners, including healthcare service providers, and a team of interdisciplinary university researchers (Figure 8.1). From the beginning, *B Sharp* was created as a community-based research project, with equal emphasis on programme development, implementation and impact assessment (Malinin et al., 2023).

The co-creation process for *B Sharp* evolved organically, with members of the team bringing deep understanding of community-engaged scholarship and design expertise to the process to align it with core tenets of a human-centred design-thinking approach. Sanders and Stappers (2008) note that the terms *co-creation* and *co-design* are often used interchangeably. We further specify the notion of these terms here, using the term co-design to describe collaborative creative processes involving an interdisciplinary team of people (including those from design and non-design disciplines) who work together throughout the project – from pre-design through to implementation, evaluation and iteration.

B Sharp relied on the expertise of professionals who worked with people with dementia and researchers with varied backgrounds to develop the pilot programme, keeping the experiences and needs of people with dementia and care partners central to the co-design process. Although people with dementia and care partners were not formal members of the steering committee, user feedback was incorporated regularly throughout the design process. During pre-design, we gathered user feedback through informal conversations and interviews, and during the later stages of prototyping, evaluation and iteration, formal user feedback was obtained through interviews, observations and focus groups. Our approach to co-design closely aligns with Giacomin's (2014) understanding that human-centred design thinking is

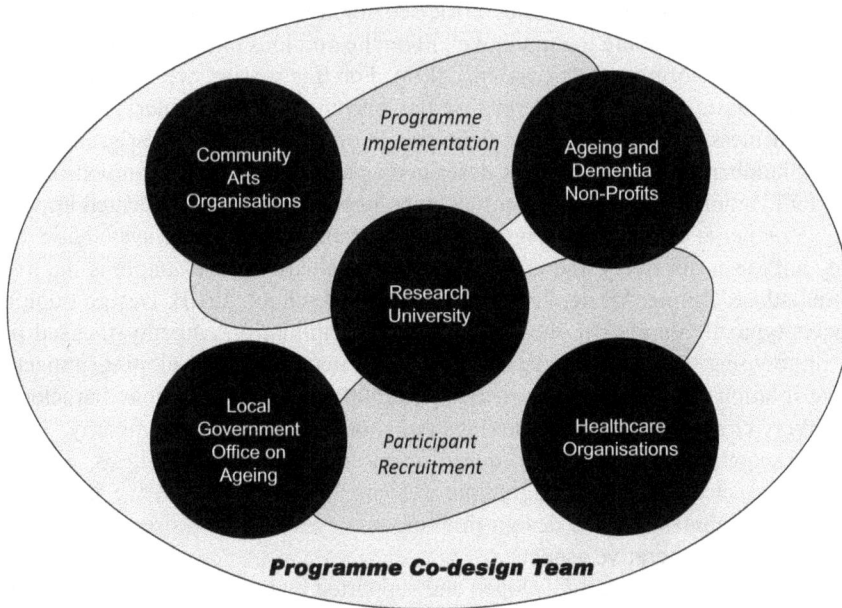

Figure 8.1 Programme co-design team with expertise in community programming, aging, dementia, occupational therapy, cognitive psychology, sociology, communications, music therapy and design

based on the use of techniques which communicate, interact, empathise and stimulate the people involved, obtaining an understanding of their needs, desires and experiences which often transcends that which the people themselves actually realised…the natural focus of the questions, insights and activities lies with the people for whom the product, system or service is intended.

(p. 7)

The steering committee met monthly to discuss and assess the programme development based on observations at events, comments from participants, interview responses and other feedback. These meetings began with discussion of observations and answered the question, 'What did we observe and what did we learn?' and moved to the questions 'What adjustments need to be made?' and 'What is working that should be kept?' These conversations highlighted expected and unexpected responses to programme components and allowed us to engage in rapid iteration with the explicit focus on empathy for participant desires, interaction and responses. Our decision-making framework focused on the values of the programme to support both care partners and people living with dementia and prioritised care. At the end of Year 1, we received a request from one care partner to continue participating after their loved one died. The co-design team asked ourselves, 'How does allowing continued participation align with the goals of the programme to support care partners sense of connection to the community?' We agreed that care partners could continue to participate after the death of a loved one precisely because it aligned with our goal to provide opportunities for community support. It seemed incongruous with our values to say they would no longer be welcome in the community and programme at precisely the time where people are most in need of emotional support from existing social ties.

Human-centred design is sometimes criticised for treating users as test subjects, over-burdening users and providing too much weight on the opinions of a small sample, ultimately limiting creativity (Norman, 2005; Salvo, 2001). For this reason, we develop Giacomin's notion through *design thinking*, a term that has become highly popularised, especially in design and business fields, although its definition is often ambiguous (Carlgren et al., 2016; Johansson-Sköldberg et al., 2013). It is described as a process to drive innovation, methods (or tools) for ideation (e.g. personas, journey mapping) and/or mindsets deemed important for creativity (Brenner et al., 2016). Design thinking is often illustrated as a systematic approach beginning with user discovery and concluding with evaluation; an example is the five-stage model: Empathise, Define, Ideate, Prototype and Test (d.school, 2010). Design thinking process models typically emphasise the value of interdisciplinarity, empathy-focused problem finding, prototyping, user/stakeholder feedback and iteration in developing impactful and innovative solutions to social problems. Brown (2008) describes common characteristics of team members engaged in design thinking: collaboration, optimism, empathy, integrative thinking and experimentalism. Our co-design team embodied these qualities, and to which we attribute the success of our programme design. For this research, we integrated both approaches into a human-centred design-thinking process that emphasises the collaborative, empathic and creative-iterative aspects.

The *B Sharp* programme was developed and supported by the *B Sharp* steering committee, which included representatives from the local County Office on Aging and the Alzheimer's Association branch, an outreach programme manager from an adult day programme, the founder of a local non-profit organisation dedicated to supporting people with dementia and care partners, the executive director of the local symphony orchestra and a public relations representative from the founding health organisation. Each steering committee member committed to a specific role and responsibility, and the group articulated a set of core values and guiding principles by which to make all decisions about the programme development, assessment and delivery.

The steering committee met ten times a year to discuss upcoming symphony events, coordinate the research and social events associated with the concerts, fundraise and recruit participants. The monthly agenda included debriefs on participant experiences, comments from post-event interviews, observations of participant experiences as well as formal and informal feedback from participants. This feedback was used by the steering committee to inform the programme and research design. As part of the pre-design phase to help sustain the programme and further understand its potential benefits for care partners and people with dementia, researchers from the local university were invited to design research methods that coordinated with the planned events. The researchers became members of the steering committee and helped to define the specific objectives, formative assessments and outcome measures. The research team included experts from the fields of psychology, sociology, music therapy, communication, occupational therapy and design and contributed to the programme design, funding and programme implementation. Applying the human-centred design thinking approach, our co-design team sought to reduce the burden on people with dementia and care partners during the co-design process by integrating feedback loops into the programme design. Specifically, the steering committee prioritised empathising with and understanding participant experiences and needs as part of the agenda each month. The steering committee, with feedback from people with dementia and care partners, identified four key aims for the *B Sharp* pilot and subsequent programmes:

- Improve quality of life (QoL) for people with dementia and care partners through arts participation.
- Expand opportunities for social interaction for people with dementia and care partners.

- Improve relationships between people with dementia and care partners.
- Increase feelings of social support and community connection among people with dementia and care partners.

B Sharp pilot: learning through prototyping and feedback loops

During the 2015 pilot, individuals with a diagnosis of mild cognitive impairment or dementia who were not in a residential nursing facility and had a care partner who was interested in taking part were recruited through dementia-focused community organisations. The inclusion criterion for the programme was diagnosed pathological memory loss and included mild cognitive impairment and a variety of dementia diagnoses. The initial participant group consisted of 44 individuals (i.e. 22 pairs). One additional dyad enrolled between the first and second concerts, resulting in a total of 23 dyads. The 23 people with dementia and their care partners (primarily spouses) received free season tickets to attend five symphonic performances spanning eight months (October to May). The people with dementia/care partner dyads were also invited to social receptions before and after performances.

The research activities associated with the pilot programme spanned ten months (September to June). Programme impacts on participants were evaluated through neuropsychological assessments with people with dementia, phone interviews with care partners approximately one week after performances and a focus group with care partners at the conclusion of the symphony season. Neuropsychological pretesting occurred approximately a month before the first concert in October and post-testing occurred one month after the final concert in May. Testing occurred at a community event space donated to the programme. The main variables of interest during the initial concert season focused on neuropsychological assessment for a number of reasons. First, neuropsychological assessment is one of the primary tools used to assess pathological aging and allowed us to verify where on the cognitive ageing continuum each person was categorised (e.g. mild cognitive impairment versus dementia). Second, as we were exploring non-pharmacological interventions, using a measure that is one of the primary tools used in pharmacological outcome studies and more medical-focused interventions (see Rinehardt study reference below) allowed us to have a better understanding of how the community-based intervention compared to medical interventions using a shared neurocognitive outcome measure (Rinehardt et al., 2010). Finally, cognitive functioning is one of the most robust predictors of quality of life in older adults, specifically in older adults experiencing pathological ageing (Stites et al., 2018). People with dementia were evaluated by trained undergraduate and graduate students using the Repeatable Battery for Assessment of Neuropsychological Status (RBANS; Randolph et al., 1998). The assessment includes 12 subtests, which yields five Index scores (immediate memory, delayed memory, attention, language and visuospatial/constructional abilities). The 'Total Score', which sums all five Index scores, was used to capture overall cognitive functioning. The RBANS was developed to assess cognitive changes in older adults and to help distinguish normal ageing and pathological ageing. The assessment includes four alternate forms (A, B, C and D) and has been widely used to serially assess changes associated with interventions and clinical trials (Wiegelmann et al., 2021).

People with dementia were administered RBANS forms A and B to evaluate cognitive performance at the beginning of the community music programme (assessment 1) and approximately ten months later at the end (assessment 8). A significant difference between pre-and post-testing on RBANS Total Scores (overall cognitive functioning) was observed for the ten participants who completed both assessments (assessment 1 and assessment 8) was observed $(p \leq .010)$. For the 15 participants who may have participated for a shorter period of time, completing the assessment either prior to the music season (assessment 1) or during the first month of concerts (assessment 2), and also completed the post-season assessment (assessment 8), a significant difference was also observed between the initial and later RBANS assessment $(p \leq .010)$. For both analyses, the assessments revealed a positive difference with an increase from beginning to end scores. Pearson correlation results in the *B Sharp* study suggested that greater participation (attendance at more events) was related to greater overall improvement in cognitive processing (RBANS Total Score) between assessments 1 and 8 $(r = .50, p = .058)$, (Davalos et al., 2019). As a reference for the results found in the *B Sharp* study, Rinehardt and colleagues (2010) used RBANS to assess deep brain-stimulation treatment effects in older adults with Parkinson's disease and 'normal' ageing controls. They found that the average change in RBANS Total score over a 12-month span associated with "normal" ageing was a 3.5% 'decrease' in Total score. In our study, of the 15 participants completing preintervention and postintervention assessment, 4 showed an average 4.25% "decrease" and the 11 who improved showed an average 10.27% 'increase' in Total score despite having diagnosed cognitive decline. Given our participants had a diagnosed progressive neurocognitive disease, our findings suggest that even in those who did not improve, the decline was relatively small and in those who improved, it was quite robust.

The week following each performance, we called caregivers for short interviews about their experiences and held 90-minute focus groups each year the month of the final symphony performance for the season. During the phone interviews and focus groups, care partners shared how they were motivated to participate in the programme to further research on dementia and that they enjoyed interacting with the student researchers. They also appreciated the social hours before and after performances and during intermission as a short reprieve from caregiving responsibilities and a time to connect with other care partners. Care partners also reported positive impacts on mood for people with dementia leading up to each performance and lasting several days after.

Programme iteration and expansion

Perhaps the most innovative aspect of this project is that *B Sharp*, and all subsequent programmes, have been designed, implemented and funded by a network of community partners. Since inception, programme designs have evolved through feedback from community partners, participants and research team members toward improving participant experiences and strengthening research methods while working toward a common goal to transform the local community to be more inclusive for people with dementia. The programme has grown iteratively based on the interest and capacity of various steering committee members to commit human capital and other resources towards evolving and expanding the programmes (Table 1).

Continuing *B Sharp*, and creating *C Sharp* and other programmes

Since the *B Sharp* pilot was seen as very successful, additional community partners connected with members of the research team to explore a programme expansion to include additional measures and other types of community activities (Figures 8.2, 8.3). A grant from the National Endowment for the Arts in 2018 funded the expansion of the *B Sharp* programme to include additional data collection and two new visual arts programmes, *C Sharp Dance* and *C Sharp Theatre*. The *C Sharp* programmes (named for their emphasis on the visual arts) mirrored the *B Sharp* programme design, providing season tickets for people with dementia/care partner dyads to either dance or non-musical theatre performances through new partnerships with local ballet and theatre groups (Malinin et al., 2023).[1] The research team added pre- and post-season QoL assessments for people with dementia and care partners, pre- and post-performance sub-tests

Table 8.1 Evolution of *B Sharp* steering committee partnership, programme teration and expansion

Date	Evolution of collaboration	Programme development, iteration and expansion
Autumn 2014	Key sponsor of Fort Collins Symphony introduced the idea of arts programming for people with dementia. New partners joining: Banner Health, Fort Collins Symphony Funding: N/A	Pre-design, inviting partners to explore idea of arts engagement programmes
Spring 2015	University research partners recruited; Arts Engagement Steering Committee formed. New Partners joining: Alzheimer's Association, Larimer County Office on Aging, Stepping Stones Adult Day Programme, Memory Café Programme, three faculty researchers Funding: N/A	Review case studies from Phoenix Symphony and Museum of Modern Art; develop programme aims
Autumn 2015	Adopted the programme name *B Sharp*; steering committee members committed to specific roles, responsibilities and monthly meetings. New Partners joining: N/A. Funding: Banner Health (2015–19); Kaiser Permanente (2015–18); Home State Bank; Crowdsource funders (2015–18)	*B Sharp* pilot
2016	New Partners joining: Museum of Art Fort Collins, two new faculty researchers Funding: International Neuroscience Network Foundation (2016–19)	*B Sharp* continues
2017	Dementia Friendly Communities of Northern Colorado becomes an officially designated non-profit organisation (501c3) making it eligible to receive new sources of funding *B Sharp* and other programs. New Partners joining: Hearts & Horses, three new faculty researchers. Funding: Rotary Club of Loveland (2017–19); Sage Benefit Advisors (2017–19); Community Foundation of Northern Colorado (2017–19); CSU Office of the Vice President for Research (2017–19); Carl and Caroline Swanson Foundation	*Mask-Making in the Moment* pilot; *B Sharp* continues
2018	New Partners joining: Columbine Health Systems, Columbine Center for Healthy Aging Funding: National Endowment for the Arts (2018–22); Canyon Concert Ballet (2018–20); Lincoln Center Fort Collins (2018–20); Open Stage Theatre (2018–20); CSU Centre for Healthy Aging (2018–21)	Redesign of *Mask-Making in the Moment*; adaptation of *Riding the Moment*™ to add care partners; *C Sharp* begins; *B Sharp* continues
2019	New Partners joining: Fort Collins Senior Center Funding: Carol Ann and Gary Hixon; Kenneth and Myra Monfort Charitable Foundation; Suzanne and Larry Pullen; Barbara and Alan Rudolph; Walta and Jim Ruff	*Gardening in the Moment; Virtual Reality Pilot; B & C Sharp* continue
2020	New Partners joining: N/A. Funding: N/A	In-person programming paused in early 2020 due to the COVID-19 pandemic
2021	Increased collaboration between Dementia Together and the research team Non-profit rebrands to become "Dementia Together" https://dementiatogether.org/New Partners joining: N/A. Funding: N/A	Creation and implementation of new virtual programming, including virtual support groups to support care partners during COVID; implementation and evaluation of a care partner communication training programme (SPECAL)
2022	New Partners joining: N/A. Funding: N/A	*B Sharp* resumes; virtual support groups and SPECAL continue

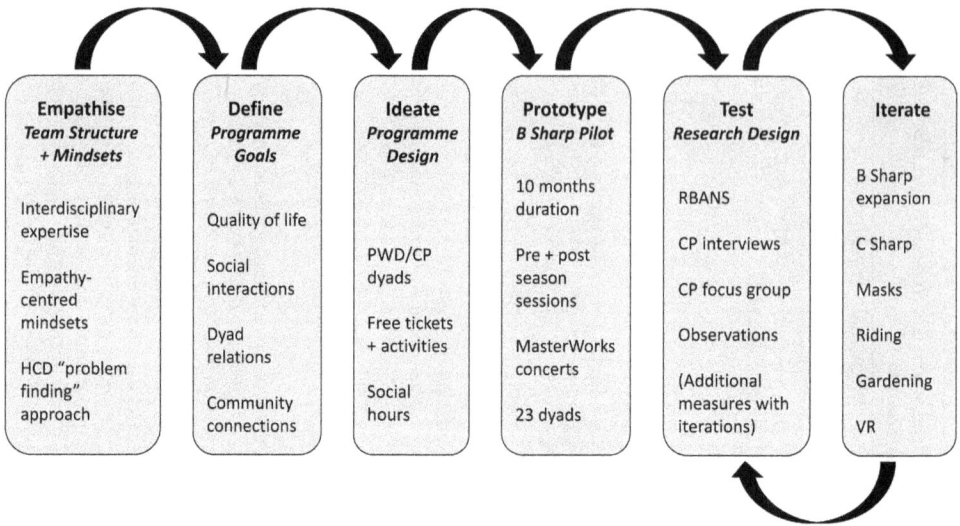

Figure 8.2 Programme co-design emphasising testing, feedback loops and iteration

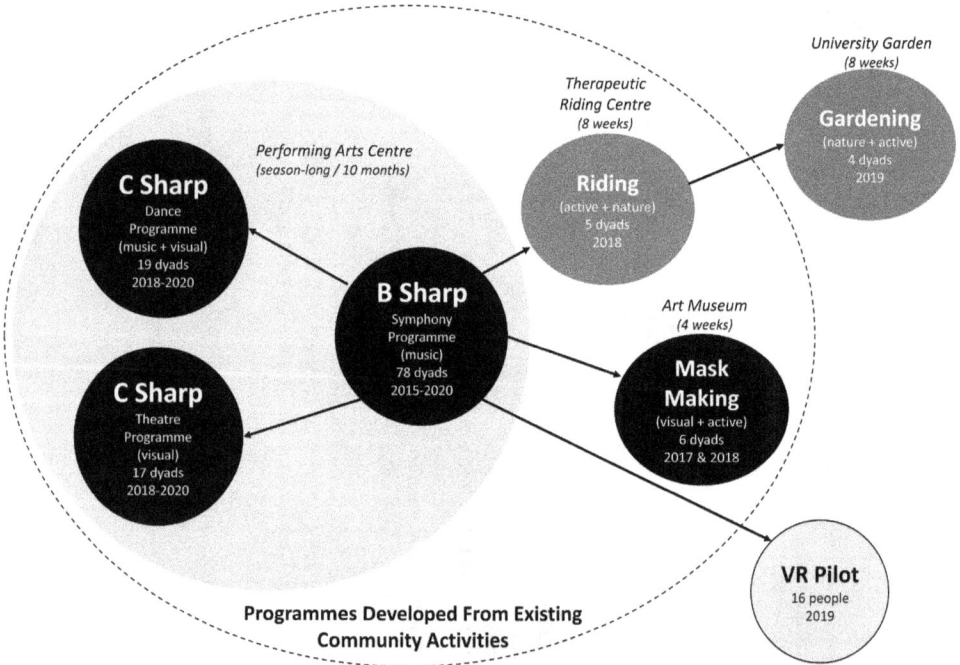

Figure 8.3 Programme evolution and expansion after the *B Sharp* pilot: from dyadic participation in season-long performing arts programmes, to four-week dyadic participation in craft, horseback riding and gardening, to exploration of remote participation using virtual reality

of the RBANS for people with dementia and mood assessments for people with dementia and care partners to explore themes that emerged from the interview data. The pre- and post-concert administration of select RBANS sub-tests were added, in addition to the pre- and post-season administrations of the full RBANS, to try to capture immediate effects of programme participation on cognition. Care partner interviews continued in *B Sharp* through spring 2019 when data saturation was reached. Many dyads stayed in that programme for several years, with care partners describing how the programme benefited relationship-building with other participants, fostered a renewed sense of dignity through a return to 'normalcy' as an engaged community member, and overall improved their feelings of positive emotions (Faw et al., 2021a; Malinin et al., 2023).

The programme expansion included collection of physiological data through wearable activity trackers (Fitbits) that also recorded sleep patterns. The Fitbits were added to be able to address the role of activity and sleep-quality associated with programme participation and to determine whether these variables might moderate the cognitive effects observed. While results from the activity tracker pilot suggested physiological benefits of programme participation, the inclusion of Fitbits proved problematic because participants found the technology confusing. The devices were often not charged properly, there were occurrences when participants lost the trackers, and the database was difficult to manage (Kurko et al., 2018; Schneider et al., 2018). Funding was secured from a university grant to collect telomere data as an alternative to the activity trackers. Telomeres are terminal DNA proteins found at the end of every cell's chromosome that serve as a biological marker of cellular ageing (Blackburn, 1991; Lansdorp, 2000; Xi et al., 2013). While telomeres tend to naturally shorten over the lifespan, research shows that lifestyle factors can slow telomere shortening and, in some cases, even lengthen telomeres (Conklin et al., 2015). The goal of incorporating telomere measures was to provide a physiological marker that might help document whether these community-based programmes had a positive effect on care partners' and people with dementia's cellular ageing.

Artistic Mask-Making (in the Moment)

Shorter, four-week programmes were developed with the goal of providing more physically interactive psychosocial activities. The first four-week expansion programme was a partnership in 2017 with a local arts museum and certified art therapist to conduct an art-making workshop in conjunction with an annual exhibit and fundraiser. The museum hosts an annual exhibit and fundraiser called *Masks*, which displays artistic masks created by community members who begin with a ceramic blank and then design and decorate their mask and return it for the exhibit. The mask-making programme involved participation by six people with dementia/care partner dyads, four of whom completed all four workshops where they designed masks based on personal memories. Like *B Sharp*, dyads participated in a social hour before and after each weekly workshop. RBANS were administered pre- and post-programme and before and after each or the four workshops during the first programme year; care partners were interviewed by phone after every workshop. Additionally, each workshop for both programme years was video recorded to facilitate observational analysis, which proved more useful than RBANS for evaluating this shorter programme. Participant feedback from the first programme year resulted in the elimination of an arts education component at the start of each workshop and inclusion of an arts therapist experienced in working with people with dementia to facilitate the mask-making activities more effectively. Results from the two programme years revealed that participation helped foster relational maintenance behaviours between people with dementia and their care partners, and it also helped dyads form new relationships with others living with dementia (Griggs et al., 2020). Future four-week programmes were distinguished from season-long programmes through emphasising shorter duration and hands-on engagement to support positive emotional experiences to bring awareness to the present moment. The phrase 'in the Moment' was added to shorter programmes modelled after the previously established community programme *Riding in the Moment*™.

Riding in the Moment™

In 2017, the research team expanded to include researchers investigating the potential of an adaptive riding programme, *Riding in the Moment (RM)*™, to improve QoL for people with dementia. The programme was created by Hearts & Horses Therapeutic Riding Center in Loveland, Colorado, to engage people with dementia in long-term care facilities. The programme occurs over eight weeks or four weeks, depending on participants' needs (Lassell et al., 2019). In 2015, an initial partnership was formed between researchers and Hearts & Horses to establish proof of concept that *RM*™ could support QoL for people with dementia in long-term care (Fields et al., 2018, 2019).

In partnership with the broader research team and the programming director at Hearts & Horses, the *RM*™ programme was expanded to study people with dementia in the community and include care partners. Proof of concept for adapting RM™ to care partners was established with positive findings for outcomes of participation, wellbeing, meaning through social connections and function in daily life (Lassell et al., 2021, 2022). During the programme, co-design began on an individual level by modifying activities based on the participant's preferences and needs from their intake form and screening assessment. For example, personalised information cards were created for each participant for volunteers to familiarise themselves with the person's preferences prior to their first session. Additionally, participants were paired with a horse based on their needs. Co-design continued across the programme with staff and volunteer debriefings after each session to further modify planned activities for the following week based on the people with dementia and care partners' responses (e.g. adding coloured reins, changing the level of challenge with an obstacle course). Since incorporating care partners, a *RM*™ manual has been produced to allow for implementation at multiple sites. Additionally, using participatory-action methods, the manual and training curriculum were created with stakeholders including care partners, therapeutic riding centres interested in implementing *RM*™, local dementia and ageing organisations and researchers (Fields et al., 2021).

Gardening in the Moment

In contrast, co-design of *Gardening in the Moment* (*GM*) occurred at the conception of the programme with stakeholders and individual participants based on their preferences and needs. *GM* arose with the need to explore the horse-nature connection (a potential mechanism of change proposed by stakeholders; Lassell et al., 2019). As such, *GM* was created to mirror *RM*™ with the aim of supporting QoL with people with dementia and their care partners. *GM* was co-designed with a local gardening educator who helped conduct the programme. Sessions were designed with opportunities to engage in gardening activities (planting, harvesting, weeding, etc.), and each dyad was paired with a volunteer throughout the programme (Lassell et al., 2021). Co-design occurred on an individual level to tailor the activities to participants' needs at intake with a history of the person's preferences, likes, dislikes and prior roles. Design followed the same iterative process of *RM*™, with planning sessions, implementing and debriefing after each session with stakeholders (volunteers and the gardening educator). Debriefing included discussions and observations of how people with dementia responded and guided refinements for planned activities in the next session. After the conclusion of the study, the local gardening educator planned to expand the gardening centre's programming to include programmes for people with dementia.

Virtual reality pilot

In 2019, we undertook a pilot study exploring the feasibility of using virtual reality (VR) to bring our performing arts programming to more diverse populations. Using a focus group co-design method, 16 participants, including people with dementia and older adults without a dementia diagnosis, engaged with two different virtual experiences: a symphonic experience modelled after the *B Sharp* programme, or a virtual college campus tour. Using feedback from participants, we changed the virtual experiences to meet their goals of greater immersion and to transcend physical limitations, i.e. instead of watching a symphony performance from the mezzanine level of a performing arts hall, participants were put centre stage in front of the conductor. Results were promising, showing that participants found VR immersive and engaging. They shared their desires for additional programme development as well as any hesitations or fears about using the technology themselves, providing an excellent starting point for additional VR programming development in the future (Faw et al., 2021b).

Programme outcomes and lessons learned

One of the strengths of the *B Sharp* programme is the collaborative spirit of non-profit agencies in Fort Collins, which enabled our community to create an arts engagement programme that was not tied to, or sponsored by, one primary organisation. This exemplary co-designed programme was initiated by a community collaborative group and funded in the first few years from a variety of community funders from local businesses, healthcare providers and individual donors. However, within the first year, it became apparent that this organisational structure would become a barrier to seeking larger funding because foundations typically look to fund programmes through the support of a single organisation. By 2016, the steering committee decided that a new non-profit organisation with a focus on supporting a variety of community-engaged programming would be the best fit as the 'parent' organization for *B Sharp*. Thus, *Dementia Friendly Communities of Northern Colorado*[2] was registered in January 2017, less than two years after the launch of the *B Sharp* programme.

During the first year, the steering committee held several discussions to identify specific roles and responsibilities (fundraising, recruitment, research coordination, logistics, etc.) necessary to fund and support the programme. In Fort Collins, all the members of the steering committee were able to commit between two and ten hours a month of their professional duties to supporting *B Sharp*. When neighbouring communities reached out with an interest to create similar programmes in their community, they found that the same stakeholder organisations did not have the human capital or ability to take on a collaborative project of this scope. Some organisations were unable to commit because of a lack of staffing while other organisations felt that formal roles in support of the programme were out of scope for their organisational mission. We have learned that even in communities with similar stakeholders and a desire to create arts engagement programmes, it typically requires a single organisation to act as a lead sponsor and director, which requires dedicated funding and staff support.

While the *B Sharp* programme had a variety of successful expansions, not all expansions were equally successful. In another community, local agencies struggled to commit staff time to manage a similar programme, and participants were difficult to recruit because many families did not want to admit they were struggling with dementia. The first *Mask-Making in the Moment* pilot revealed what adaptations an art education and creation programme requires to support people with dementia and care partners. Despite improvements in the second year, the *Mask-Making* programme was discontinued due to difficulties recruiting participants. Across many programmes, participant recruitment was a challenge. Over-recruitment proved an important strategy due to the progressive nature of dementia and the age of participants. People with dementia with more advanced disease were often frustrated by the RBANS and mask-making and care partners were saddened to see their partner struggle. Despite this, most dyads persisted in attending the programmes, motivated by the research component and social connection with other care partners. University infrastructure, such as clinical Alzheimer's disease research centres, can play an important role to help leverage community partnerships supporting recruitment, easing the burden on individual researchers or community stakeholders.

Finally, outcomes from our programme underscore the value of practising continual learning and adaptation through processes of 'rapid iteration'. For example, ongoing feedback from participants revealed a variety of surprises about the programme design. The time of symphony performances, 7:30pm, was a concern for care partners because of sundown syndrome, thus other programmes were designed with this in mind. Despite the late *C Sharp* start time, we found participants looking forward to performances for a day or two ahead of concerts, staying past the performance to socialise with other participants, and perking up to attend concerts even on days when care partners thought participants with dementia might not be feeling up to going out. The steering committee and research team were also pleasantly surprised to learn that participating in the programme, including the research component, increased motivation to participate, as one participant shared regarding her involvement in the *B Sharp* programme and the level of investment she felt from the community:

> They mention [*B Sharp*] in the [symphony] printed programme, and at every concert. And I think, 'Someone cares about us. Someone is trying to help us.' It's a feeling of someone doing something for this disease and trying to solve it. ... It's been a nice thing. It's like someone giving me a gift. It's like a present.
>
> (Faw et al., 2021a, p. 7)

Conclusion

This chapter details our journey of co-designing the *B Sharp* programme and expanding community offerings to accommodate different participant interests and community needs. It highlights the importance of interdisciplinary collaboration, of iteration and feedback loops throughout the co-design process and of the successes and challenges in enacting an ambitious programme to address care partners and people with dementias' needs and interests. One of the remarkable aspects of this co-design effort was that each member of the steering committee agreed to take responsibility for one specific task (e.g. fundraising, recruitment of participants, organising the social events) which made it possible to stand up a programme that no one organisation owned. This was only possible because the leaders of each participating organisation were bought into the value of the programme and gave permission for their staff to officially participate in the steering committee and to take responsibility for discrete tasks. The steering committee was also essential because all decisions for how to shape the programme were made within the group, referenced the values and goals set at the beginning of the project, and sought input and expertise from all participants. We believe that our experiences document the great potential for co-design research to address important community needs and create sustainable programmes.

Notes

1 See Malinin et al., 2023 for additional details about the program evaluation procedures and results.
2 Name changed to *Dementia Together* in 2021.

References

Bienvenu, B., & Hanna, G. (2017). Arts participation: Counterbalancing forces to the social stigma of a dementia diagnosis. *AMA Journal of Ethics*, *19*(7), 704–712. https://doi.org/10.1001/journalofethics.2017.19.7.msoc2-1707

Blackburn, E. H. (1991). Structure and function of telomeres. *Nature*, *350*(6319), 569–573.

Brenner, W., Uebernickel, F., & Abrell, T. (2016). Design thinking as mindset, process, and toolbox. In W. Brenner & F. Uebernickel (Eds.), *Design thinking for innovation* (pp. 3–21). Springer.

Brotons, M., & Marti, P. (2003). Music therapy with Alzheimer's patients and their family caregivers: A pilot project. *Journal of Music Therapy*, *40*(2), 138–150. https://doi.org/10.1093/jmt/40.2.138

Brown, T. (2008). Design thinking. *Harvard Business Review*, *86*(6), 84–95.

Carlgren, L., Rauth, I., & Elmquist, M. (2016). Framing design thinking: The concept in idea and enactment. *Creativity and Innovation Management*, *25*(1), 38–57. https://doi.org/10.1111/caim.12153

Conklin, Q., King, B., Zanesco, A., Pokorny, J., Hamidi, A., Lin, J., Epel, E., Blackburn, B., & Saron, C. (2015). Telomere lengthening after three weeks of an intensive meditation retreat. *Psychoneuroendocrinology*, *61*, 26–27. http://dx.doi.org/10.1016/j.psyneuen.2015.07.462

Cooper, C., Mukadam, N., Katona, C., Lyketsos, C. G., Ames, D., Rabins, P., & Livingston, G. (2012). Systematic review of the effectiveness of non-pharmacological interventions to improve quality of life of people with dementia. *International Psychogeriatrics*, *24*(6), 856–870.

Davalos, D. B., Luxton, I., Thaut, M., & Cross, J. E. (2019). B sharp-The cognitive effects of a community music program for people with dementia-related disorders. *Alzheimer's & Dementia: Translational Research & Clinical Interventions*, *5*, 592–596. https://doi.org/10.1016/j.trci.2019.08.004

Dschool. (2010). *An introduction to design thinking process guide*. Hasso Plattner Institute of Design, Stanford University. https://s3-eu-west-1.amazonaws.com/ih-materials/uploads/Introduction-to-design-thinking.pdf

Faw, M. H., Buley, T., & Malinin, L. H. (2021b). Being there: Exploring virtual symphonic experience as a salutogenic design intervention for age-related cognitive decline. *Frontiers in Psychology*. https://doi.org/10.3389/fpsyg.2021.541656

Faw, M. H., Cross, J., Luxton, I., & Davalos, D. (2021a). Surviving and thriving: Exploratory results from a multi-year, multidimensional intervention to promote well-being among caregivers of adults with dementia. *International Journal of Environmental Public Health*, *18*(9), 4755. https://doi.org/10.3390/ijerph18094755

Fields, B., Bruemmer, J., Gloeckner, G., & Wood, W. (2018). Influence of an equine-assisted activities program on dementia-specific quality of life. *American Journal of Alzheimer's Disease and Other Dementias*, *33*(5), 309–317. http://doi.org/10.1177/1533317518772052

Fields, B., Peters, B. C., Merritt, T., & Meyers, S. (2021). Advancing the science and practice of equine-assisted services through community-academic partnerships. *Human-Animal Interaction Bulletin*, *9*(2), 30–44.

Fields, B., Wood, W., & Lassell, R. (2019). Impact of a dementia-specific program of equine-assisted activities: Providers' perspectives. *Quality in Ageing and Older Adults*, *20*(2), 37–47. http://doi.org/10.1108/QAOA-10-2018-0047

GBD 2019 Dementia Forecasting Collaborators. (2022). Estimation of the global prevalence of dementia in 2019 and forecasted prevalence in 2050: An analysis for the global burden of disease study 2019. *The Lancet. Public Health, 7*(2), e105–e125. https://doi.org/10.1016/S2468-2667(21)00249-8

Giacomin, J. (2014). What is human centered design? *The Design Journal, 17*(4), 606–623. https://doi.org/10.2752/175630614X14056185480186

Gillis, K., Stifkens, K., Lahaye, H., & Van Bogaert, P. (2021). Developing an effective strategy to implement non-pharmaceutical interventions amongst residents with dementia in residential care facilities: Caregivers' perspectives. *Alzheimer's & Dementia, 17*, e053127. https://doi.org/10.1002/alz.053127

Griggs, A., Faw, M., & Malinin, L. H. (2020). The art of love: Using arts engagement as a promoter of relational maintenance in couples with dementia. In K. Afary & A. M. Fritz (Eds.), *Communication research on expressive arts and narrative as forms of healing: More than words*, (pp. 213-240). Lexington Books.

Johansson-Sköldberg, U., Woodilla, J., & Çetinkaya, M. (2013). Design thinking: Past, present and possible futures. *Creativity and Innovation Management, 22*(2), 121–146. https://doi.org/10.1111/caim.12023

Kurko, S. A., Darwin, M. L., Davalos, D. B., & Cross, J. E. (2018, April 16). *The association between physiological health and cognition in those with cognitive impairments*. Poster presented at the Celebrate Undergraduate Research and Creativity 2018, Colorado State University.

Lansdorp, P. M. (2000). Repair of telomeric DNA prior to replicative senescence. *Mechanisms of Ageing and Development, 118*, 23–34. https://doi.org/10.1016/S0047-6374(00)00151-2

Lassell, R., Fields, B., Busselman, S., Hempel, T., & Wood, W. (2019). A logic model of a dementia-specific program of equine-assisted activities. *Human-Animal Interaction Bulletin, 9*(2), 22–54. https://doi.org/10.1079/hai.2021.0022.

Lassell, R., Fields, B., Cross, J. E., & Wood, W. (2022). Dementia care partners' reported outcomes after adaptive riding: A theoretical thematic analysis. *Quality in Ageing and Older Adults*. http://doi.org/10.1108/QAOA-01-2022-0007

Lassell, R., Wood, W., Schmid, A. A., & Cross, J. E. (2021). A comparison of quality of life indicators during two complementary interventions: Adaptive gardening and adaptive riding for people with dementia. *Complementary Therapies in Medicine, 57*, 102658. http://doi.org/10.1016/J.CTIM.2020.102658

Lepp, M., Ringsberg, K. C., Holm, A.-K., & Sellersjo, G. (2003). Dementia - Involving patients and their caregivers in a drama programme: The caregivers' experiences. *Journal of Clinical Nursing, 12*(6), 873–881. https://doi.org/10.1046/j.1365-2702.2003.00801.x

Mabire, J. B., Gay, M. C., Charras, K., & Vernooij-Dassen, M. (2022). Impact of a psychosocial intervention on social interactions between people with dementia: An observational study in a nursing home. *Activities, Adaptation and Aging, 46*(1), 73–89. https://doi.org/10.1080/01924788.2021.1966574

Malinin, L. H., Faw, M., & Davalos, D. (2023). Performing arts as a non-pharmacological intervention for people with dementia and care-partners: A community case study. *Frontiers in Psychology, 14*, 1149711. https://doi.org/10.3389/fpsyg.2023.1149711

Moniz-Cook, E., Vernooij-Dassen, M., Woods, B., Orrell, M., & Network, I. (2011). Psychosocial interventions in dementia care research: The INTERDEM manifesto. *Aging and Mental Health, 15*(3), 283–290. https://doi.org/10.1080/13607863.2010.543665

Near, M, Schneider, B., Darwin, M., Davalos, D., & Cross, J. (2018, April). *Feasibility of the Fitbit in research involving people with dementia and mild cognitive impairment*. Poster presented at the Celebrate Undergraduate Research and Creativity Symposium, Fort Collins, CO.

Norman, D. A. (2005). Human-centered design considered harmful. *Interactions, 12*(4), 14–19.

Phoenix Symphony. (n.d.). *Phoenix Symphony education and community health and wellness programs*. The Phoenix Symphony. Retrieved May 14, 2022, from https://www.phoenixsymphony.org/education-and-community/health--wellness-programs

Randolph, C., Tierney, M. C., Mohr, E., & Chase, T. N. (1998). The Repeatable Battery for the Assessment of Neuropsychological Status (RBANS): Preliminary clinical validity. *Journal of Clinical and Experimental Neuropsychology, 20*(3), 310–319. https://doi.org/10.1076/jcen.20.3.310.823

Rinehardt, E., Duff, K., Schoenberg, M., Mattingly, M., Bharucha, K., & Scott, J. (2010). Cognitive change on the Repeatable Battery of Neuropsychological Status (RBANS) in Parkinson's disease with and without bilateral subthalamic nucleus deep brain stimulation surgery. *The Clinical Neuropsychologist, 26*(2), 370–371. https://doi.org/10.1080/13854046.2012.662797

Salvo, M. J. (2001). Ethics of engagement: User-centered design and rhetorical methodology. *Technical Communication Quarterly, 10*(3), 273–290. https://doi.org/10.1207/s15427625tcq1003_3

Sanders, E. B. N., & Stappers, P. J. (2008). Co-creation and the new landscapes of design. *Co-Design, 4*(1), 5–18. https://doi.org/10.1080/15710880701875068

Stites, S. D., Harkins, K., Rubright, J. D., & Karlawish, J. (2018). Relationships between cognitive complaints and quality of life in older adults with mild cognitive impairment, mild Alzheimer disease dementia, and normal cognition. *Alzheimer's Disease & Associated Disorders, 32*(4), 276–283. https://doi: 10.1097/WAD.0000000000000262

Thomas, J. M., & Sezgin, D. (2021). Effectiveness of reminiscence therapy in reducing agitation and depression and improving quality of life and cognition in long-term care residents with dementia: A systematic review and meta-analysis. *Geriatric Nursing, 42*(6), 1497–1506. https://doi.org/10.1016/j.gerinurse.2021.10.014

Walton, J., & Bartleet, B. L. (2021). *Health and wellbeing: An overview of current literature. [pdf] Commissioned by the Queensland Symphony Orchestra.* Creative Arts Research Institute, Griffith University. https://www.qso.com.au/uploads/QSO-Health-and-Wellbeing-Report.pdf

Wiegelmann, H., Speller, S., Verhaert, L. M., Schirra-Weirich, L., & Wolf-Ostermann, K. (2021). Psychosocial interventions to support the mental health of informal caregivers of persons living with dementia–a systematic literature review. *BMC Geriatrics, 21*(1), 1–17. https://doi.org/10.1186/s12877-021-02020-4

Wilhelm, L., & Wilhelm, K. (2020). Music-based interventions with informal caregivers of adult care recipients: An integrative review. *Music and Medicine, 12*(3), 177–187.

Xi, X., Li., C., Ren, R., Zhang, H., & Zhang, L. (2013). Telomere, aging and age-related disease. *Aging: Clinical and Experimental Research, 25*(2), 139–146. https://doi.org/10.1007/s40520-013-0021-1

Part 2
Design interventions

Introduction

Designing interventions to support mental health and wellbeing

Geke Ludden, Kristina Niedderer, Vjera Holthoff-Detto and Tom Dening

Setting the scene for Part 2

Designers have historically been interested in improving the world around them and the lives of the people in it. Consequently, their interest in designing for health and wellbeing is not new. In 1971, in his book Design for the Real World Victor Pananek wrote about how design should contribute to healthcare by designing better solutions for health and care (Papanek, 1971, pp. 138):

> *Surely blood pressure can be taken more easily and more comfortably for anxiety-prone patients. Urinalysis can be a gamble. One commonly used device works like a hydrometer, but because the scale inside the tube is printed on a piece of paper that is not firmly fixed, such readings are completely meaningless. (...) The discomfort, pain, and puzzlement of a small baby that is teething is really pathetic. After experiencing 4.5 million years of this (according to Robert Ardrey), we have developed one toy: a plastic tube filled with water that can be frozen. It gives the baby comfort for about five minutes, by which time it has warmed up and is therefore no longer soothing. Surely, we can do better than that.*

What is interesting about this quote is that Papanek clearly has the wellbeing of patients in mind. He criticises the suboptimal functionality of the products that are used pointing to the pain and discomfort they cause people. Since 1971, the role of design in changing care has increased significantly. Recent advances in the philosophy and organisation of care as well as related technological developments have expanded perspectives on care and broadened the possibilities to deliver more inclusive and humane solutions to promote wellbeing. Ongoing transitions in the organisation of care; moving care from the hospital to the home; and an increasing focus on preventative health and on self-management of patients add to the complexity of designing for health and wellbeing and promoting autonomy and responsibility of patients and people. Roles of patients, formal and informal carers change, as they are asked to adapt to evolving practices that involve new ways of doing things, new kinds of devices and services making use of new technologies. For designers in this domain, it means that they will work in and for increasingly complex situations that often involve multidisciplinary teams. While this is true for the complete healthcare domain, this also holds for the field that is the focus of this book: design for dementia, mental health and wellbeing. In many countries, people are ageing in place, this means that many people live at home with dementia and need appropriate care in this environment. In mental healthcare, we see a rise in people who suffer from psychological distress and need care and healthcare systems have to find new ways to accommodate this increase in demand.

The developments and transitions outlined above inevitably lead to a high demand for innovation. This part of the book has a specific focus on the design of interventions, where we define

DOI: 10.4324/9781003318262-12

interventions in a broad way in line with Simon (1996, p. 111) as anything that aims to change an existing state into a preferred one. Interventions can and will be complementing traditional approaches but can also change them. They can both support those living with dementia and mental illness as well as those offering support. They can therefore be processes and services but also new ways of working and tangible products (often devices using some form of technology) that can be used in these new ways of working. In line with the definition of health that Huber and colleagues (Huber et al., 2011) have proposed and that emphasises the ability to adapt and self-manage in the face of social, physical and emotional challenges, the chapters in this section show how the design of interventions for mental health and wellbeing covers all aspects of human life. Making sure that we can adapt to physical challenges by altering the places we inhabit, offering support in the interactions we have with other people (not in the least during moments of distress) and allowing for seamless interactions with the products and services that surround us.

In the Papanek quote above, he clearly describes with a variety of terms the (actual vs. the desired) user experience of products used in healthcare. Emphasising that in this domain both the experience of patients (and their family) and that of those caring for them is important. For designers, it comes natural to start from identifying people's needs, wants, wishes, dreams and aspirations, as we have also introduced in Chapter 1 of this book. In evaluating the outcomes of design processes, design researchers often put people's subjective experiences first, arguing that when a person is happy using a product it surely is successful. In contrast, in the healthcare domain evaluation is mostly about establishing effects on certain health-related (often objectively measured) outcome measures (Smits et al., 2022). Smits et al.'s (2022) review also found that in the fields of both design and healthcare, wellbeing is seen to encompass a broad range of factors until now, which has led to uncertainty on how to create wellbeing through design. Only the recent discussion of wellbeing by Niedderer et al. (2022) has attempted to integrate the different aspects of wellbeing into a holistic definition as elaborated on in the introduction to this volume. To further bridge the fields of design and health and to capitalise on the role of design in changing care, we need more thorough evaluations of design solutions that consider both the subjective experiences of people as well as effects on wellbeing. Health-related outcome measures will have to be used if an intervention will be used in clinical practice.

As the chapters in this section show, the field of design is taking on the challenge of evaluating design interventions to arrive at evidence-based design solutions. Both, in design processes that are increasingly value-based and in evaluation methods, the field is taking huge steps ahead.

Chapter overview in Part 2

The chapters in Part 2 of the book cover approaches and methodologies to designing for dementia, mental health and wellbeing as well as case studies introducing the development of innovative interventions. While the larger part of this section discusses design for dementia, it also discusses the wider area of mental health where innovative interventions aimed at (self-management of) individuals and at psychosocial interactions can be found. Together, the chapters cover a wide range of interventions, crossing the breadth of the design space and including design of environments, services and (digital) products.

The section starts off with a number of chapters showcasing and outlining research and practices in design for dementia. In Chapter 9, Paul Rogers discusses design for dementia from an overarching perspective as well as in detailed cases that reveal and compare best practices in the field. While arguing how the demand for effective health and social care services will continue to increase, he shows how design for dementia projects funded by the UK Research and Innovation body is contributing to making improvements to the lives of people with dementia and their carers. The chapter highlights just how many design-researchers are working in dementia-related contexts, including the LAUGH project as an example of a project that focuses on improving wellbeing for people in later stages of dementia. LAUGH and the HUG product that was developed from it is further described by Cathy Treadaway in Chapter 10. Treadaway discusses the importance of physical touch in dementia care and describes the design and implementation of HUG in dementia care environments. It also discusses how the Compassionate Design Methodology was used as the guiding principle behind developing HUG, outlining that loving kindness for the individual should be central when designing for people with cognitive impairment while incorporating sensory properties, connecting to others and personalisation are key guiding principles.

We move from a Western European to an Indian perspective on dementia care with the work of Vivek Kant and colleagues in Chapter 11. This chapter presents an example of the development of a digital health intervention, a mobile application for supporting dementia caregivers in Indian families. It shows how, in India, dementia is a social problem and how in this context a focus on creating awareness and support for informal caregivers is important. The design process took a multi-stakeholder perspective, including professionals, care providers and people with dementia and their families, both, in the design and evaluation phases.

Chapter 12 adds another part of the world: North America. In this chapter, Jodi Sturge describes and compares models for dementia villages in the Canadian and Dutch contexts, and how the original Dutch innovation was adopted and adapted for the Canadian context. It is an interesting comparison of how a relatively new dementia care model was implemented in two different countries, discussing what their differences might mean to the people who live there. Sturge calls for more evaluative studies into how such villages and the elements in them work to improve quality of life. Eventually, this is envisaged to lead to a set of evidence-based design principles for the implementation of the dementia village model.

In Chapter 13, Michael Craven contributes to this call for more evaluative approaches by summarising techniques and methods used in the Designing for People with Dementia (MinD) project. Craven discusses how these methods were developed and used with people with dementia. Mirroring the definition of wellbeing we have introduced in Chapter 1 (with its three components of emotional, social wellbeing and agency), the AIR model is introduced that describes Activities, Internal World of the Individual with dementia and Relationships. It can be used as a guiding principle for the design and evaluation of interventions, acknowledging that the three components of AIR are interrelated and there can be positive or negative influences on any and each of the components that can affect the whole system.

The next chapters consider how mindful design as an approach can be used in design for dementia and in the wider field of mental health. In Chapter 14, Niedderer and colleagues explore the integration of mindfulness theory and practices within design with the aim of embedding mindfulness in the lives of people with dementia. From their analysis of existing interventions, these researchers distil six categories of mindful design and a framework that can provide guidance for designers on how to use mindfulness in designing and evaluation. It can also assist people with dementia, carers and care professionals in choosing appropriate interventions to enhance wellbeing. For those designers who want to include (and evaluate) mindfulness in a design education context, Bosse and Wölfel add a further tool with their Mindful Design Evaluation Scale in Chapter 15. They also introduce the Visual Mindful Design cards, that are based on the constructs underlying the Mindful Design Evaluation Scale and that help adhere to Mindful design criteria during design processes. These tools can be valuable for designers in the wider field of mental health and wellbeing. Focusing on compassion as a value, Geke Ludden and her colleagues in the Compassionate Technology project elaborate on what it means to design for this value that is of utmost importance for (mental) healthcare. They discuss their explorations in this area in relation to other value-based design and design for compassion methods and approaches and describe a case of an innovate product that was designed to be part of a therapeutic journey and improve the compassionate interaction between client and care professional.

Finally, in Chapter 17, we travel all the way to Australia where the co-design work of Jordan McKibbin and colleagues is situated. Their work is again a good example of including the social component of care, focusing on multi-generational wellbeing. The chapter describes the development of an intergenerational play service that could counter social isolation and associated mental health problems for older adults. Using co-design sessions to inform the service design process led to a service that made use of existing public spaces while fostering local support networks.

Summary

This part of the book brings together perspectives on how to design for better mental health and wellbeing by connecting people across generations as well as to their (social) environment. It also shows more specific cases on design for dementia and design of (e-)mental health interventions for specific user groups. It does so by bringing together contributions from different parts of the world (from the Global North mostly but including Indian and Australian perspectives), thereby showing how important this topic is to people around the world while different contexts and cultures require different solutions. This does not stand in the way of learning from each other, but it requires being sensitive to the context in which insights and interventions are arrived at. In terms of the types of interventions, which the different chapters describe, we indeed see that interventions can be services and systems, analogue and digital products and environments. While many are advocating for digital health interventions as an emerging area where design can have a large role, the examples described here show that there needs to be a balance between providing tangible solutions as important elements in our physical environment (and in connection with our bodies) and making use of ICT innovation.

Importantly, many of the chapters transcend the cases that are discussed: (1) they show what methods and approaches can be used in the design processes that lead to interventions for dementia, mental health and wellbeing; (2) they elaborate on how co-design methods are a part of these processes; and (3) they discuss how we can and should evaluate the outcomes of such processes. We will elaborate on these three points here since they are of utmost importance to further the field.

When it comes to design processes, we see that many of the contributors to this part of the book have introduced frameworks, models and approaches that aim to clarify their work and make adoption by others easier. Some of the models seem to be very much connected. For example, looking at the Compassionate Design Methodology from Chapter 10 and the AIR model described in Chapter 13, we see that both introduce connecting to others (Relationships in AIR) as important for people with dementia as well as paying attention to the inner world of the person (personalisation). Furthermore, compassion as an underlying value in mental healthcare is discussed in Chapter 10 as well as in Chapter 16, each discussing design for compassion approaches. It is good that while we bring these chapters together, we also reflect on the use of similar constructs to see if we come to common understandings in designing for mental health and wellbeing.

Further, when it comes to using co-design methods as part of the design process, we see that co-design of interventions is common practice, at least for the contributors to this section. What is striking is the difference in scale of co-design projects, the field has yet to find a golden standard for when and how many people to involve in developing interventions.

On the point of evaluation of outcomes of design processes, the chapters in this part show that design researchers are taking steps but there is also still work to do. To be of value in changing care for the better, designers could adopt more thorough evaluation practices. This doesn't necessarily mean that we should run randomised controlled trials for every intervention. However, it does mean that we should be clear about what we evaluate and that we use and develop evaluation methods that are recognised within the field of application. In Chapter 13, Michael Craven adequately describes how a range of methods for evaluation can be used in design for health and wellbeing while also showing how co-design can be a part of the evaluation phase of design processes. In Chapter 15, Bosse and Wölfel add to the evaluation methods, outlining the development of their Mindful Design Evaluation Scale, while Ludden et al explain how they are developing a Compassionate Technology scale in Chapter 16. All offer examples of evaluation tools that can be used to measuring people's subjective experiences with some objectivity.

References

Huber, M., Knottnerus, J. A., Green, L., van der Horst, H., Jadad, A. R., Kromhout, D., et al. (2011). How should we define health? *BMJ, 343*, d4163. https://doi.org/10.1136/bmj.d4163

Niedderer, K., Holthoff-Detto, V., van Rompay, T. J. L., Karahanoğlu, A., Ludden, G. D. S., Almeida, R., Losada Durán, R., Bueno Aguado, Y., Lim, J.N.W., Smith, T., et al. (2022). This is me: Evaluation of a board game to promote social engagement, wellbeing and agency in people with dementia through mindful life-storytelling. *Journal of Aging Studies, 60*. https://doi.org/10.1016/j.jaging.2021.100995

Papanek, V. (1971). *Design for the real world: Human ecology and social change*. Random House.

Simon, H. A. (1996). *The sciences of the artificial* (3rd ed.). MIT.

Smits, M., Kim, C., van Goor, H., & Ludden, G. (2022). From digital health to digital well-being: Systematic scoping review. *Journal of Medical Internet Research, 24*(4), e33787. https://doi.org/10.2196/33787

9 Designing for dementia

Examining design-led approaches and innovations

Paul A. Rodgers

Introduction

Dementia is the umbrella term used to describe the symptoms that occur when the brain is affected by a number of conditions, most commonly Alzheimer's disease. Currently there is no cure for the 130+ kinds of dementia. The illness has a profound impact on society and those directly affected by it. Symptoms of dementia include loss of memory, mood changes communication problems, and people affected will typically experience a decline in the ability to talk, read and write. Dementia is progressive, meaning that the symptoms will gradually get worse. A person in the later stages of dementia will have problems carrying out everyday tasks of daily living and will become increasingly dependent on other people.

The massive scale of the challenges surrounding dementia and how we best care for people affected by it is illustrated in the fact that someone in the world develops dementia every three seconds. This means there are over 50 million people worldwide living with dementia today and this number is predicted to double every 20 years, reaching 82 million in 2030 and 152 million in 2050. The estimated worldwide cost of dementia is $818 billion US dollars, which represents 1.09% of global Gross Domestic Product (GDP). This figure includes costs attributed to informal care (unpaid care provided by family members and friends), direct costs of social care (provided by community care professionals and in residential home settings), and the direct costs of medical care (the costs of treating dementia and other conditions in primary and secondary care). If dementia were a country, it would be the world's 18th largest economy.[1]

In the UK, there are around 850,000 people living with dementia and this number is projected to rise to 1.6 million by 2040. The total cost of care for people with dementia in the UK is £34.7billion. This is set to rise sharply over the next two decades, to £94.1billion by 2040. In addition to these startling figures, a further 700,000 people act as 'informal carers'" in the UK (Alzheimer's Research UK,2015). Informal carers in the UK are unpaid, untrained and often have no formal networks of support. Informal carers shore up significant gaps in health and social care services. In the complex system of dementia care and support, the contributions of these informal carers are often overlooked. Unpaid carers supporting someone with dementia save the UK economy £13.9 billion a year, with two-thirds of the cost of dementia being paid by people living with dementia and their families.

The emotional impact of caring, however, can be even more debilitating. Informal carers regularly speak of social isolation and marginalisation and of being unable to pursue activities that were once integral to them and gave their lives meaning. As a result, the psychological impact of dementia cannot be overstated. Dementia erases significant elements of a person's being, which contributes to an ongoing sense of grief without closure or 'ambiguous loss' (Boss & Yeats, 2014) that can affect carers as much as those diagnosed with the condition.

DOI: 10.4324/9781003318262-13

It is clear then that the demand for effective health and social care services will continue to increase into the future. Responding to these challenges will require innovative ways of supporting people with dementia to live well from the early stages of their diagnosis. People will need highly effective forms of support from the point of diagnosis to come to terms with this life-altering event to ensure that they remain connected to their community and are able to live well. This chapter will examine design-led responses by showcasing a range of creative design interventions (e.g. products, spaces and services) that have been developed to challenge well-formed attitudes and opinions, commonly-held beliefs and ways of thinking and acting in the health and social care of people living with dementia. The chapter will also shine a strong light on how contemporary design thinking, making and doing are at the forefront of imagining future visions of dementia health and social care across a range of design disciplines including product design, service design, architecture, textile design, interaction design and graphic design.

Design's response

In recent years, design researchers have undertaken a wide range of projects with aims such as developing new products, services, strategies and environments that will enhance the health and wellbeing of people living with dementia, their carers and caregivers. In these projects, design researchers have focused on creating environments, objects and technologies to support person-centred dementia care. As some of the chapters in the first part of this book show, many design research projects use interdisciplinary co-design methods and tools to establish new knowledge and to develop user-centred design interventions to improve quality of life for people living with dementia and their family members.' These designed interventions look to promote individuals' abilities in three key areas:

1. Cognitive ability: improved by promoting the use of familiar and recognisable surroundings and activities that respond to individuals' deepest and earliest memories.
2. Social ability: addressed through the design of artefacts and services that create opportunities for individuals and caregivers to interact more easily in activities of daily living.
3. Physical ability: promoted through design which unobtrusively compensates for disabilities such as mobility and vision, which are prevalent amongst people living with dementia.

(Timlin & Rysenbry, 2010)

This chapter examines the diverse approaches and innovations of over 10,000 UK Research and Innovation[2] funded projects via Gateway to Research,[3] the repository of publicly funded research and innovation in the UK. This search was carried out to locate and identify information about publicly funded design and dementia research projects in the UK. The search, which focused on design and dementia projects, shows that five of the seven UKRI funding councils have funded this research over the time period 2015 to 2025 (Figure 9.1).

From Figure 9.1 we can see that almost three quarters of the design and dementia projects funded in the UK since 2015 have been funded by the Medical Research Council (MRC) and the Economic and Social Research Council (ESRC). The ESRC is the UK's largest organisation for funding research on economic and social issues. The ESRC supports research which has an impact on business, the public sector and civil society. They have an annual budget of around £202 million and they support around 4,000 researchers in academic institutions and independent research institutes at any one time. The MRC funds research at the forefront of science to prevent illness, develop therapies and improve human health. The MRC supports research across the biomedical spectrum, from fundamental lab-based science to clinical trials,

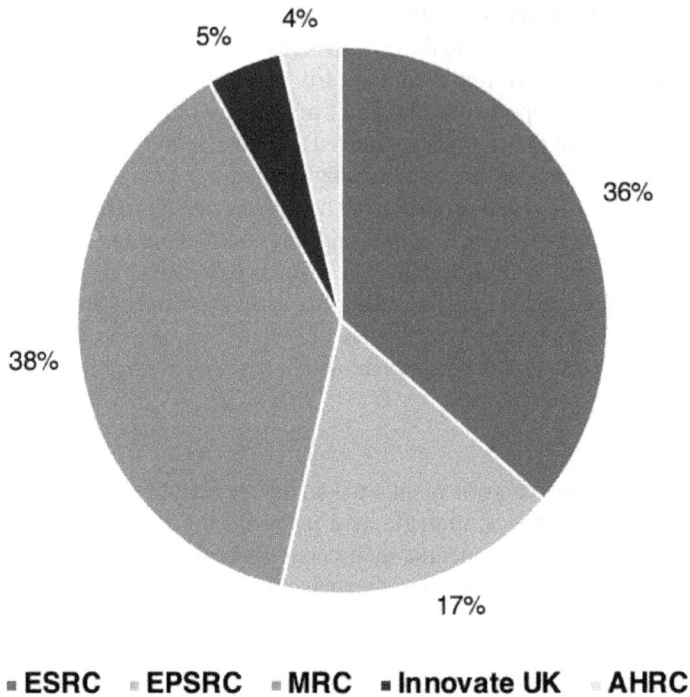

Figure 9.1 Design and dementia projects by funding council

and in all major disease areas. Working closely with the National Health Service (NHS) and UK health departments, the MRC supports research that is likely to make a real difference to clinical practice and the health of the population. In 2017/18 the MRC's research expenditure was £814 million. The other funders who have supported design and dementia research projects in the UK during this time period are the Engineering and Physical Sciences Research Council (EPSRC) (who support research to benefit society and the economy), the Arts and Humanities Research Council (AHRC) (who support research in subjects from philosophy and the creative industries, to art conservation and product design to address some of society's biggest challenges, such as tackling modern slavery, exploring the ethical implications of artificial intelligence and understanding what it is to be human) and Innovate UK (who support business-led innovation through the development and commercialisation of new products, processes and services).

Figure 9.2 shows the distribution of funded design and dementia projects across UK universities. Here, we can see that University College London (UCL) has attracted the highest number of funded projects than any other university in the UK. The majority of these projects are based in UCL departments such as psychiatry, neurology, behavioural sciences and epidemiology and public health dealing with issues such as empowering better end-of-life dementia care, the impact of multicomponent support groups for those living with rare dementias and lifestyle factors (i.e. sleep and physical activity) in dementia and cognitive impairment in England and China. The University of Edinburgh, Imperial College London and University of Manchester come next for the highest number of funded projects. In terms of more design-related research, projects such as 'navigating everyday adaptations, equipment and technology at home for people with dementia: a focussed design ethnography' (University of Manchester), 'interaction,

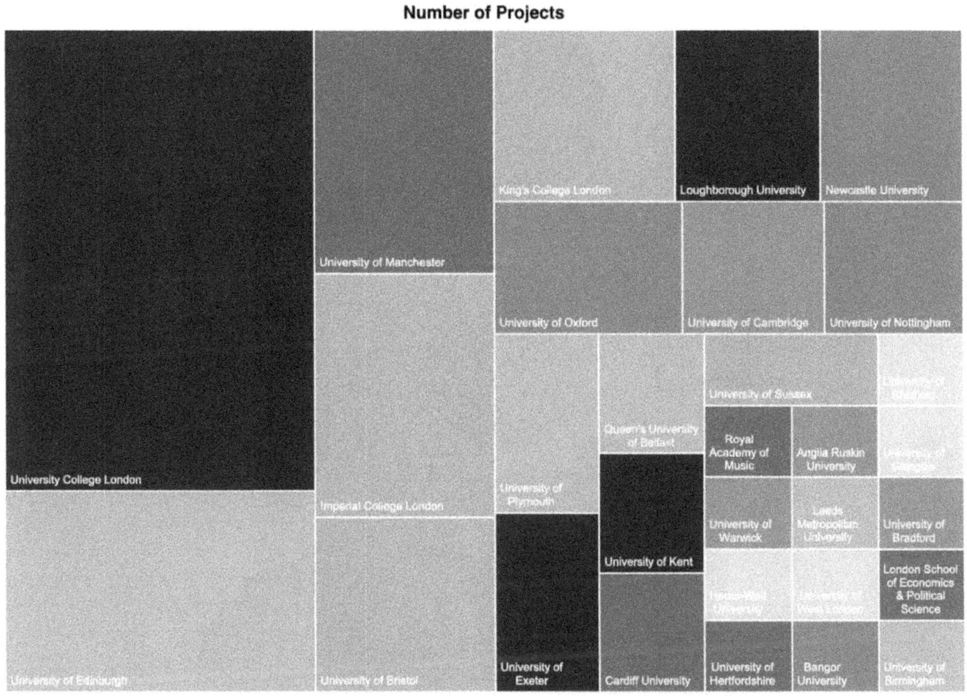

Number of Projects

Figure 9.2 Number of design and dementia projects by UK university

dementia and engagement in arts for lifelong learning' (Newcastle University) and 'dementia and the art of caring: new opportunities for creative practitioners in the ageing economy' (Queen's University of Belfast) can be found.

Figure 9.3 shows the distribution of funded design and dementia projects across the UKRI's UK regions. Here, we can see that London (31 projects) and Scotland (12 projects) make up almost 40% of all UKRI-funded design and dementia projects in the UK between 2015 and 2025.

Figure 9.4 illustrates the wide-ranging number of disciplines that are involved in design and dementia research in the UK. Over 20 university departments, including subject areas and disciplines ranging from arts and humanities to aerospace engineering, psychiatry to sociology and social policy and neurology to law, are represented. This research covers wide-ranging subjects that cover virtual reality for cognitive evaluation of dementia, real-time radio remixing for people with mild to moderate dementia who live alone, and legal decision-making processes in dementia.

In terms of the focus of the design and dementia projects funded over the period 2015 to 2025, we can see in Figure 9.5 a selection of the design and dementia projects (title), the aim of each project (Theme 1), the methods or approach used (Theme 2) and the key outcomes (Theme 3). The design and dementia projects were analysed taking a content analysis approach (Crowley & Delfico, 1996), which was chosen because of its ability to process large amounts of data with relative ease in a systematic manner. Content analysis is a useful research tool used to determine the presence of certain words, themes or concepts within qualitative data (i.e. text). Content analysis allows researchers to quantify and analyse the presence, meanings and relationships of words, themes or concepts.

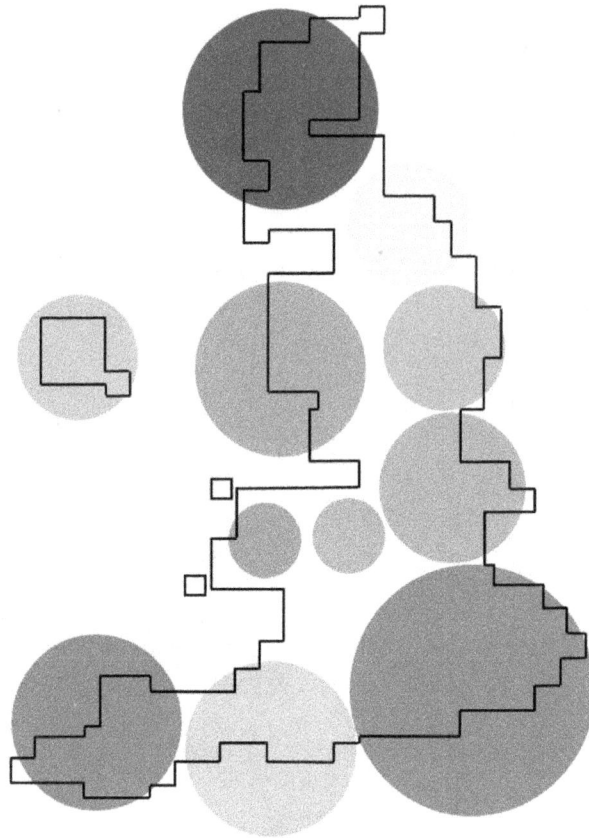

Figure 9.3 Number of design and dementia projects by UK region (larger dots represent higher number of projects)

For example, the key aim of the first project was related to navigating everyday adaptations via a focused design ethnography with a view to designing and developing 'better' technologies/ equipment. From Figure 9.5, a range of clear patterns emerge that cover the aim of each project, the methods or approach used in each project and the key outcomes of each project (Table 9.1).

Patterns that emerge amongst the aims of these design and dementia projects include work that seeks to adapt everyday home equipment and technology for people with dementia, socially assistive robots for rehabilitation, programmes/services that empower better end-of-life dementia care, physical activity to promote social connectivity and wellbeing in older adults living with dementia, understanding the eating and drinking experiences of people living with dementia in care homes and investigating the implementation, take-up and use of an online personalised platform for those who care for people with dementia.

In terms of the methods used, we can see that there is a wide range of both qualitative and quantitative research approaches and tools used such as ethnography (Lariviere, 2018), experimental methods (Bramble et al., 2011), computational modelling, conversational analysis, mixed methods (Windle et al., 2016), interviews (Samsi Manthorpe, 2020), creative practice including design-led research (Rodgers, 2022), empirical investigations, arts-based methods and feasibility studies.

Design and Dementia Projects by Department

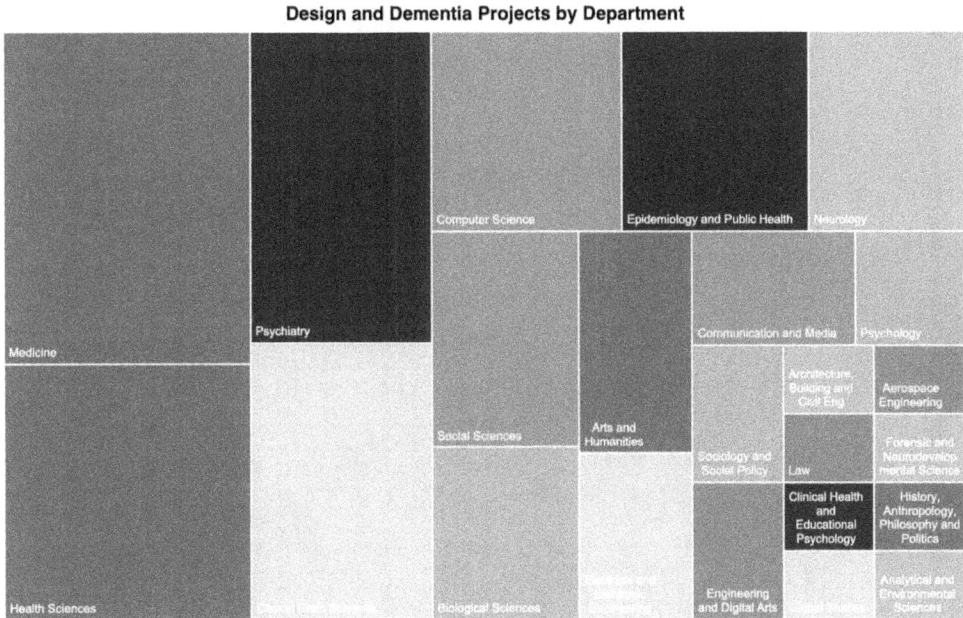

Figure 9.4 Design and dementia projects by department

The outcomes of these selected design and dementia projects include quotidian equipment and technology for domestic dwellings such as air-quality adaptations for people living with dementia, socially assistive robots for dementia rehabilitation, communication technologies for dementia-inclusive communities, peer-to-peer mentorship programmes, multisensory culture boxes to support the health and wellbeing of people living with dementia in care homes, toolkits to improve access and diagnosis of dementia, computational modelling of care needs, music interventions, personalised VR experiences and off-the-shelf AI-based voice technologies (e.g. Amazon Echo, Google Home) for formal and informal carers.

Design and dementia projects: disciplines, aims and results

Up to this point, this chapter has dealt with design-led dementia projects that have been funded in the UK. The paper now moves from solely UK-based work on designing for dementia to a view on work from all over the world. As such, the next part of this chapter will focus in greater detail on 18 design-led projects from design researchers based all over the world describing original work that highlights the significant aims, results and outputs that design-led research projects are delivering in dementia health and social care contexts. The 18 design-led projects include pioneering work from design researchers based in the UK, Germany, the Netherlands, Belgium, Australia, Canada, Mexico and Brazil spanning a range of design and other disciplines including product design, textile design, interaction design, graphic design, music, psychology, human-computer interaction (HCI) and the social sciences (Table 9.2). These 18 contemporary design-led projects, detailed in the recent book *Design for People Living with Dementia* (Rodgers, 2022), show how design thought and action are contributing to addressing stigma surrounding dementia, helping to overcome isolation, raising greater awareness and understanding

#	Project Title	Theme 1 - Aim	Theme 2 - Method(s) / Approach	Theme 3 - Key Outcome(s)
1	Navigating everyday adaptations, equipment and technology at home for people with dementia: A focussed design ethnography	adaptations	ethnography	technology, equipment
2				
3	Air quality home adaptations for people living with Dementia.	adaptations		better air quality
4	Socially Assistive Robots and Sensory Feedback for MCI/Dementia Rehabilitation	rehabilitation		robots
5	Empowering Better End of life Dementia Care (EMBED-Care Programme)	empower		better end of life care
6	Coherent ultra-wideband radar for biosensing in dementia	biosensing		radar
7	Imaging early blood-brain barrier dysfunction in dementia	imaging		
8	Deep and Frequent Phenotyping: combinatorial biomarkers for dementia experimental medicine	phenotyping	experimental	biomarkers
9	Virtual Reality for Cognitive and Psychomotor Evaluation of Dementia	evaluation		VR
10	Music in Mind Remote - award winning dementia music therapy programme	music therapy		music
11	Robotics to enhance independence & safety for dementia patients in the home	independence and safety		robots
12	Examining low and high communication technologies for dementia-inclusive community programming	communication		technologies
13	The Contribution of Physical Activity to Social Connectivity and Wellbeing in Older Adults Living with Dementia	social connectivity and wellbeing	physical activity	
14	Co-Developing a Peer-to-Peer Mentorship Program (P2MP) for People Living with Dementia	mentorship		peer/peer programme
15	iPAD - Defining measures of proximity to symptom onset in the GENetic Frontotemporal dementia Initiative	proximity measures		measures of proximity
16	Establishing computational behavioural models for the detection of early dementia from speech	detection	computational modelling	computer models
17	The impact of multicomponent support groups for those living with rare dementias	support		support groups
18	Understanding the eating and drinking experiences of people living with dementia and dysphagia in care homes from multiple perspectives.	eating and drinking experiences		greater understanding
19	Lifestyle Factors in Dementia and Cognitive Impairment in England and China: The Role of Sleep and Physical Activity	lifestyle factors	physical activity	
20	The APPLE Tree programme: Active Prevention in People at risk of dementia through Lifestyle, Behaviour change and Technology to build RESilIEnce	build resilience		technologies
21	Using multisensory culture boxes to promote public health guidance and to support the wellbeing of people with dementia in care homes.	support		multisensory culture boxes
	Development and evaluation of a toolkit to improve access and diagnosis in memory services for British Urdu speaking population	improve access and diagnosis		toolkit to improve access and diagnosis
22				
23	DETERMIND: DETERMinants of quality of life, care and costs, and consequences of INequalities in people with Dementia and their family carers	quality of life		care
24	Identifying and mitigating the individual and dyadic impact of COVID19 and life under physical distancing on people with dementia and carers (INCLUDE)	mitigating		
25	Prevention of dementia by targeting risk factors	prevention		
26	Assisted Living for People with Dementia	assisted living		
27	Supporting the impact of dementia in rural Wales	support		
28	Legal Decision-Making in Dementia: A Conversation Analytic Study	legal decision making	conversational analysis	
29	Negotiating Changes in Friendships in the Context of Dementia	Negotiating Changes in Friendships		
30	Modelling dementia progression based on machine learning and simulations	modelling dementia progression	machine learning	simulations
31	Computational modelling of care needs in the rare dementias	care	computational modelling	computer models
32	Predicting post-stroke dementia from CT neuroimaging and other biomarkers	predicting		biomarkers
33	Acoustic signal processing applications for the support of dementia sufferers	support	acoustic signal processing	
34	Interaction, Dementia and Engagement in Arts for Lifelong Learning (IDEAL)	engagement and interaction		arts
35	Modelling dementia progression based on machine learning and simulations	modelling dementia progression	machine learning	simulations
36	Cognitive Stimulation Therapy (CST) for dementia: International implementation in Brazil, India and Tanzania (CST-International)	implementation	cognitive stimulation therapy	
37	How does specialist dementia nursing work? A mixed methods study of UK Admiral Nursing	nursing	mixed methods	
38	Investigating kinship care in dementia: an ethnography of families in Andalucia	kinship care	ethnography	
39	Sharing the diagnosis of dementia in the post-Covid clinic: patient and practitioner perspectives	sharing	interviews	
40	Music Interventions for Dementia and Depression in ELderly care: International cluster-randomised trial (MIDDEL)	depression		music interventions
41	Personalised VR experience for patients with dementia within a secure psychiatric setting	personalisation		personalised VR experiences
42	Advanced signal processing and MRI to assess cerebrovascular health in small vessel disease and dementia	assessing	Advanced signal processing	
43	Managing selfhood in dementia: Interrogating the operationalisation of identity work & its relationship with media representations.	managing selfhood		
44	Dementia and the Art of Caring: New Opportunities for Creative Practitioners in the Ageing Economy	care	creative practice	sharing stories
45	Exploring and supporting everyday life with a rare dementia - understanding symptoms, developing strategies and sharing stories	support		
46	The role of sleep in protecting against amyloid and glial pathology in dementia	lifestyle factors		
47	Managing Selfhood in Dementia: Interrogating the operationalisation of identity work in the context of aging, environment and lifestyle	managing selfhood		
48	Linking genetic, epidemiology and metabolic phenotyping in dementia in the context of aging, environment and lifestyle	lifestyle		
49	Semi-automated personalised VR experience for patients with dementia in a secure psychiatric setting	personalisation	VR	personalised VR experiences
50	Natural Language Processing based Knowledge Base and Chatbot for People with Dementia and Caregivers	communication	computational modelling	Robots
51	The persistence, causes, and consequences of sleep disturbances in people with dementia living in care homes	lifestyle factors		
52	Is 'elderspeak' always inappropriate? An empirical investigation of the use of elderspeak in dementia care	communication	empirical investigation	
53	Understanding the linguistic, pragmatic and relational determinants of effective communication in dementia care in Wales.	communication		
54	PREADAPT: Identification of personalised inflammatory profiles of aging and senescence which are modified specifically by risk factors of dementia	personalisation		
55	Social and Psychological factors Affecting primary Care planning Effectiveness for people with dementia and other long term conditions.	care		
56	The Arts and Dementia: how might the arts contribute to the creation of more inclusive ageing societies?	inclusivity	arts	greater inclusion
57	Counselling People with Dementia: a feasibility study investigating the potential for accessible therapy delivered through a social enterprise model	counselling	feasibility study	
58	A qualitative study into the care & support experiences of individuals from African Caribbean backgrounds with diagnosis of dementia, living in Wales	care	qualitative study	accessible therapy

Figure 9.5 Selection of design and dementia projects content analysis process

Table 9.1 Selection of design and dementia project themes (aims, methods, outcomes)

Theme 1: Project aim(s)	Theme 2: Methods used	Theme 3: Key outcome(s)
Adaptations	Ethnography	Home equipment
Lifestyle factors	Experimental	Socially assistive robots
Rehabilitation	Computational	Communication technologies
Support	Conversational analysis	Mentorship programmes
Care	Mixed methods	Multisensory culture boxes
Communication	Interviews	Toolkits
Personalisation	Design-led methods	Computational modelling
Engagement	Empirical methods	Music interventions
Empower	Feasibility studies	Personalised VR experiences

of the positive contributions people living with dementia can bring to society while challenging some of the most commonly held assumptions in dementia health and social care.

There are different types of dementia, but all have a similar effect on the individual affected. In the majority of cases, the progression of dementia is slow and changes manifest themselves over time. However, the progress of dementia can be simplified into three stages, namely early, mid and late, although it can be difficult to pinpoint with accuracy where one stage begins and ends. Figure 9.6 shows these 18 design research projects and highlights the stages of dementia where each of the designed interventions is intended to be used. Here, we can see that the majority of the 18 design-led projects focus on the early and mid (moderate) stages of dementia with only a couple dedicated to the later or more advanced stages of dementia.

In the early stages of dementia, a person will slowly develop changes in their abilities and behaviour. They may not be vocal about problems and will often cover up gaps or lapses in memory. As such, the onset of dementia can be difficult to pinpoint. Very often, it is only diagnosed retrospectively, and recognition that someone is in the early stages of dementia can be challenging. An early indicator is difficulty in remembering recent events. Care for a person at this stage should be supportive to allow them to retain their independence and connections to their family and friends. In this vein, Robertson et al.'s (2022) *Interactive Textiles for Well-being in Dementia-friendly Communities* brings people living with dementia together and has led to individuals offering each other help, encouragement and support that has ultimately created a safe space for them to discuss dementia and the new challenges facing them. Winton and Rodgers' (2022) *Designed with DeMEntia* work rejects commonly held assumptions and preconceived ideas about what people living with dementia are capable of and instead highlights positive aspects such as their ability to learn new things, develop new knowledge and skills and participate in new creative ventures, including the design of new projects, products and events. On a slightly different tack, Brankaert and den Ouden (2022) suggest that 'warm technology' offers an alternative way of supporting people living with dementia in an era of diminishing health and social care resources. Their work presents nine factors that can benefit designers when developing products and services for people living with dementia. Similarly, Wilkinson and Hendriks' (2022) work focuses on 'designing for one' that concentrates on an individual's capabilities, wishes and interests. In their work, they have developed a list of 12 factors that influence empathetic relationships between a designer and a person living with dementia that forms the basis of a hyper-personalised 'designing for one' co-design approach.

Independence is the focus of Beh et al.'s (2022) work that looks at how technology (virtual assistants) can help people living with dementia live independently at home for longer. Their work found that using non-stigmatising technology created a balance between assistance when it is timely and assistance when it is requested, leading to a greater feeling of independence

Table 9.2 18 Design-led projects, disciplines, aims and results

Design project	Aim(s)	Results/outputs
Interactive Textiles (Robertson et al.)	Greater wellbeing; Social connectivity; Creativity; New relationships/experiences	Interactive textiles; Positive emotions and engagement; Enhanced relationships; Safe space
Textile Memories (Danckwerth)	Greater participation; equal involvement; greater carer involvement	Wearable technologies (enhancements); More equal involvement; Greater involvement of relatives/carers
Designed with DeMEntia (Winton & Rodgers)	Challenge preconceived ideas; Highlight creative potential of PLWD; Unlock latent skills	PLWD learn new skills, Develop new knowledge; Participate in creative ventures; Public design exhibitions
Technology and Design (Brankaert & den Ouden)	A more person-centred and inclusive design process; Discover which 'design aspects' are important when designing technology for people living with dementia	Nine factors that can benefit design for PLWD in two categories – (i) 'artefact aspects' and (ii) 'functional aspects'
Nurturing Experiences (Treadaway)	Give pleasure and improve PLWDs' quality of life; Promote greater opportunities for playful experiences and nurturing activities in dementia health and social care	Award-winning HUG by LAUGH product; An academic research concept, through testing, development and into the market
Designing for One (Wilkinson & Hendriks)	Greater reciprocity; Mutual benefits for both designers and PLWD	12 factors that influence empathetic relationships between a designer and PLWD that form a hyper-personalised 'desiQninQfor one' co-design approach
Dementia Architecture (van Buuren, van Del)	A 'research through design' approach in their designing of typological floor plans of inpatient residential health care facilities for people living with dementia	A design workshop that produced a typological floor plan for an inpatient residential health care facility for PLWD in the Netherlands that offers greater social cohesion
Virtual Assistants (Beh et al.)	To explore the usefulness of technology in supporting the everyday activities of PLWD; To support PLWD with self-management	Virtual assistants that lead to greater independence, enhanced enjoyment and increased confidence for PLWD
Caregiving Relative (Schreiber & Curlis)	To simplify and improve everyday life in a domestic environment for PLWD: Address issues using participatory design methods to empower PLWD	A number of "Dementia Things"– which can be either tangible products or take the form of a new service or social practice
Paradise Room (Jakob)	To inform and support carers, care-home staff and healthcare practitioners on how to install a multi-sensory space that will improve the quality of care of PLWD	The first-ever guidebook advising on the design of sensory rooms for PLWD; Key design principles to foster a more holistic approach when designing with PLWD
Parlours of Wonder (Manchester & Rumble)	Inclusive spaces that emphasise rights, dignity, consistency and thoughtfulness in institutions of care where PLWD are welcome and feel involved	Designing a new 'space' in a care setting working closely alongside care staff to disrupt current assemblages of care in their care home settings
Social Change through the Curriculum	Bring together design students and PLWD in care homes to co-design and co-write publications focused on their life experiences	The 'Perspectives Program' builds effective relationships and intergenerational exchange between PLWD and design students through publication of their life stories

(Continued)

Table 9.2 (Continued)

Design project	Aim(s)	Results/outputs
Dementia Services (Carey)	To better understand the hidden experiences of caring for PLWD	Visualisations (Carer Maps) of the carers' individual experiences and the relationships between the public services they encountered along the way
Trigger Memories (Maya Rivero)	A light-hearted approach to reminiscence therapy helping caregivers recreate historical periods by dressing up with fashion and clothing of 1950s Mexico.	Designed reminiscence material such as clothing, household appliances, beauty products, furniture, aromas, music and movies from the past for PLWD
Dementia Rehabilitation (Aride & Couto)	Form new domains of collective creativity and provide a good quality of life and resilience to PLWD	Two designed outcomes – (i) multi-functional magnetised modules and (ii) living mandala used for occupational therapy and yOga classes respectively
MemoryBox (Nayer & Nayer)	To address social isolation, loneliness and boredom amongst PLWD	"MemoryBox" - a personalised media intervention that provides pre-recorded video messages from family members, photographs, videos and music for PLWD
Shared Tablet Interactions (Favilla *et al.*)	To create a range of two-person (dyad) tablet interactions bundled as apps to support 'better visits' for family members and carers for PLWO	The tablet application (app) promotes enriched social interactions, moments of insight, opportunities for conversations, reminiscence and enjoyment for PLWO
Everyday Sounds (Campbell et al.)	Help family members to connect through conversations and discover things about each other through engaging in collective storytelling and reminiscing	Recorded sounds for stimulating memories and conversation between PLWD and their informal (family) carers in their homes

Early	Mid	Late
Interactive Textiles (Robertson *et al)*		
Textile Memories (Danckwerth)		
Designed with DeMEntia (Winton & Rodgers)		
Technology and Design (Brankaert & den Ouden)		
		Nurturing Experiences (Treadaway)
Designing for One (Wilkinson & Hendriks)		
Dementia Architecture (van Buuren, van Delden & Mohammadi)		
Virtual Assistants (Beh *et al)*		
Caregiving Relative (Schreiber & Cürlis)		
Paradise Room (Jakob)		
Parlours of Wonder (Manchester & Rumble)		
Social Change through the Curriculum (Hannan et al)		
Dementia Services (Carey)		
Trigger Memories (Maya Rivero)		
Dementia Rehabilitation (Aride & Couto)		
MemoryBox (Nayer & Nayer)		
	Shared Tablet Interactions (Favilla *et al)*	
Everyday Sounds (Campbell *et al)*		

Figure 9.6 Eighteen designed interventions and the three progressive stages of dementia

for people living with dementia. Schreiber and Cürlis' (2022) interdisciplinary design project, *Dementia Things*, developed a series of generative tools to spark the imagination, invite personal and emotional reflection and encourage speculation and dreams in domestic settings for people living with dementia and their family members. Designing and making collaboratively features in a lot of early-stage dementia work, and this is true in Hannan et al.'s (2022) *Perspectives Program* that brings together design students and people living with dementia in care homes to co-design and co-write publications focused on their life experiences, and the collective reading of these stories. Carey's work (2022), which included several years' research undertaken in collaboration with *Newcastle Carers*, highlights different individual aspects of dementia care, illustrating that no single 'user pathway' exists in health and social care and that carers experience particular issues with finance, stress, bewilderment and guilt, and these are always in different guises and permutations.

In the mid (moderate) stages of dementia, an individual will experience memory lapses and confusion may become more obvious. Short-term memory becomes impaired and the person living with dementia will often ask many repetitive questions. They may also be anxious about when events are happening, become more forgetful and develop difficulties in finding words or remembering names. It is common in the mid stages of dementia that the person living with dementia will fail to recognise some people or confuse someone known to them with someone else. During this stage, a major challenge facing people living with dementia, their family members and carers is managing everyday life. A person living with dementia may need frequent reminders about appointments or how to complete basic everyday tasks. Gradually, the tasks of daily living will begin to become more difficult, and they may need help or encouragement with eating, dressing or going to the toilet. A person living with dementia may become more socially withdrawn and less comfortable in group situations, which may ultimately lead to them becoming more socially isolated. In the mid stages of dementia, the person can become more confused about where they are and wander off and become lost. In some situations, this can present a real risk to the person living with dementia and those around them, such as forgetting to light the gas on a stove, trying to drive or leaving an iron on. Therefore, the level of care a person requires at this stage of living with dementia increases. Danckwerth's (2022) work on 'wearable enhancements' (WE) highlights the importance of adaptation in order not to overstrain people living with dementia. Adaptation in an architectural context is highlighted in van Buuren et al.'s (2022) work that has resulted in floor plans for residential health care facilities for people living with dementia in the Netherlands that offer greater social safety, shared, common and private spaces and a wider sense of community. How a care home might offer greater sensory qualities to improve residents' experiences, support their abilities and individual needs, as well as assist the daily work of care practitioners, provides the focus for Jakob's (2022) work. This topic is continued in Manchester and Rumble's (2022) *Parlours of Wonder* work that designs inclusive spaces where people living with dementia are welcome and feel involved alongside more cognitively able older people, care workers, volunteers and children and teachers from local primary schools. Their work foregrounds rights, dignity, consistency and thoughtfulness in planning and running institutions of care and activities within them.

Taking a global perspective, Maya Rivero's *Trigger Memories* (2022) describes work based in Mexican care centres for people living with dementia where staff designed and developed a suite of reminiscence material, adopting a light-hearted approach to reminiscence therapy, that included information about local textiles, clothing, radio, television, beauty supplies, flavours, aromas, music and movies from the past. Likewise, Aride and Couto's work (2022), based on a 14-month field study conducted at the Centro de Atividades Bem Viver nursing home in Brazil, established new forms of collective creativity to stimulate the cognitive, motor, behavioural and social skills of people living with dementia so that they could experience holistic and integrated care with respect to their singularities and complexities. Addressing the issue of social isolation, loneliness and boredom amongst people living with dementia in Melbourne, Australia, Nayer and Nayer (2022) developed *MemoryBox* – a device that provides pre-recorded video messages from family members, personal photographs, videos and music that has resulted in family members reporting positive changes in their loved ones' motivation and wellbeing after *MemoryBox* trials. Campbell et al.'s (2022) *Everyday Sounds* work also utilises recorded sounds for stimulating memories and conversations between people living with dementia and their informal (family) carers in their homes that has led to family members connecting again through conversations and discovering things about each other through engaging in collective storytelling and reminiscing.

In the late stages of dementia, a person will ultimately become dependent on other people for nursing care. Memory loss extends to older memories, and a person may not be able to determine their function.of familiar objects or recognise people who are close to them.

There is a gradual and increasing loss of speech. People living with dementia, at this stage, can become restless, agitated and have a tendency to want to search for someone or something. Some people can have less control of their emotions and become restless, particularly if they feel threatened. It is common for a person to become increasingly immobile, often starting to shuffle when they walk or becoming more unsteady on their feet. In the late stages of dementia, a person's care requirements dramatically increase. At this stage, a person living with dementia will need daily, if not full time supervision. Dementia will limit their ability to communicate verbally and they will need high levels of assistance with activities such as bathing and dressing, which can no longer be carried out independently. When levels of dementia care and assistance increase, it is imperative that the person is constantly reminded of who they are and consulted about what they are doing to lessen the feeling that they have no control over the situation.

Despite a person no longer being able to communicate verbally, it is still possible to share significant experiences and to communicate using other methods. Treadaway's (2022) work (see also Chapter 10) emphasises a compassionate approach to dementia care, where holding someone's hand, a smile, the scent of a fresh flower, the sound of a loving voice, or the feel of an animal's fur can all communicate where words fail. Treadaway's *HUG by LAUGH®* product has been developed to give pleasure and improve the quality of life of people living with dementia, giving users a reciprocal experience of being hugged who are near the end of their lives and need comfort and reassurance. Similarly, for people living with moderate-to-advanced forms of dementia, Favilla et al.'s (2022) work creates a range of two-person (dyad) tablet interactions bundled as apps to support 'better visits' for family members and carers, which has resulted in enriched social interactions, moments of insight, opportunities for conversations, reminiscence and enjoyment by encouraging non-verbal forms of expression for people with speech aphasia or advanced dementia and their family members.

Conclusion

In the UK, there are close to one million people living with dementia and this number is projected to rise to 1.6 million by 2040. The total cost of care for people with dementia in the UK is £34.7 billion, which will rise sharply over the next two decades. In addition to these massive numbers, a further 700,000 people act as 'informal carers' in the UK (Alzheimer's Research UK, 2015). Unpaid, untrained and often with no formal networks of support, informal carers shore up significant gaps in health and social care services. It is estimated that unpaid carers supporting someone with dementia save the UK economy £13.9 billion a year, with two-thirds of the cost of dementia being paid by people living with dementia and their families. The emotional impact of caring can be even more debilitating. Informal carers regularly speak of social isolation and marginalisation, and this impact cannot be overstated. Dementia erases significant elements of a person's being, which contributes to an ongoing sense of grief without closure or 'ambiguous loss' (Boss & Yeats, 2014) that can affect carers as much as those diagnosed with dementia.

Because dementia currently has no cure, there is a real need for carefully designed interventions (e.g. products, services, spaces and systems) that enable people to live as well as possible with dementia. The hope is that this chapter shines a strong light on what and how various forms of design research can do for people living with dementia in the years ahead. This chapter highlights the increasing number of design researchers working in dementia-related contexts. This includes design researchers from a wide range of design disciplines including product design, service design, experience design, architecture, information design, co-design and user-centred design that are working with people living with dementia, their formal and informal carers and their family members. Many of the design-led projects included in this chapter are undertaken in collaboration with researchers in other disciplines such as health and social care, nursing, occupational therapy, sociology, engineering and computer science, and others, highlighting the range of design research for change interventions in dementia care and the essential role these interventions play.

Notes

1 https://www.alzint.org/about/dementia-facts-figures/dementia-statistics/
2 UK Research and Innovation is a non-departmental public body of the Government of the United Kingdom that directs research and innovation funding, funded through the science budget of the Department for Business, Energy and Industrial Strategy.
3 https://gtr.ukri.org

References

Alzheimer's Research UK. (2015). *Dementia in the family - The impact on carers*. Retrieved August 13 2020, from https://www.alzheimersresearchuk.org/about-us/our-influence/policy-work/reports/carers -report/

Aride, A., & Couto, R. (2022). Products and strategies for dementia rehabilitation and prevention in nursing homes. In P. A. Rodgers (Ed.), *Design for people living with dementia* (pp. 201–212). Routledge.

Beh, J., Pedell, S., de Kruiff, A., & Reilly, A. (2022). Alexa, what day is it again? Virtual assistants empowering people living with dementia at home. In P. A. Rodgers (Ed.), *Design for people living with dementia* (pp. 108–120). Routledge.

Boss, P., & Yeats, J. (2014). Ambiguous loss: A complicated type of grief when loved ones disappear. *Bereavement Care, 33*(2), 63–69.

Bramble, M., Moyle, W., & Shum, D. (2011). A quasi-experimental design trial exploring the effect of a partnership intervention on family and staff well-being in long-term dementia care. *Aging and Mental Health, 15*(8), 995–1007. https://doi.org/10.1080/13607863.2011.583625

Brankaert, R., & den Ouden, E. (2022). Design for people living with dementia: Considerations and qualities for technology and design. In P. A. Rodgers (Ed.), *Design for people living with dementia* (pp. 51–64). Routledge.

Campbell, S., Frohlich, D., & Alm, N. (2022). Exploring the role of everyday sounds to support people living with dementia. In P. A. Rodgers (Ed.), *Design for people living with dementia* (pp. 237–248). Routledge.

Carey, D. (2022). Super/normal: Designing dementia services around wicked assets. In P. A. Rodgers (Ed.), *Design for people living with dementia* (pp. 176–188). Routledge.

Crowley, B. P., & Delfico, J. F. (1996). *Content analysis: A methodology for structuring and analyzing written material*. United State General Accounting Office (GAO), Program Evaluation and Methodology Division.

Danckwerth, J. (2022). Textile memories: Designing wearables technology for people living with dementia. In P. A. Rodgers (Ed.), *Design for people living with dementia* (pp. 25–38). Routledge.

Favilla, S., Pedell, S., Murphy, A., & Beh, J. (2022). Evaluating shared tablet interactions co-created for people living with moderate-to-advanced dementia. In P. A. Rodgers (Ed.), *Design for people living with dementia* (pp. 225–236). Routledge.

Hannan, J., Raber, C., & Peterson, M. (2022). Connecting design students with people living in long-term care: Driving social change through the curriculum. In P. A. Rodgers (Ed.), *Design for people living with dementia* (pp. 163–175). Routledge.

Jakob, A. (2022). "Paradise room" – How the sensory room can become a desirable destination for residents in care homes. In P. A. Rodgers (Ed.), *Design for people living with dementia* (pp. 133–149). Routledge.

Lariviere, M. J. (2018). *An ethnography of the everyday practices of people with dementia and their informal carers with assistive technologies and telecare in community-based care* (PhD Thesis). University of East Anglia.

Manchester, H., & Rumble, H. (2022). Parlours of wonder: Designing intergenerational spaces of encounter. In P. A. Rodgers (Ed.), *Design for people living with dementia* (pp. 150–162). Routledge.

Maya Rivero, A. (2022). Trigger memories through material culture in Mexican people living with dementia. In P. A. Rodgers (Ed.), *Design for people living with dementia* (pp. 189–200). Routledge.

Nayer, K., & Nayer, K. (2022). MemoryBox – Using digitised memories to improve the quality of life of people living with dementia. In P. A. Rodgers (Ed.), *Design for people living with dementia* (pp. 213–224). Routledge.

Robertson, L., Lim, C., & Moncur, W. (2022). Interactive textiles for well-being in dementia-friendly communities. In P. A. Rodgers (Ed.), *Design for people living with dementia* (pp. 13–24). Routledge.

Rodgers, P. A. (2022). *Design for people living with dementia*. Routledge.

Samsi, K., & Manthorpe, J. (2020). *Interviewing people living with dementia in social care research*. NIHR School for Social Care Research.

Schreiber, C., & Cürlis, D. (2022). Making the fuzzy end even fuzzier: The role of the caregiving relative in participatory design processes with people living with dementia. In P. A. Rodgers (Ed.), *Design for people living with dementia* (pp. 121–132). Routledge.

Timlin, G., & Rysenbry, N. (2010). *Design for dementia: Improving dining and bedroom environments in care homes*. Helen Hamlyn Centre, Royal College of Art, ISBN 978-1-907342-27-1.

Treadaway, C. (2022). Designing nurturing experiences for people living with advanced dementia. In P. A. Rodgers (Ed.), *Design for people living with dementia* (pp. 65–76). Routledge.

van Buuren, L., van Delden, L., & Mohammadi, M. (2022). Dementia architecture: Designing typological floor plans using the 'research through design' approach'. In P. A. Rodgers (Ed.), *Design for people living with dementia* (pp. 91–107). Routledge.

Wilkinson, A., & Hendriks, N. (2022). The emergence of empathy: Through designing for one. In P. A. Rodgers (Ed.), *Design for people living with dementia* (pp. 77–90). Routledge.

Windle, G., Newman, A., Burholt, V., Woods, B., O'Brien, D., Baber, M., … Tischler, V. (2016). Dementia and Imagination: A mixed-methods protocol for arts and science research. *BMJ Open*, *6*(11), e011634. https://doi.org/10.1136/bmjopen-2016-011634, PubMed: 27807080, PubMed Central: PMC5129039.

Winton, E., & Rodgers, P. A. (2022). Designed with DeMEntia: Building long-lasting collaborative care. In P. A. Rodgers (Ed.), *Design for people living with dementia* (pp. 39–50). Routledge.

10 Reducing anxiety with a HUG

Cathy Treadaway

Caring touch

Our propensity to thrive is linked to our ability to maintain social connections and feel part of a community. Medical anthropology has shown ways in which the human body has evolved to enable social communication and respond positively to it. The pharynx, larynx, inner ear and facial muscles, all used in interpersonal communication, are intricately connected to the autonomic nervous system via the vagus nerve. These parts of the body provide an essential neural feedback loop that can moderate sympathetic stress responses that are physically experienced in the body as 'anxiety' (Porges, 2011). Human touch is also deeply connected to social communication and emotional wellbeing and is thought likely to have evolved from early communal grooming practices, which can be observed in primates (Dunbar, 2010). Preening, grooming and care practice have the adaptive advantage of cementing relationships to promote safety. To touch, hold, stroke, nurture and care for others are innate human behaviours that need to be expressed and acknowledged if an individual is to thrive and live well.

The physiological benefits of human caring touch are well proven. Research has shown that caring touch can relieve physical as well as psychological pain (Jiang & Qin, 2008 cited in Tai et al., 2011). Physiological processes stimulated by touch include the release of endorphins and hormones, including oxytocin (sometimes known as the 'cuddle hormone') (Dunbar, 2010). This has a positive impact on mood, lowering blood pressure and activating the parasympathetic nervous system to relieve stress. Studies have shown the positive benefits of touch on a range of social behaviours including stimulating generosity, trust, enhancing performance and bonding (Tjew A Sin & Koole, 2013). Nevertheless, not everyone likes to be touched, and there are also wide cultural differences that delineate the location and nature of socially acceptable touch. Our unique lived experiences prime how we accept or recoil from a touch from another person. If we have a bad experience of human touch, we are likely to remember, and it will affect how we receive or reject it in the future despite our innate predisposition to benefit from it.

There is a wide body of research to evidence ways in which health is detrimentally affected when people are touch deprived (Linden, 2015). In studies with newborn babies, those who receive little skin-to-skin contact have been found to fail to thrive. Premature babies who have either been neglected in orphanages or kept in incubators with little staff contact are reported in a number of studies to have a wide range of developmental problems, physical, psychological and behavioural, that can last into adult life (Hobson, 2004; Linden, 2015). Problems arising from deprivation can be reversed via therapies that involve handling infants for 20–60 minutes a day. 'Kangaroo care' (Bailey, 2012), a touch therapy in which premature babies are nursed by the mother skin to skin for the first 14 days of life, has been shown to have health benefits that last through childhood (Feldman et al., 2014). This and other forms of touch stimulation therapy

DOI: 10.4324/9781003318262-14

are used routinely in hospitals around the world to improve the health outcomes of premature infants (Linden, 2015).

Harlow, a behavioural scientist, conducted a series of experiments on macaque monkeys in the 1950s that have illuminated the importance of comforting touch. His work explored the behavioural theory of attachment and showed that infants have an innate need to touch and cling to something for emotional comfort (Harlow & Harlow, 1962). In his experiments, two groups of baby rhesus macaque monkeys were separated from their mothers at birth. The first group was placed in isolation cages containing a soft textile cloth surrogate mother providing no food and another one made of wire holding a bottle with milk. The results of the study showed that, when stressed, the baby monkeys preferred the cloth surrogate mother whether or not it provided them with nourishment. Although food is an essential requirement for survival, when placed in stressful situations it was the nurturing comfort of soft skin-to-skin care that they craved. Without a real mother to snuggle up to, the padded textile form provided an alternative comforter. Harlow was influenced by the work of psychologist John Bowlby, whose research on nurturing touch highlighted its importance on emotional development in childhood, leading to better relationship attachments in later life (Suomi et al., 2008).

Human touch has been shown to be vital for wellbeing, and its deprivation can negatively impact psychological health. During the global pandemic, many people found themselves living in isolation in a state of 'touch poverty' (von Mohr et al., 2021). Despite the technological benefits of online communication, the lack of physical interpersonal human touch (hugs, hand-holding, etc.) became a source of frustration and distress for many people and featured heavily in media reports. Those who live alone, and in particular people living with dementia or cognitive impairment, were negatively affected, with many experiencing a marked decline in their condition.

Dementia, anxiety and agitation

Dementia is a condition that affects an estimated 55 million people globally, with numbers of those diagnosed increasing rapidly due to an ageing population and negative lifestyle factors (WHO, 2022). The term 'dementia' is used to describe a group of symptoms that result from a range of different degenerative diseases affecting the brain. These symptoms can include memory loss, confusion, changes in cognition, mood, perception and behaviour, often resulting in communication difficulties. Not everyone experiences dementia in the same way. The gradual neurodegenerative nature of the condition results in a person becoming increasingly withdrawn from a world that they no longer recognise, remember, or feel a part of. Inevitably, many people living with dementia experience high levels of anxiety, agitation and depression. They often do not know why they feel as they do and are unable to articulate the reasons for their anxiety and distress.

The way that anxiety is expressed is often misunderstood. In acute dementia care and hospital contexts, anxiety is often perceived by staff as so called 'challenging behaviours' which may include shouting, aggression, disinhibition, wandering and sleep disturbances. Communication with caregivers, family members and health professionals can become difficult, and relationships strained as a result. This can leave a person living with dementia feeling increasingly isolated and distressed. Anti-psychotic and anti-anxiety medication is often used in these situations, although there is a growing appreciation that this may be detrimental to a person's quality of life. Side effects from drugs can include drowsiness, often resulting in falls, or apathy leading to a person's withdrawal from engaging with the world. Effective non-drug-based therapies are needed to help treat anxiety and agitation, to maintain a person's quality of life. Research studies are revealing the benefits of a variety of therapeutic approaches involving touch (Kim & Buschmann, 1999).

Touch Therapy is an approach that has been used in care practice since the 1950s and involves caring physical touch that is outside of a health practitioner's procedural tasks, for example: face-touching, head-touching, hand-holding, placing an arm around the patient's shoulders. A review of studies cited by Cai and Zhang (2015) found that simple expressions of human kindness through hand-touching have a positive impact on the recipient's quality of life and can reduce agitation in people living with dementia. Unfortunately, safeguarding practices in many countries have resulted in interpersonal touch being actively discouraged or prohibited. Similarly, during the COVID-19 pandemic, social-distancing measures to mitigate virus transmission have meant that many people, especially those living alone, have been deprived of physical touch from another person.

Animal therapies provide an alternative to human touch and have been found to be very beneficial with care home residents (Pitheckoff et al., 2016). Smoothing the fur on a rabbit, cat or dog has been shown to lower blood pressure and reduce anxiety, and in some residential care homes, social care activity providers bring alpacas and other animals for residents to hold and stroke. Although some care homes keep pets, not everyone enjoys having animals around; some are afraid of them or may suffer allergic reactions. However, furry fabrics and soft toys, when touched and cuddled, have a similar soothing psychological effect as stroking animals. Teddy bears and soft dolls are not only beneficial as comforters for children but are continued to be used by some people into adult life. Many adults keep childhood soft toys, and, for some, hugging a teddy or cushion can bring comfort in moments of stress and anxiety. In very young children, soft toys are objects that enable a baby to transition from dependence on maternal care to self-care and awareness (Winnicott, 1953; 1971; Bollas, 1979). The soft physical form and the tactile experiences they provide may evoke emotional memories of being held in their parents' arms, stimulate a sense of security and reduce anxiety. For this reason, children become very attached to their comforting object and will need it at bedtime to sleep peacefully. In adult life, even when the transitional object (teddy bear/doll) is relegated to a bedroom shelf or chair, it may retain deep emotional significance for its owner (Kenning & Treadaway, 2017).

Research supports the therapeutic benefit of using teddy bears in treating anxiety, agitation and low mood in people of all ages. Tai and colleagues (2011) found that touching a teddy bear mitigates the negative effects of loneliness, stimulates positive emotions, reduces stress, helped people to develop prosocial behaviour and provided compensation for the lack of human touch. Touching and holding teddy bears has also been found to help individuals suffering from low self-esteem and anxiety (Koole et al., 2014).

Objects such as teddy bears, dolls and soft toys can provide emotional significance, reassurance and comfort to people living with mid to late dementia even though memories associated with them may be lost (Mitchell & O'Donnell, 2013; Tanner, 2017). There is an increasing acknowledgement in the care sector of their therapeutic benefit. However, fears of some healthcare professionals that they may be perceived as infantilising sometimes inhibit their use. Person-centred care approaches, which prioritise the needs and preferences of the individual person living with dementia over societal expectations, are challenging these attitudes at last (Mitchell, 2016).

HUG: designing for therapeutic touch

There is a clear need for well-designed tactile comforting therapeutic products to help alleviate anxiety in dementia care and other mental health contexts. Finding the right approach, designing appropriately for age and with materials and technologies that stimulate optimal comforting responses is vital. Additional sensory features such as sound, vibration and warmth can be added

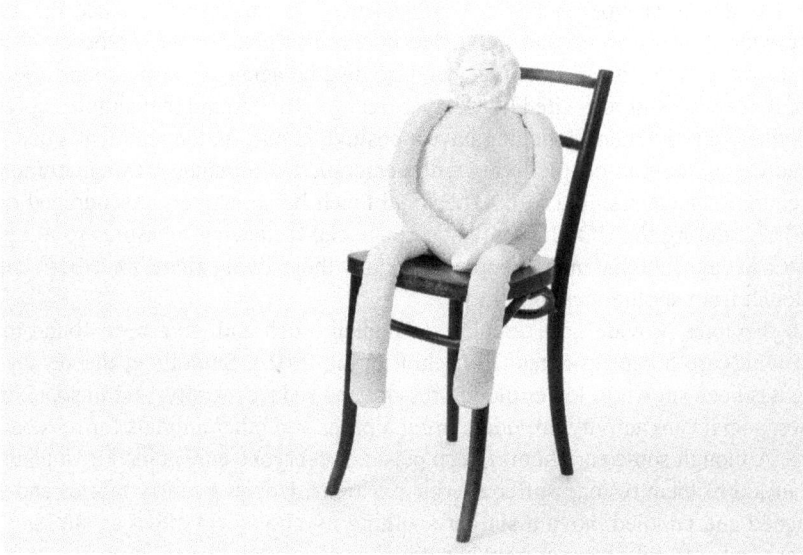

Figure 10.1 HUG (www.hug.world)

to objects by embedding electronics, microcontrollers and sensors. Haptic jackets can simulate an affectionate embrace, and soft toys are now commercially available that respond autonomously to being stroked. Although the rich benefits of interpersonal human touch cannot be replaced by such products, they do have a role to play in some contexts when human contact is restricted (when people are lonely or isolated) or prohibited (such as during the pandemic). The following section describes research that has led to an award-winning therapeutic device, HUG, which is now being used to help reduce anxiety for people living with dementia in care homes and hospitals in the UK.

HUG is a soft comforter with weighted extended arms and legs that can be worn around the body to simulate the experience of both giving and receiving a hug (see Figure 10.1). The product has a soft furry cushion-like body, which contains an electronics module that simulates a human beating heart and can be programmed to play a personalised music playlist. The product is underpinned by six years of academic research and has been commercialised with support from Alzheimer's Society UK. The HUG prototype product was one of six outputs developed during LAUGH interdisciplinary research at Cardiff Metropolitan University 2015–2018. LAUGH research sought to understand how to design playful hand-held objects to support the wellbeing of people living with advanced dementia and involved an international interdisciplinary team of researchers including designers, technologists, health care professionals and psychologists. The research used interpretive qualitative methodologies informed by grounded theory and participatory approaches. It tested out a Compassionate Design methodology which places loving kindness for the individual living with dementia at the heart of the design process and focuses on designing for sensory stimulation, personalisation and connection (Treadaway et al., 2018, 2020a).

People with lived experience of dementia were included at all stages of the project. At the outset, a group of people living with early-stage dementia contributed their experiences through focus group activities. People living with advanced dementia, their families and carers were involved throughout, contributing as experts by experience as the project developed. Other experts, including professional carers, psychologists, medics, medics and occupational therapists also contributed their dementia expertise. Six bespoke playful object prototypes were developed and evaluated during the research project, one of which was HUG (Treadaway et al., 2019b).

The first prototype of HUG was developed for a woman who was in the later stage of the disease and on end-of-life care. Once the life and soul of the care home in which she resided, she had become withdrawn, unable to communicate verbally, was largely bed-bound, fell frequently and would sleep for most of the day. Her carer advised the research team that, in her opinion, what this person really needed was a hug. The design team developed the first HUG prototype, informed by findings from a series of participatory workshops with dementia experts (Treadaway et al., 2019a). The HUG prototype was created in soft plush fabric with long weighted limbs designed to wrap around the body to form an embrace. The design aimed to replicate the sensory experience of both giving and receiving a hug. The size, shape and weight of HUG replicated that of a small child. Internal electronics provided the sensation of a calming beating heart to emotionally signal the need for the object to be nurtured by its owner. A small MP3 player and speakers were integrated into the cavity of the HUG prototype, since music has been shown to have profound emotional benefits for people living with dementia and can soothe and relax people who are anxious (Särkämö, 2018).

When the prototype of HUG was given to the person it was designed for, her body language immediately indicated that she was enjoying the sensation (Figure 10.2). She visibly relaxed and nestled her head onto the soft furry object, holding it close to her body. The research evaluation process took place in three stages: after one week, a month and three months. The impact on her was profound, and after three months she was no longer spending most of the day in bed but was up and socialising with other residents. She regained some language, her general health improved, and she had no further falls. The resident lived for another nine months with a much improved quality of life.

Evaluating the benefits of HUG

The success of the HUG prototype led to funding support for a much larger study in which 40 HUGs were evaluated by people living with advanced dementia, in both residential care and National Health Service (NHS) hospital contexts. LAUGH EMPOWERED involved a research team that included designers, medical professionals and the care industry. The study was government funded and involved two partner organisations: a care home provider and an NHS hospital. Twenty participants were recruited for the study in each context (N=40). The data collection, reporting and analysis were conducted in the care home context by a senior consultant occupational therapist and in the hospital context by the university research team in collaboration with a consultant gerontologist and a multidisciplinary team comprising occupational therapists, nurses, speech and language therapists, dieticians and psychologists. An adapted Pool Activity Level (PAL) tool (Pool, 2012) and Bradford Dementia Well-being Profile (Bradford Dementia Group, 2008) were used in the care home study to collect participant data at baseline, three months and six months after residents had been given a HUG. These tools identified the participants' cognitive and functional abilities, assessed their personal wellbeing, and provided guidance on how to introduce HUG to each person in an appropriate manner. The university research team also conducted semi-structured interviews with family members and staff to illuminate the findings. Unfortunately, the hospital study was undertaken during the pandemic when staff were experiencing severe stress and time pressures. Consequently, it was only possible to collect post hoc qualitative data for the NHS study once the pandemic restrictions eased. This was undertaken by the university researchers via semi-structured interviews with members of the multidisciplinary team who had worked directly with patients who had been prescribed a HUG.

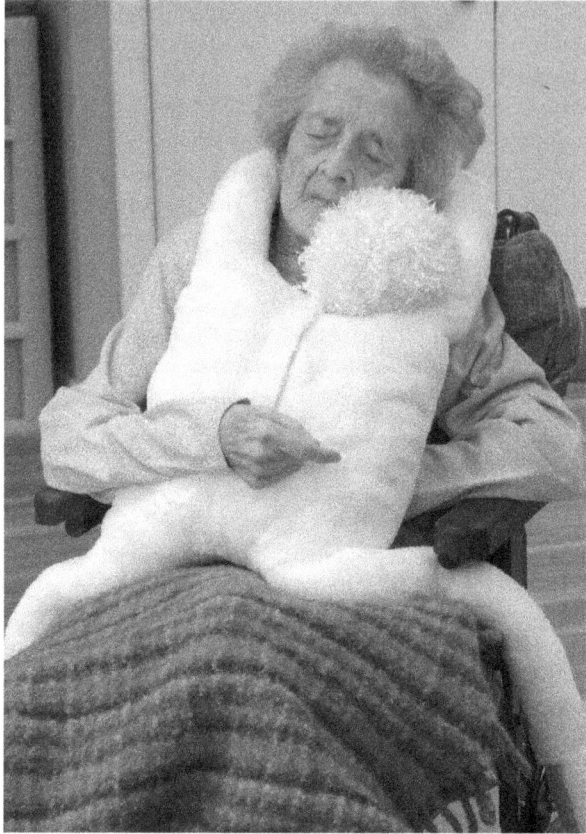

Figure 10.2 Person with the first HUG prototype

The care home study findings corroborated the first LAUGH HUG evaluation: 87% of residents who used HUG over the six-month study showed an increase in their wellbeing. Of those for whom wellbeing improved, over half increased their functional and cognitive ability as defined by the PAL tool (Treadaway et al., 2020b). This result is particularly significant given the degenerative nature of the condition. Simply maintaining the cognitive and functional ability of someone living with dementia over six months might be considered a positive result, but the collected PAL data also evidenced an improvement for some.

Personal testimonies of staff and family members corroborated the data. There were heart-warming stories about residents who had enjoyed the tactile and sensory benefits of using the product. One resident, who had been thought unlikely to respond to HUG due to her perceived aggressive behaviour, experienced a profound change. She became calmer, less anxious and exhibited fewer moments of aggression and distress. Other residents saw HUG as a companion or perceived it to be a baby needing care and attention. One resident enjoyed having HUG to help her sleep in bed, as she missed the physical presence of her husband at night and felt lonely in the care home. Care staff commented on how residents found the tactile experience of HUG soothing and explained how they would sometimes involve care staff in the embrace with HUG. Safeguarding fears and employment regulations frequently inhibit staff from showing physical affection to residents in care. The limbs of HUG are long and weighted to enable it to be wrapped around and worn on the body and are made from soft padded plush fabric. The end of each limb has a satin pad, reminiscent of the smooth ribbon edge of a classic woven woollen blanket. This satin pad provides a different tactile sensation when stroked and feels pleasant against the smooth skin of a person's face or palm of the hand. Staff found that they could use HUG as an intermediary object to give a person a hug, fulfilling the person's emotional need without human contact.

HUG's simulated heartbeat is clearly palpable when it is held against the body in an embrace. The regular pulsating vibration was found to be an additional soothing sensory feature of HUG's design. The tactile sensation also signified to the user that HUG had a heart, was breathing and needed to be cared for. The concept behind the design emerged from one of the key themes arising from the LAUGH research – our innate human need to nurture and be nurtured. The design concept aimed to stimulate the instinctive behaviours of cradling, cuddling, hugging and giving care. For many of the residents in the study, HUG became a surrogate baby, rekindling memories of nursing a small child and providing opportunities to stimulate conversations with caregivers and visitors. One woman who had been a teacher would collect HUGs together in the care home, in a playful re-enactment reminiscent of gathering school children for a class. Another resident found great comfort in soothing HUG on her lap. She enjoyed the weight of the object and stroking its soft furry body, which reminded her of a pet cat she had once owned. The woman was visually impaired, so the tactile sensation and weight of HUG were particularly important.

The NHS hospital study corroborated many of the findings from the care home study regarding the tactile sensory benefits of HUG (Treadaway et al., 2023). The NHS study took place over a six-month period during which time HUG was prescribed to 20 patients on the Stroke Rehabilitation Centre and Dementia wards. Patients were selected for inclusion in the study if they had a diagnosis of dementia or post-stroke cognitive impairment and were suffering from anxiety. All participants and their families completed NHS IRAS (Integrated Research Application System) approved ethical consent forms, prior to being prescribed a HUG as an alternative to anti-anxiety medication. It should be noted that patients who are admitted to the hospital with dementia are often in crisis and very anxious. This may be due to comorbidities that require them to be hospitalised or because the progression of their dementia has reached a critical stage, and they need specialist medical care. Patients who experience a stroke are often particularly anxious due to the sudden onset of the condition and subsequent cognitive impairment. Anti-anxiety medication is problematic for both sets of patients due to conflict with other drugs administered or because their sedative effect makes patients more prone to falls. An elevated sense of anxiety is often expressed by a patient in aggressive or agitated behaviour, negative attitudes or withdrawal. The introduction of HUG as a therapeutic aid needed a sensitive approach from staff and time spent with the patients introducing it. When this happened, patients were found to be more relaxed, less anxious and happier. Not all patients offered HUG accepted it. However, when it was accepted, HUG made a significant impact on their hospital experience by reducing anxiety, increasing their willingness to cooperate with medical procedures, take prescribed medication, eat, drink and engage in activities of daily care such as washing and dressing. Staff also noted that HUG helped with communication, reduced agitation, alleviated distress and the need for extra staff attention when a patient felt lonely.

The physical tactile experience of HUG was noted as being particularly beneficial to patients. When patients have had a stroke, their proprioceptive sense of body position in space can be affected, leading to a sensation of falling and increased anxiety. One doctor noted that a patient who was experiencing this found the sensation diminished and he felt 'grounded' again once he was given HUG. Several doctors commented that they observed that the heartbeat soothed distressed patients and helped them relax.

Patients who had been living alone during the pandemic were particularly anxious. An occupational therapist described how one visually impaired female patient, who was particularly distressed on admission to the hospital, found intense emotional release and comfort using HUG.

> I popped the arms and legs round so she could feel the weight and feel the pressure on her and she literally burst into tears and howled, it was so sweet! And this was during the first wave of the pandemic, so she'd lacked any sort of proper physical comfort and I think her crying was like a release. You know, because 'oh, this is what I needed'.

From design concept to manufactured product

The LAUGH EMPOWERED research found that HUG can make a significant contribution in a person's care by fulfilling a basic human need to feel socially connected and loved. It also provides a nurturing experience that can bring meaning and purpose to a person's life. For some of the HUG users, the product has been life changing, giving pleasure, companionship and a reason to keep living (see www.hug.world for case studies and video evidence). The underpinning LAUGH research investigated the importance of hand use and touch to support the wellbeing of people living with advanced dementia. It explored fundamental human needs and found nurturing touch to be particularly significant in supporting their wellbeing.

The Compassionate Design methodology (depicted in Figure 10.3) that was used throughout the project guided the design process, ensuring that loving kindness for the individual was placed at its heart (Treadaway et al., 2018). In addition, designing to incorporate sensory properties, connect the user to others and the wider world they experience, and the facility to personalise the product are key design considerations when designing for users with cognitive impairment. The sensory properties aim to keep the user 'in the moment' with rich tactile experiences that are not reliant on memory nor place cognitive load on the user. HUG has a physical weight and tactile presence that is designed to evoke implicit emotional memories of holding a child, baby,

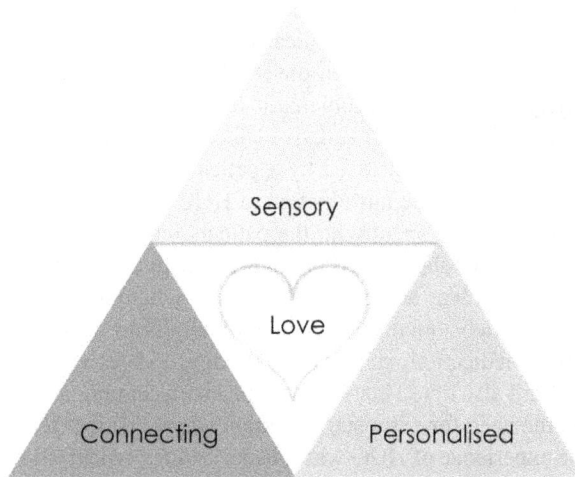

Figure 10.3 Compassionate Design methodology places loving kindness for the user central to the design process and focuses the designer's attention on personalisation, sensory stimulation and potential to connect the user with others and the world around them. (Download the free publication from https://www.laughproject.info)

or pet. Its weighted limbs provide the sensory experience of receiving a cuddle, and the heart-beat arouses the desire to nurture it. The music player enables the product to be personalised with sounds that can stimulate emotional responses and memories.

The final chapter of the research project involved design amendments, prior to manufacture of the product, so that its benefits could be experienced by many others. These included a change to the body of HUG to facilitate washing and ensure compliance with NHS infection control guidelines, changes to the construction of the head to make it easier to manufacture, improvements to the electronics to make it easier to upload sound files to the MP3 player, and longer battery life. The process of making HUG commercially available was supported by Alzheimer's Society UK (through their Accelerator Award programme) and Cardiff Metropolitan University, who helped to establish the HUG by LAUGH Ltd. spinout business in 2020. The product was launched commercially in October 2021 and is now being used by individuals in care homes and hospitals in the UK and around the world.

Although HUG was initially conceived as a product for people living with advanced dementia, it is already having a much wider application. It has been used to help people receiving end-of-life and palliative care, for people living with a variety of medical conditions, and is used by children as well as adults. The LAUGH research has contributed important insights into the benefits of affective touch and social connection to support the wellbeing of people who are cognitively impaired or living with dementia. Tactile experiences have been shown to provide important channels of communication and stimulation that can reduce anxiety and bring comfort to those who are no longer verbal or coming towards the end of their lives. HUG provides comforting tactile experiences that help people feel loved, valued and secure, as evidenced in case studies and testimonials on the HUG by LAUGH website (www.hug.world).

Acknowledgments

LAUGH (Ludic Artefacts Using Gesture and Haptics) was funded by the UK Arts and Humanities Research Council (2015–2018) Grant number: AH/M005607/1 (www.laughproject .info acc. 16.05.22.)

LAUGH EMPOWERED research was funded by Welsh Government SMART Expertise grant ref: 2018/COL/012/80839 (2018–2021) Cathy Treadaway (Academic Lead Investigator), with partners: Sunrise Senior Living Ltd. led by Jackie Pool and NHS Llandough Hospital, Cardiff and Vale University Health Board (CAVUHB) led by Dr Ben Jelley.

Alzheimer's Society 'Service Users Reporting Panel' (Cardiff) and Dementia Voices contributed to the LAUGH and LAUGH EMPOWERED studies.

Alzheimer's Society – Accelerator Award grant funding for HUG by LAUGH (2021).

References

Bailey, S. (2012). Kangaroo mother care. *British Journal of Hospital Medicine*, *73*(5), 278–281.

Bollas, C. (1979). The transformational object. *International Journal of Psycho-Analysis*, *60*(1), 97–107.

Bradford Dementia Group. (2008). *The Bradford well-being profile*. University of Bradford. Retrieved May 16, 2022, from https://www.bradford.ac.uk/repos/health/Bradford-Well-Being-Profile-with -cover-(3).pdf

Cai, F.-F., & Zhang, H. (2015). Effect of therapeutic touch on agitated behavior in elderly patients with dementia: A review. *International Journal of Nursing Sciences*, *2*(3), 324–328.

Dunbar, R. I. M. (2010). The social role of touch in humans and primates: Behavioural function and neurobiological mechanisms. *Neuroscience and Biobehavioral Reviews*, *34*(2), 260–268.

Feldman, R., Rosenthal, Z., & Eidelman, A. (2014). Maternal pattern skin to skin contact enhances child physiologic organization and cognitive control across the first 10 years of life. *Biological Psychiatry*, *75*(1), 56–64.

Harlow, H. F., & Harlow, M. K. (1962). Social deprivation in monkeys. *Scientific American*, *207*, 136–150.

Hobson, R. P. (2004). *The cradle of thought: Exploring the origins of thinking*. Pan. Retrieved May 16, 2022, from https://www.bbc.co.uk/news/uk-wales-50237366 https://www.bbc.co.uk/programmes/p0974ckg https://www.itv.com/news/central/2022-03-31/hug-dolls-to-help-patients-with-dementia-at-derbyshire-care-home

Kenning, G., & Treadaway, C. (2017, January). Designing for dementia: Iterative grief and transitional objects. *Design Issues*, *34*(1), 42–53. Special Issue on Mortality. https://doi.org/10.1162/DESI_a_00475

Kim, E. J., & Buschmann, M. T. (1999). The effect of expressive physical touch on patients with dementia. *International Journal of Nursing Studies*, *36*(3), 235–243.

Koole, S. L., Tjew, A.-S. I. N., M., & Schneider, I. K. (2014). Embodied terror management: Interpersonal touch alleviates existential concerns among individuals with low self-esteem. *Psychological Science*, *25*(1), 30–37. https://doi.org/10.1177/0956797

Linden, D. J. (2015). *Touch: The science of hand, heart, and mind*. Penguin Books.

Mitchell, G. (2016). *Doll therapy in dementia care*. Jesica Kingsley.

Mitchell, G., & O'Donnell, H. (2013). The therapeutic use of doll therapy in dementia. *British Journal of Nursing*, *22*(6), 329–334.

Pitheckoff, N., Mclaughlin, S. J., & De Medeiros, K. (2016). Calm . . . Satisfied . . . comforting: The experience and meaning of rabbit-assisted activities for older adults. *Journal of Applied Gerontology*, *37*, 1564–1575.

Pool, J. (2012). *The pool activity level PAL instrument for occupational profiling*. Jessica Kingsley.

Porges, S. W. (2011). *The polyvagal theory: Neurophysiological foundations of emotions, attachment, communication, and self-regulation*. W.W. Norton.

Särkämö, T. (2018). Music for the ageing brain: Cognitive, emotional, social, and neural benefits of musical leisure activities in stroke and dementia. *Dementia (London, England)*, *17*(6), 670–685.

Suomi, S. J., Van Der Horst, F. C. P., & Van Der Veer, R. (2008). Rigorous experiments on monkey love: An account of Harry F. Harlow's role in the history of attachment theory. *Integrative Psychological and Behavioral Science*, *42*(4), 354–369.

Tai, K., Zheng, X., & Narayanan, J. (2011). Touching a teddy bear mitigates negative effects of social exclusion to increase prosocial behavior. *Social Psychological and Personality Science*, *2*(6), 618–626.

Tanner, L. (2017). *Embracing touch in dementia care*. Jessica Kingsley.

Tjew, A., Sin, M., & Koole, S. L. (2013). *That human touch that means so much: Exploring the tactile dimension of social life. In-mind magazine*, *17*. VU University Amsterdam.

Treadaway, C., Fennell, J., Prytherch, D., Kenning, G., Prior, A., & Walters, A. (2018). *Compassionate design: How to design for advanced dementia*. Cardiff Metropolitan University. ISBN 978-0-9929482-8-3. Retrieved December 12 2023, from https://www.laughproject.info/wp-content/uploads/2018/04/Compassionate-Design_toolkit.pdf

Treadaway, C., Fennell, J., Prytherch, D., Kenning, G., & Walters, A. (2019a). Designing for well-being in late stage dementia. In R. Coles, S. Costa, & S. Watson (Eds.), *Pathways to well-being in design: Examples from the arts, humanities and the built environment*. pp. 186-202. Routledge.

Treadaway, C., Fennell, J., & Taylor, A. (2020a, September 4). Compassionate design: A methodology for advanced dementia. In K. Christer, C. Craig, & P. Chamberlain (Eds.), *6th International conference on Design4Health* (pp. 19–25). Sheffield Hallam University.

Treadaway, C., Pool, J., & Johnson, A. (2020b). Sometimes a hug is all you need. *Journal of Dementia Care*, *28*, 32–34.

Treadaway, C., Seckam, A., Fennell, J., & Taylor, A. (2023). HUG: A compassionate approach to designing for wellbeing in dementia care. *International Journal of Environmental Research and Public Health*, *20*(5), 4410. https://doi.org/10.3390/ijerph20054410

Treadaway, C., Taylor, A., & Fennell, J. (2019b). Compassionate design for dementia care. *International Journal of Design Creativity and Innovation, 7*(3), 144–157.

Von Mohr, M., Kirsch, L. P., & Fotopoulou, A. (2021). Social touch deprivation during COVID-19: Effects on psychological wellbeing and craving interpersonal touch. *Royal Society Open Science, 8*(9), 210287–210287.

Winnicott, D. W. (1953). Transitional objects and transitional phenomena. *International Journal of Psychoanalysis, 34*(2), 89–97.

Winnicott, D. W. (1971 [1991]). *Playing and reality.* Routledge.

World Health Organization. (2022). Retrieved May 16, 2022, from https://www.who.int/news-room/fact -sheets/detail/dementia

Links to videos about HUG

BBC News (31 October 2019) Dementia device 'kind of brought my mum back'. https://www.bbc.co.uk/ news/uk-wales-50237366 [accessed 16 May 2022]

BBC One (16 February 2021). The One Show. https://www.bbc.co.uk/programmes/p0974ckg [accessed 16 May 2022]

Itv News (31 March 2022) 'Hug dolls' to help patients with dementia at Derbyshire care home. https:// www.itv.com/news/central/2022-03-31/hug-dolls-to-help-patients-with-dementia-at-derbyshire-care-home [accessed 13 May 2024]

11 DCare

Empowering dementia caregivers in Indian families in informal care settings

Vivek Kant, Rishi Tak and Manish Asthana

Introduction

In low-income and highly populated countries like India, dementia is expected to grow over the coming decades as a sizeable population starts to age (World Health Organisation, 2012). In India, the care provision for people with dementia is currently inadequate, largely disconnected, scarce, expensive and not suited to meet the needs of a majority of low-income families (Choudhary et al., 2021; Kumar et al., 2019; Ravindranath & Sundarakumar, 2021). The reasons could be due to a lack of dementia awareness as well as the low priority given to dementia as a public health challenge (Sathianathan & Kantipudi, 2018). This gives rise to a lack of knowledge toward dementia care and demands for the importance of improved informal care and self-care (for caregivers) in large sections of society. In order to achieve this, there is a need for design solutions that aim to address the caregiving ecology of dementia in India to improve social health (e.g. Guisado-Fernández et al., 2019; also Sachdev, 2022; Vernooij-Dassen & Jeon, 2016 for social health).

The proposed app *DCare* can be a helpful tool in the early stage of dementia for caregivers to prepare themselves for better caregiving , along with understanding dementia as a disorder in a better manner); while at a later stage, personalised activities and reminiscence could be a huge help in maintaining and improving social bonds between the caregiver and the person with dementia (PWD). Apart from this, the idea of community-building and finding a network of local caregivers can help people open up and learn from each other's experiences.

This chapter is divided into five sections. The first section is the main introduction. The second section introduces the challenge of Indian dementia care. The third section refers to these themes to develop the *DCare* app from the initial conceptualisation to the final product through two rounds of intermediate usability testing. The article concludes with the fourth section in terms of generalisations and challenges related to the app in the broader Indian caregiving ecology.

Dementia and the Indian ecology of caregiving: themes and challenges

While dementia is a global problem (World Health Organisation, 2012), the Indian care ecology presents some significant challenges along four interrelated themes: (a) lack of awareness, (b) dementia as a social problem, (c) support for caregivers and family and (d) digitalisation and healthcare in India (Chakravorty et al., 2021; Lieber et al., 2020; Muhammad et al., 2021; Ravindranath & Sundarakumar, 2021; Srivastava et al., 2021).

DOI: 10.4324/9781003318262-15

a) Lack of awareness

Dementia is often misdiagnosed or not diagnosed at all, due to the lack of awareness of the disorder in India (Kumar et al., 2019). At other times, dementia diagnosis is misunderstood due to family members comprehending it as the onset of old age. While this aspect is changing in metropolitan cities, such as Mumbai and Delhi, the challenge still exists in several smaller cities in India. Therefore, in India, a major problem is diagnosis and a proper care journey for PWD. In addition, the outward symptoms of dementia include memory loss, emotional distress and apathy, among others. As a result, caregivers who are not apprised about the manifestations of these symptoms can end up exacerbating the emotional distress and the decline in the general wellbeing of the PWD, or they may not be able to provide appropriate care given certain symptomatic manifestations. Thus, a major theme for dementia in India is the lack of awareness of dementia and associated symptoms that need to be comprehended in designing for this sector.

b) Dementia as a social problem

A major theme in India is that dementia is a social problem. This is because the family unit often includes grandparents, parents and children living in one household. The multi-generational family is a common sight in India (Chakravorty et al., 2021; Lieber et al., 2020). In most cases, the PWD remains with their families as the idea of strong family support often exists. Therefore, in India, homecare situations are quite prominent as opposed to residential care facilities; i.e. the PWD is at home and cared for by family members. In homecare situations, in most cases, a woman, either the wife of the PWD, the daughter-in-law or even the eldest daughter (if staying together), takes up the role of the caregiver. In addition, in larger cities such as Mumbai and Delhi, there are several startup clinics and centres that provide short-term services to the PWD by visiting them at their residences. In most cases, these visits by external caregivers supplement the existing care routines of family members. In the family unit, along with being a cognitive challenge, dementia also becomes a distributed social challenge for the entire family. In most cases, the lack of awareness of dementia, as well as the social stigma attached to it in many cases, exacerbates the problem. Thus, dementia has to be seen not only as perceived by the members of the family but also the social milieu.

c) Communication and support for caregivers and PWD

Communication difficulties between the PWD and those who care for them occur frequently (Sinha et al., 2020). These challenges may begin with the PWD's reluctance to participate in daily social interactions. Frequently repeated questions by PWD and changes in their behaviour can be tiring and irritating for caregivers. Often, the lack of replies gives an impression that the conversation is being ignored by the PWD. This becomes progressively frustrating for the PWD and stressful for the caregivers and those who are close to them and who are making an effort to have 'a pleasant communication' with the PWD.

Studies on residential care reveal how the way PWD (people with dementia) are treated by the caregivers (family members or care professionals) may directly affect how the PWD is misinterpreted, positioned in a negative sense and ultimately treated. Thus, this state of affairs is not because of the outcome of dementia but the ways in which the behaviour emerges as a by-product of the interactions between PWD and their families. Sometimes the manner in which PWD are given inappropriate social treatment and their behaviours misinterpreted could be the result of stereotyping due to the lack of awareness of dementia as a disease and its care requirements. Thus, connecting caregivers and more organically and interactively could be explored to curb social isolation and encourage effective social bonding.

d) Digitalisation and healthcare in India

In this chapter, we have focused on the mobile phone app as the digital solution because of the following reasons. Digital aids are quite prominent in dementia care worldwide and range from interactive products to virtual reality experiences.[1] In India, there is an added challenge for digitalisation. Due to a resource-constrained ecology, digitalisation in the form of computers or other technologies such as AR/VR never reached a cohesive mass. In contrast, the mobile phone served as a major channel through which digitalisation could progress. The mobile phone serves as the first audio-visual, communication and entertainment device that caters to the social, economic and personal relations of Indians. The mobile has seen a plethora of apps and digital watches, as well as social media pages for ailments and WhatsApp network groups for caregiving. Therefore, in order to comprehend how digitalisation can help PWD in India, the mobile phone should be taken as an important consideration and vehicle for supplementing care relations.

Design process for supporting dementia care in India

The primary goal of the design process (Fig.11.1; corresponding to the double diamond process, Design Council, 2022) was to support family members of PWD using ICT to encourage prosocial behaviour so as to spend quality time with the PWD. This could be enabled by improving social interactions of PWD with caregivers by exploring multiple interaction opportunities to motivate, encourage and facilitate social encounters that are vital in providing person-centred care.

The secondary goal is to improve awareness about dementia care and have a better understanding of the disorder, which can challenge the stigmatisation and barriers to diagnosis and care. The global action plan for dementia from the WHO reports (World Health Organisation, 2012) that dementia is underdiagnosed worldwide and usually reported at late stages. As a result, there is a need for better solutions that can improve the quality of life of PWD and their caregivers.

User studies, insights and personas

The design process started with developing an understanding of users.[2] Our main focus was on home caregivers. The key idea in this phase was to understand the caregiving experience from varying perspectives. Therefore, we first focused on three different caregiving agencies and four families, along with one neurologist and one neuropsychologist. In all cases, one researcher conducted the interviews to minimise variability. This study was conducted during the COVID-19 pandemic; therefore, all the user studies and the evaluations were conducted online through teleconference. Interview sessions could easily last between one to one and a half hours. Insights from the user studies (see Box 11.1) were used to develop personas.

The caregiving agencies were situated in metropolitan cities of Mumbai (one in-home, one residential) and Delhi (one in-home). These agencies were selected from these major cities as

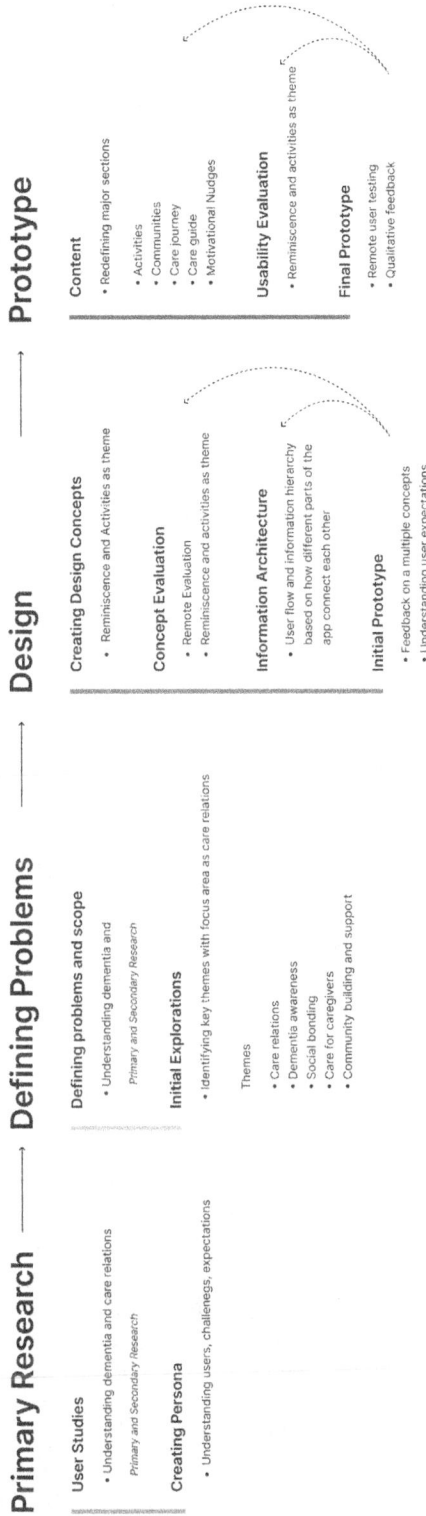

Figure 11.1 Detailed overview schematic of the design process. Image by the authors

Box 11.1 Summary of insights from the field study

(F = Families, C = Caregivers, N = Neurologist/neuropsychologist)

1 Families who opted to provide care at home usually relied on instructions from the professional caregivers and suggestions about activities to follow. [F][C]

2 Family members sometimes find it hard to commit enough time to spend with the PWD due to other commitments at work and with family members, even if they want to. [F][N]

3 Family members are often worried about leaving the PWD on their own, and sometimes find it hard to understand the PWD's mood. [F][C][N]

4 PWD like doing childhood hobbies or revising memories over and over again. [F][C][N]

5 Talking about new topics is hard, yet caregivers find it tedious to talk about past memories repeatedly. [F][C]

6 Although some people liked to engage in activities, some didn't, and getting them to participate can be hard at times. [C][N]

7 It's hard to handle the unexpected behaviour of PWD at times. [F][C]

8 It can be hard for external caregivers to build trust with PWD when they first meet. [F][C]

9 Change in the schedule of PWD can leave them agitated and worried. [F][C]

10 Therapies keep PWD engaged during the sessions and help them feel calm and content after the therapy as well. [F][C][N]

11 Family members usually bring PWD to be diagnosed at a late stage when the condition is quite severe. [N]

12 It is hard to slow the progression of dementia, and as it becomes more severe, providing care can become extremely hard. [F][C][N]

13 Reminiscence about the recent past (one or two days ago) could help PWD engage and build confidence. [N]

14 PWD are usually not encouraged to do activities/therapies alone and like companionship with personal contact, to keep them motivated during the activity. [F][C][N]

in urban areas there is a more widespread awareness of dementia as a problem. Amongst these agencies, we initially started with four caregivers [C] who were ready to share their insights. Of these, three were involved throughout the duration of the project and were interviewed multiple times and also provided feedback on the prototypes in later stages of the design process. In the case of families [F], we interviewed five members from four different families – two from one family and one each from the remaining three families. In all the families, the primary caregivers were interviewed. In addition, one neurologist and one neuropsychologist [N] provided a wealth of general knowledge and trends based on families and caregiver challenges based on their past experiences throughout the duration of the project.

It is noteworthy that all the participants from the care-giving centres, as well as the neurologist and neuropsychologist, agreed to be a part of the study but were not ready to sign a consent form to that effect. They were willing to share their insights and viewpoints; however, they were not ready to sign any paperwork. This is because they considered 'signing anything' as official and they did not want to claim anything in an official capacity. This state of affairs was present despite the researcher explicitly guaranteeing anonymity and confidentiality. However, they were able to provide insights based on informal discussions. In the case of family members, the reasons were similar. Despite these challenges, all participants provided in-depth insights throughout the project regarding caregiving, PWD behavioural changes, social interactions, the impact of social environment on their quality-of-life, therapeutically successful methods and instruments used.

Initial explorations and framing the design problem

Based on the user insights, some key themes were identified that served as the design goals: empathise with PWD, encourage active involvement and establish dialogue. Based on the possibilities, we focused on a mobile app, *DCare*, for initiating conversations, reminiscing and sharing experiences, self-care and reflection for caregivers, as well as dementia care awareness. Solutions, such as mobile apps, which are easily customisable and have a wide reach can be useful for a larger segment of caregivers.

There are existing apps that focus on dementia awareness, facilitating therapies, activities and maintaining a daily schedule (reminders etc.) with the possibility of being used by both PWD and caregivers. However, in the current case, the caregivers did not possess such apps. They were connected to each other through WhatsApp groups created by a common health consultant or neuropsychologist, as this was the preferred mode of digital interaction in this sector.

Some of the existing apps focus on all the possible aspects related to dementia like therapy, insurance, counseling, activities, among others, which not only increase the complexity of the solution but also dilute the overall solution at times. Based on the interviews and the generic themes of dementia in India, a few key aspects of the app are highlighted:

1. Creating a journey for dementia care (app grows and learns from caregiver experiences) – track experiences, dynamic prompts, personalised suggestions.
2. Getting informed about dementia in a *progressive* manner – this included care suggestions and advice based on the experience, the underlying symptoms of PWD and issues faced in providing efficient care by the caregivers, thus, making it a personalised care awareness by exposing the caregivers to the right information at the right time.
3. Encouraging social bonding, not just therapies – the app will encourage social behaviours through nudges and features targeted to bring caregivers and PWD together at various touchpoints over the course of caregiving. For example, the app could nudge users to spend some time with caregivers on a daily basis by setting up target hours in a week to spend with caregivers. Findings from the user studies suggest that collaborative activities, daily or weekly, could help caregivers and PWD to come together and create/do something which initiates conversations, improving the social interactions that could be useful for both PWD and caregivers. Sharing the results and experiences of such activity in the community would help users to be encouraged and establish social recognition for the caregivers.
4. Care for caregivers – it is important for caregivers to be conscious of their own psychological, emotional and physical wellbeing in order to provide healthy caregiving and improve the quality of life for both PWD and caregivers. Understanding the caregiver's emotional state and stress levels would allow the app to provide necessary suggestions to overcome caregiver challenges.
5. Community – there are many active dementia groups on social networks such as Facebook where people share their stories and caregiver experiences. People provide strong emotional support and caregiving suggestions; this motivates the caregivers and helps them understand

that they are not alone in this journey. Such communities provide strong emotional support. One of the features could be finding caregivers locally to connect with them in the physical world.

Design concept and information architecture

A number of central ideas was discussed based on insights from the user studies. We finalised on a design concept that kept activities at the central idea. The major highlight of this concept was to provide new engagement for caregivers and PWD through activities on the platform as well as suggestions to spend time together. Apart from engagement, having nudges like activity points (AP) and activity reminders could also be motivators for caregivers to attempt the activities with PWD. The activities could be done together in group sessions to share more experiences across the community of caregivers. After the design concept, the information architecture was defined.

Initial prototype

The initial prototype had five main sections ranging from content to care journey (a–e). All these five sections were developed in greater detail. In addition, two main aspects of Care guide for non-English-speaking caregivers and motivational nudges, which (f–g) that were included in the prototype, are also discussed.

a) Content

The home section provides information to help the caregiver engage with the app. This includes personalised recommendations from each of the other sections (Activities, Community, Care journey, Care guide). This also houses dynamic information like achievements, therapist appointments and recommendations. Another noticeable emphasis was prioritising messages over notifications to allow caregivers to connect with each other.

b) Onboarding

The app begins by asking the language preference of the first-time users. Once this is done, the onboarding starts, and the caregiver journey begins. Here, the primary information such as care experience, the purpose of using the app, and dedicated time spent with PWD is collected. This information is supposed to help in curating personalised experiences based on the preferences and care experiences of the caregiver. This personalisation could be useful in suggesting care activities and the dementia knowledge sources that were recommended, as well as helping people to connect with other community members on the app.

c) Activities

This section was designed to have daily activities, suggestions based on PWD and caregiver experiences of doing the activity. Such preferences could be personalised by taking feedback after each activity to help suggest similar activities in the future. Apart from being a medium for interaction, the activities could also accommodate various dementia therapies that are already being used. The focus in this project was more towards how activities will be conducted rather than designing new activities or exploring the published literature to assess how effective they are. Therefore, activities like drawing/creating art from the pool of activities, which are usually recommended by doctors, were chosen for the app. These activities could be in the real world outside the app, with physical interactions, and need not have any reliance on the app.

A key challenge in creating new activities is to decide how long the platform would take to create new activities, which could then be used by caregivers. This might question the value of the activities when created at such a large scale and might challenge the business viability in the long run. One of the ways to address this challenge is to crowdsource the activities from independent developers by giving them guidelines on the criticalities of designing activities for caregivers and PWD. These activities would later be validated by experts before they could be launched on the app platform.

In order to accommodate a wide variety of categories, the categories can be mainly categorised in terms of therapeutic and non-therapeutic activities. Therapeutic activities are the ones which are focused on targeting a particular type of activity. These could be physical, cognitive, behavioural, communicative, among others, conducted with the caregivers in the physical space using prompts from the app, such as colouring; while the non-therapeutic activities include less-directed activity, such as simply spending time outdoors. To keep the community linked and establish interactions with other caregivers, daily activities are proposed so that users can follow the guided activity regime. These would allow the caregivers to share results of common activities and bond over the results created by the people they care for.

d) Community

From the user feedback, it was observed that finding fellow caregivers and sharing experiences was not always the preferred way for Indian families, especially when there are significant differences in demographics, culture, language and the way people share stories. Moreover, the idea of bringing people in close geographies together to encourage physical interactions was used as the central idea for the community section of the app. Apart from geography, other factors were also considered to recommend caregivers to find and connect with other users on the platform. These factors could include the level of care experience, similar interest in activities, among others. Allowing users to find local caregivers could also be the first step towards creating a healthier offline community of caregivers, like local chapters, who could meet for different workshops and dementia awareness events.

e) Care journey

From the primary and secondary research, it was observed that apart from activities, reminiscence was the most adopted way to go for the caregivers to spend quality time with PWD, and most of the interventions discussed in the secondary research revolved around this idea. There were two major aspects that were required to make reminiscence an easily adaptable feature. One was an easy creation of memories. This could come through direct upload of significant pictures, instances or stories, both past and present moments, from activity sessions. The second was to have a different view for the caregivers and PWD to reminisce; i.e. caregivers would be interested in more detailed ways of visiting previous events while PWD might respond to a simpler interface. It was therefore decided to offer both complex and simpler modes of reminiscence aimed at caregivers and PWD respectively.

f) Care guides

From primary research, it was observed how important it was for caregivers and PWD to have access to the right information about dementia from the early stage based on personalised recommendations and distribution of information in an effective manner to be easily consumed. Another highlight was language support. During the study, it was observed that most information on dementia and related care was in the English language, which restricted the use for non-English-speaking caregivers. Therefore, major spoken languages were included, and the user was allowed to choose the language for the app in the setting references stage.

g)   Motivational nudges

These are the triggers (or notifications) that would encourage and motivate the users to use the app through prompts, incentives, reminders, achievements, etc. These could be through completing activities (Activity Points), reminders about new activities, suggested articles, achievements on sharing memories (Memory Points). It was observed that motivation to achieve these milestones and reward points might fade away if they are attained too easily by caregivers or if there was no potential use of these points in the in future. Therefore, the earned points and rewards could be planned to be used in buying/obtaining dementia care-related products or services.

Evaluation of preliminary prototype

Three caregivers (two male, one female) from two families were recruited for the preliminary feedback on the ideas through known connections and the help of neuropsychologists. Once they agreed to participate, the meeting links were sent to the users. One of the users reported that they liked the idea of how the emotions were tracked and used for caregivers for an in-depth journey of past events. However, the users found the representation too detailed for the caregivers to revisit them with the PWD and therefore had to be simplified. This encouraged the need to have an alternate view to revisit the memory which was later embedded as a dedicated mode for revisiting memories called 'reminiscence mode'. Over discussion with other users and participants, it was observed that the term 'reminiscence' might turn out to be a little complex (although precise) for people to remember and use. Therefore, the 'reminiscence mode' was later then termed as 'Memory Lane'. This turned out to be easier to remember than the word 'reminiscence'.

Participants also found ideas for motivational nudges through activity points and care points interesting. This also led to a discussion on how these points could be used and how caregivers could be motivated to earn more points. Therefore, a couple of potential use cases were identified. One was to use these points to avail offers with dementia-related services like psychologist fees or buying dementia-care–related products like fall detection devices, PWD location monitoring, among others. The concept of developing a community allowing users to connect to caregivers in nearby localities and connect with people with similar demographics cultural backgrounds turned out to be the most interesting use case for people to find caregivers around. This feature was the result of observations from the various dementia support groups that one of the authors joined on Facebook to understand the kind of experiences, feelings and the general mood.

Improvements in prototypes

After the preliminary set of ideas, the observations about missing affordances were identified based on the questions asked by the users when they had doubts. As a result, for the final design, the user interface (UI) layout was designed keeping the principles of Google's Material Design Language in mind. In order to improve the visual properties and keep the inclusivity of users in mind, web accessibility tests and colour blindness tests were also conducted on the interface designed. This was important to make sure the elements of the interface are easily identifiable. To ensure legibility, we used the standards of Web Content Accessibility Guidelines 2.0 (WCAG2.0). For contrast, we used the Figma A11y-Color Contrast Checker.

Second evaluation

Since the designs were done remotely, a similar approach to that used in the preliminary evaluation was adopted, where users were invited to participate using a link. However, this approach was not able to monitor user interactions while using the app. Therefore, for this phase of the study, we explored possible solutions to have such evaluation and eventually adopted a remote testing tool Loopback™ which allowed observers (designers/evaluators) to see how the participant was interacting on the screen while using the app and their behaviour in physical space could also be observed through the front camera and microphone on their phones.

We engaged two new caregivers and one neuropsychologist who agreed to participate in this second evaluation. Since the number of participants was fewer, we decided to have qualitative feedback from the participants to validate the other data. The feedback was taken with a set of questions common for each participant to record their own experience and usefulness of the app. The users were also asked to navigate the app for the first five minutes on their own and then were asked to open an activity, see the details and finish the activity by uploading a picture (clickables were designed to replicate the live app behaviour).

The evaluation was conducted with two key ideas as central:

1. The inclination towards adopting such products with the available features, along with validating the claim that having such a system can bring caregivers and PWD closer.
2. The usability of the app.

In order to further understand usability, the user was asked to open a particular activity and perform the interaction until the activity was completed and saved into memory. We also noticed the points where the user hesitated/took time/was confused when asked to think aloud while performing the task. Most of the participants saw value in using the app if customised new and interesting activities were shared on a regular basis which could be used for interacting with PWD.

Another appreciated feature of the app was the ease in finding local caregivers and forming a community/companionship with fellow caregivers. There were no significant challenges that were faced while navigating the app. However, one of the users highlighted that having too many options on the home page led to a confusion of choice and presumed direction. Most of the users could navigate through the app even without much external assistance. Participants also liked the idea of progressive onboarding in each section when visiting for the first time. Based on the feedback, the final screens were designed (Figure 11.2 a & b).

Discussion and conclusion

This chapter has described the design of the *DCare app* to support Indian home caregivers and the families of PWD. The Indian caregiving ecology reflects the lack of dementia awareness and the unique challenges of caregiving in Indian families. The task of caregiving exacts its toll both mentally and physically. Therefore, the design of the app was based on user studies and subsequent evaluations. A few final themes can be gleaned from the app journey that will be helpful for the future development of digital health working with the Indian caregiving ecology.

a) Value and lifetime of the application

Feedback from experts suggested that *DCare* could be a valuable aid at an early stage of dementia when caregivers are new to the role of caregiving. If the app could help them prepare more

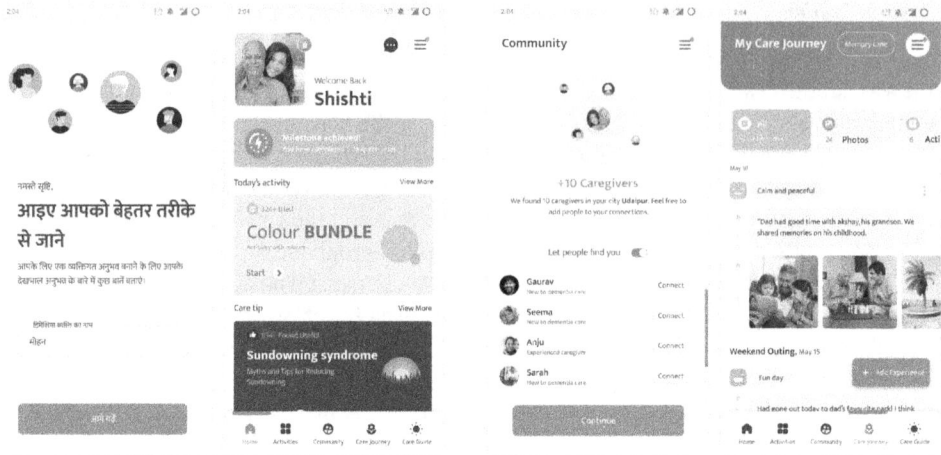

Figure 11.2 Composite images of the final screens. Designs by the author

effectively, this could have great benefits. The purpose of putting activities at the centre was to provide support and stimulation for caregivers, which might lead them to use the app for a longer period of time.

b)   Content

The knowledge available on the topic of dementia is vast and the amount of research that is being done is extensive. This might be both an advantage as well as a disadvantage. Before the content is made available to the user, material from various sources needs to be verified to be published on the app. Another challenge would be bringing new updated activities, which might not be a feasible solution in the long run for a few stakeholders. Therefore, collaborations with independent developers could be of huge help.

c)   Supporting caregiving in the early and mid-stages of dementia

Dementia has a very broad spectrum of cognitive, behavioural, psychological symptoms, and thus it is hard to design and develop a common solution. As a result, the app is most suitable for early to mid-stage dementia. At an early stage, it could help the caregivers adjust mentally and psychologically to their tasks, while at a later stage, activities and reminiscence could be valuable to maintain the social bond between the caregiver and PWD.

d)   Development

Since the app heavily relies on learning from the experiences of caregivers, PWD behaviour, as well as changes in symptoms through activities, it requires the use of machine learning to understand such changes in behaviour to recommend suitable content to the caregivers. Due to the lack of such apps targeting caregivers, there is a need for mobile healthcare applications that build on a strong application of interaction design and digital analytics.

In conclusion, the major contribution of the app in the care domain is the personalised experience which is the core requirement of any dementia-related support. In the future, augmenting the use of the app with smart wearables will be able to enhance the use and recommendation of the app on a larger scale. This will help caregivers understand the emotional wellbeing of PWD and help them connect with each other more effectively.

Supplementary material

The final screens can be viewed as a working prototype at the following link: https://bit.ly/3QEeFPy.

Acknowledgements

The authors would like to thank all the participants involved in the study and the conceptualisation and development of the work. These wonderful people have taken the time to show us a slice of their life and the challenges of living with dementia in India. We are very grateful to them.

Notes

1 Many such experiential products and technologies are being researched and developed globally. These include, i) interactive products such as *Turnaround* (Houben et al., 2020) and *SwayTheBand* (Morrissey, McCarthy & Pantidi, 2017) that facilitate collaborative turn-taking, often around the milieu of music; ii) audio-visual interfaces such as *SmartPyramid* (Huber, Berner, Uhlig, Klein, & Hurtienne, 2019), *PicGo* (Lee et al., 2014) and *CIRCA* (Astell et al., 2010); iii) virtual reality experiences (García-Betances, Jiménez-Mixco, Arredondo & Cabrera-Umpiérrez, 2015); iv) tangible devices such as *Dementia Soundboard* (Houben et al., 2019) and *Laugh Toolkit* ('Design for Dementia – LAUGH Project', 2022); iv) exercise games such as *Mobiassist* (Unbehaun et al., 2018) that aid in collaborative motion sessions.
2 The study was provided ethical clearance through the Institutional Review Board, Indian Institute of Technology Bombay (IITB-IRB/2021/017).

References

Astell, A. J., Ellis, M. P., Bernardi, L., Alm, N., Dye, R., Gowans, G., & Campbell, J. (2010). Using a touch screen computer to support relationships between people with dementia and caregivers. *Interacting with Computers*, *22*(4), 267–275.

Chakravorty, S., Goli, S., & James, K. S. (2021). Family demography in India: Emerging patterns and its challenges. *SAGE Open*, *11*(2). http://doi.org/10.1177/21582440211008178

Choudhary, A., Ranjan, J., & Asthana, H. (2021). Prevalence of dementia in India: A systematic review and meta-analysis. *Indian Journal of Public Health*, *2*(2), 152.

Design Council. (2022). *Framework for innovation: Design council's evolved double diamond*. Retrieved August 2, 2022, from https://www.designcouncil.org.uk/our-work/skills-learning/tools-frameworks/framework-for-innovation-design-councils-evolved-double-diamond/

Design for Dementia - LAUGH Project. (2022). *Design for dementia*. LAUGH Project. https://laughproject.info/

García-Betances, R. I., Jiménez-Mixco, V., Arredondo, M. T., & Cabrera-Umpiérrez, M. F. (2015). Using virtual reality for cognitive training of the elderly. *American Journal of Alzheimer's Disease and Other Dementias*, *30*(1), 49–54. http://doi.org/10.1177/1533317514545866

Guisado-Fernández, E., Giunti, G., Mackey, L. M., Blake, C., & Caulfield, B. M. (2019). Factors influencing the adoption of smart health technologies for people with dementia and their informal caregivers: Scoping review and design framework. *JMIR Aging*, *2*(1), e12192–e12192.

Houben, M., Lehn, B., van den Brink, N., Diks, S., Verhoef, J., & Brankaert, R. (2020). *Turnaround: Exploring care relations in dementia through design*. Presented at the Extended Abstracts of the 2020 CHI Conference on Human Factors in Computing Systems. Association for Computing Machinery, pp. 1–8. http://doi.org/10.1145/3334480.3382846

Huber, S., Berner, R., Uhlig, M., Klein, P., & Hurtienne, J. O. R. (2019). *Tangible objects for reminiscing in dementia care*. Presented at the Proceedings of the Thirteenth International Conference on Tangible. Embedded, and Embodied Interaction. Association for Computing Machinery, pp. 15–24. http://doi.org/10.1145/3294109.3295632

Kumar, C. S., George, S., & Kallivayalil, R. A. (2019). Towards a dementia-friendly India. *Indian Journal of Psychological Medicine, 41*(5), 476–481.

Lee, H.-C., Cheng, Y. F., Cho, S. Y., Tang, H.-H., Hsu, J., & Chen, C.-H. (2014). *Picgo: Designing reminiscence and storytelling for the elderly with photo annotation*. Presented at the Proceedings of the 2014 Companion Publication on Designing Interactive Systems. Association for Computing Machinery, pp. 9–12. http://doi.org/10.1145/2598784.2602769

Lieber, J., Clarke, L., Timæus, I. M., Mallinson, P. A. C., & Kinra, S. (2020). Changing family structures and self-rated health of India's older population (1995–96 to 2014). *SSM - Population Health, 11*. https://doi.org/100572–100572.

Morrissey, K., McCarthy, J., & Pantidi, N. (2017). *The value of experience-centred design approaches in dementia research contexts*. Presented at the Proceedings of the 2017 CHI Conference on Human Factors in Computing Systems. Association for Computing Machinery, pp. 1326–1338. http://doi.org/10.1145/3025453.3025527

Muhammad, T., Balachandran, A., & Srivastava, S. (2021). Socio-economic and health determinants of preference for separate living among older adults: A cross-sectional study in India. *PLoS One, 16*(4), e0249828. http://doi.org/10.1371/journal.pone.0249828

Ravindranath, V., & Sundarakumar, J. S. (2021). Changing demography and the challenge of dementia in India. *Nature Reviews. Neurology, 17*(12), 747–758.

Sachdev, P. S. (2022). Social health, social reserve and dementia. *Current Opinion in Psychiatry, 35*(2), 111–117. http://doi.org/10.1097/YCO.0000000000000779

Sathianathan, R., & Kantipudi, S. J. (2018). The dementia epidemic: Impact, prevention, and challenges for India. *Indian Journal of Psychiatry, 60*(2), 165–167.

Sinha, S., Prasad, I., & Prasad, P. (2020). Dementia and the challenges of caregiving: A personal account. *Economic and Political Weekly, 55*(14).

Srivastava, S., Thalil, M., Rashmi, R., & Paul, R. (2021). Association of family structure with gain and loss of household headship among older adults in India: Analysis of panel data. *PLoS One, 16*(6), e0252722. http://doi.org/10.1371/journal.pone.0252722

Unbehaun, D., Vaziri, D., Aal, K., Li, Q., Wieching, R., & Wulf, V. (2018). *MobiAssist - ICT-based training system for people with dementia and their caregivers: Results from a field study*. Presented at the Proceedings of the 2018 ACM Conference on Supporting Groupwork. Association for Computing Machinery, pp. 122–126. http://doi.org/10.1145/3148330.3154513

Vernooij-Dassen, M., & Jeon, Y.-H. (2016). Social health and dementia: The power of human capabilities. *International Psychogeriatrics, 1*, 1–3.

World Health Organisation. (2012). *Dementia: A public health priority*. World Health Organisation. https://www.who.int/publications/i/item/dementia-a-public-health-priority

12 The adaptation of the dementia village model

Comparing design features of a Dutch and Canadian dementia village

Jodi Sturge

Introduction

Without a cure for dementia, and limited treatment interventions (Gauthier et al., 2016), there is a focus on providing care that supports quality of life and living well with dementia (Vernooij-Dassen & Jeon, 2016). The COVID-19 pandemic further highlighted the vulnerability of people with dementia with additional health risks brought on by social isolation and challenges in recalling measures to decrease the chance of infection (Vernooij-Dassen et al., 2020; Wang et al., 2020). Dementia is a syndrome that includes a range of symptoms often associated with challenges in cognitive functioning, such as speech, spatial and temporal impairments. Dementia mainly occurs in older adults; however, it can develop in younger people, affecting more women than men (Livingston et al., 2020). Experts predict that, due to an overall ageing population, over 152.8 million people worldwide will experience some form of dementia by 2050 (Nichols et al., 2022). This global trend will lead to significant public health, social and economic concerns for people living with dementia, their families and society (Gilbert et al., 2019). To best support people with dementia, there is a movement toward a dementia-friendly society and designs promoting orientation, safety and intuitive usability (World Health Organization, 2021). Several studies have shown how environmental factors and designs can influence persons with dementia (Marquardt et al., 2014). For instance, environments for people with dementia should include features that facilitate orientation and wayfinding, limit noise and distracting sounds and avoid confusion by avoiding mirrors and shiny materials (Fleming & Purandare, 2010). Persons with dementia can also have age-related impairments such as problems with vision and hearing, which make the environmental design necessary. Therefore, there is a need to design care models that reflect the diverse needs of people with dementia, where each person is unique in their personality, life story, needs and preferences.

Dementia Villages: a dementia care innovation

The Netherlands has been leading the re-design of dementia care through the creation of small-scale, home-like environments, including the well-known dementia village (Pedro et al., 2020; Verbeek et al., 2009; Vinick, 2019). A dementia village is considered a pioneering, experimental health care model (Chrysikou et al., 2018; Haeusermann, 2018) that, as described on the founding agency's website, is a place for 'normal life for people living with severe dementia' (The Hogeweyk, 2023). The first dementia village, known as The Hogeweyk, opened in 2009 in Weesp, a small town approximately 30 kilometres south of Amsterdam in the Netherlands. The Hogeweyk model was designed to increase the quality of life of people with dementia by creating an environment focused on physical activity, social interaction and autonomy, including amenities found in most neighbourhoods (Chrysikou et al., 2018). Due to the novelty of the model, the site hosts

DOI: 10.4324/9781003318262-16

several delegations from around the world. The model has since been replicated and adapted in Canada, Denmark, France, Italy, Norway and the United States (Geuna, 2020). One example of a dementia village inspired by the Dutch model is the Langley Village (The Village, 2023). The Langley Village, located 50 kilometres from the Vancouver international airport in Langley, British Columbia, Canada, is known to be Canada's first dementia village.

A few academic reflections have described site visits and impressions of the dementia village in the Netherlands (Jenkins & Smythe, 2013; Morgan et al., 2019), including the architectural typology (Chrysikou et al., 2018); plus, a few qualitative studies of Dutch-inspired dementia villages in Australia (Tierney et al., 2022), Germany (Haeusermann, 2018) and Denmark (Hansen et al., 2021; Kielsgaard et al., 2021; Peoples et al., 2020). A common finding among these international studies is the need for community and meaningful engagement opportunities within and beyond the village. However, neither of these studies reflected how the model was translated into a different context. Therefore, this chapter describes some similarities and differences between the design features of two dementia villages, one in the Netherlands and one in Canada.

Site visit observations

This chapter is based on observations made during site tours of both sites. The first site tour took place at the Hogeweyk in April 2019. The tour was scheduled in the morning for a half-day site visit hosted by one of the founders of the care concept. The second visit to the Langley Village site occurred two years later, in October 2021. This site visit was an overnight stay arranged by the executive director of the Langley Village. During both visits, a walking tour of the site was provided by both representatives, where we visited most of the spaces in the village, including the residents' homes, grocery stores and cafes. As visitors, we were permitted to take photos of the environment but no photos of the residents. Based on observations and photos from the site tours, the characteristics of these villages are presented in five themes: 1) first impressions, 2) size and layout, 3) architecture and design, 4) café spaces and 5) grocery store.

1)   First impressions

One of the most comparable features of these two sites is their physical location. Both locations are tucked away in residential areas. To visit the Hogeweyk, I arrived by train at Weesp and walked 15 minutes to the site. The most convenient way to get to the Canadian site was by car. However, a bus stop was located less than a ten-minute walk from the site. Despite being located in residential areas, both villages are gated communities that keep the residents inside the Village for their safety. The Hogeweyk is enclosed by a continuous brick wall, while the Langley Village is enclosed through a combination of structures, including a two-storey building and high wooden fences. Upon arriving at the sites, both had a receptionist at the site entrance to greet guests and family members and prevent residents from leaving the site unsupervised. Both sites had a quiet atmosphere and natural features, such as trees. Compared to the Dutch model, the Langley Village feels more spacious with a better overview of the site, possibly because it is surrounded by large cedar trees, which are typical of British Columbia. In both villages, staff did not wear uniforms but wore name tags to designate them as staff members. However, as the Canadian village tour happened during COVID-19, staff and visitors were more distinguishable where they had to wear masks, but residents did not. Vehicle access was limited to commercial deliveries and emergency services at both sites. For relatives visiting the Village, their vehicles were parked outside the perimeter of the Village.

The cost of living in the Villages is comparable – approximately 5,000 euros per month in the Netherlands and 4,800 – 5,200 euros ($6,000–7,000 Canadian dollars) at the Village. Therefore, living in a dementia village is cost-prohibitive for most people in the Netherlands and Canada without a government subsidy.

2) Size and layout

The Hogeweyk is home to 152 residents with dementia who live in clusters of six residents in 23 small houses and have open access to village amenities such as a grocery store, hair salon and cafe (Chrysikou et al., 2018; Glass 2014). Services such as meals, social events and adult day services allow the facility to integrate into the community as a support hub for residents and those in the broader community (Glass, 2014). In the early days of operation, care was organised by grouping residents into seven lifestyle choices determined by the provider: i) homey, simple life, ii) Christian, iii) craftsman, iv) arts and culture, v) aristocracy, (vi) Indonesian and (vii) urban (Glass, 2014). These lifestyle themes have since changed to reflect the backgrounds of the residents.

In comparison, Langley Village is a smaller model with a capacity of 78 residents who reside among six single-storey houses. The Village includes several amenities for residents, including a cafe, activity rooms, a hair salon and a general store. Unlike the Dutch Village, the houses are designated by the level of care (ranging from assisted living to long-term care) instead of a lifestyle. However, in the Canadian Village, each resident had a private washroom; in the original model, residents had a shared toilet and washroom. Resident rooms in both sites have views of outdoor spaces, and residents are encouraged to bring their furniture to customise their space and make their rooms their own. Most resident rooms are for single occupancy. However, there are limited rooms available for couples. Furnishings throughout both villages are more of a home-like style than institutional.

3) Architecture and design

As expected, the architecture is dramatically different between the two sites. The housing architecture in Hogeweyk resembles housing in the outside Dutch society. As seen in Figure 12.1a, the architecture of the housing units and buildings in the Hogeweyk is similar to the colour and material of housing architecture and street design seen throughout the Netherlands. The houses are made of brick with garden spaces and metal fences and are arranged along pathways that resemble streets made of brick. The street signage in the Hogeweyk reflects Dutch public space; street signs are on metal plates with a blue background and white text.

In comparison, the cottage style and the colour choices of the houses in Langley Village (Figure 12.1b) are less similar to the typical housing style and public space that are seen throughout British Columbia. The resident homes in Langley Village are arranged along a wide, meandering roadway that is not typical of a streetscape outside the Village, and the paint colour (e.g. bright pink) is not common beyond the Village. The landscape architecture, such as a rock garden enclosed by a fence, is a style more typically seen in holiday resorts than in typical neighbourhoods or villages. In addition, the type of asphalt and the sidewalks are unique to the Village and not typical of other residential spaces in the surrounding area. In comparison, there were no typical street signs on the Canadian site. However, there was clear signage with arrows (illuminated at night) pointing the way to various locations in the Village.

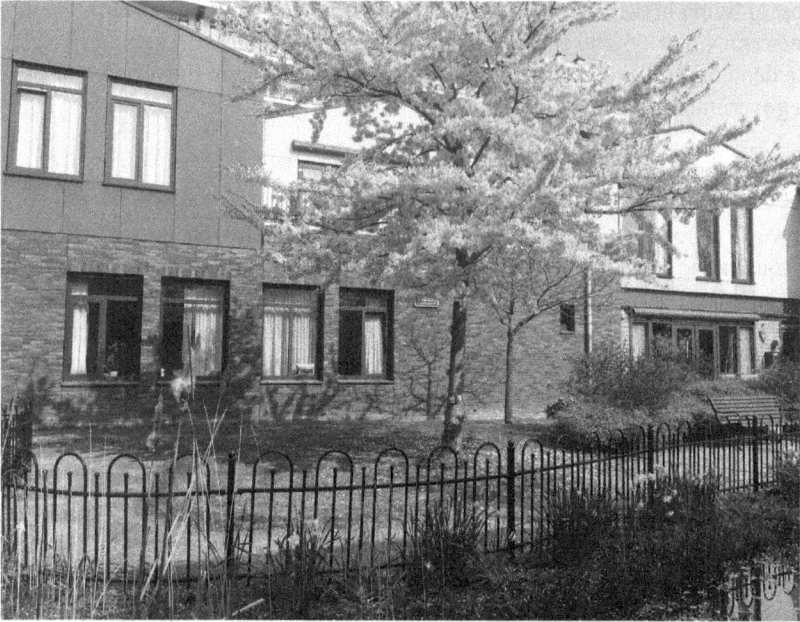

Figure 12.1a Example of housing typology in Hogeweyk

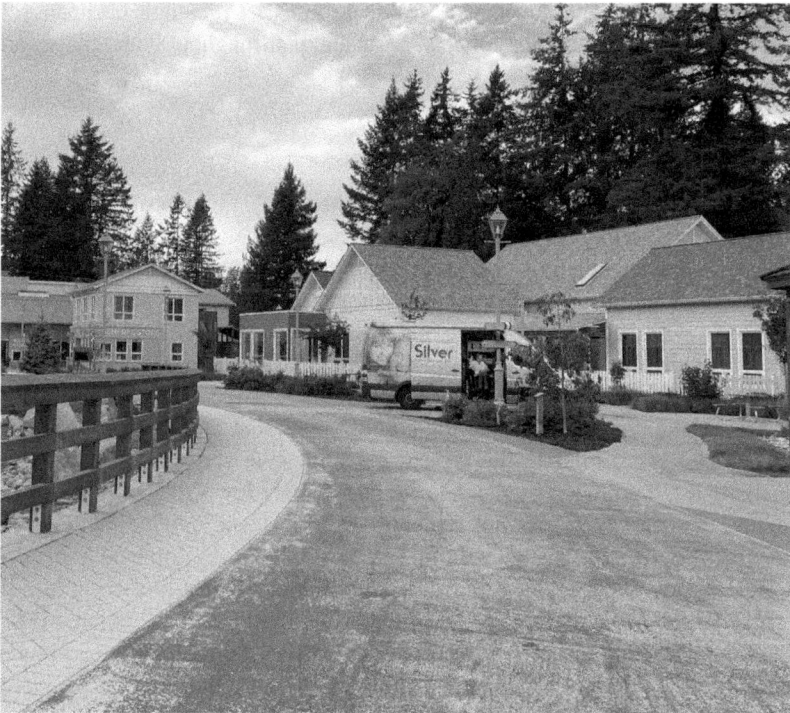

Figure 12.1b Example of housing typology in Langley Village

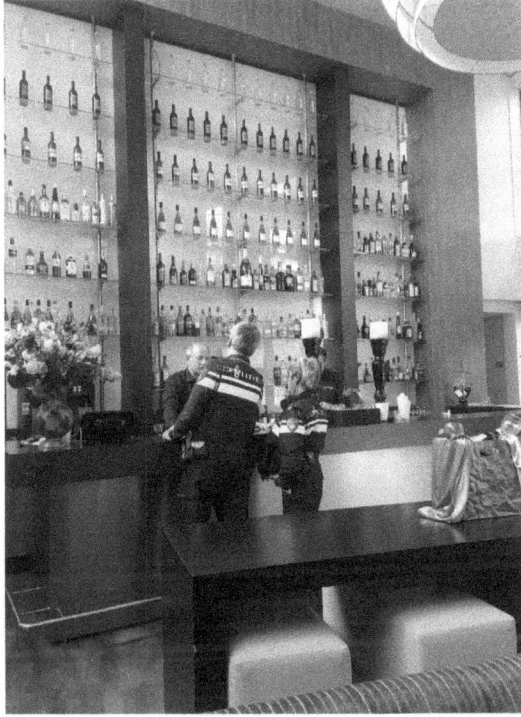

Figure 12.2a Cafe counter space in Hogeweyk

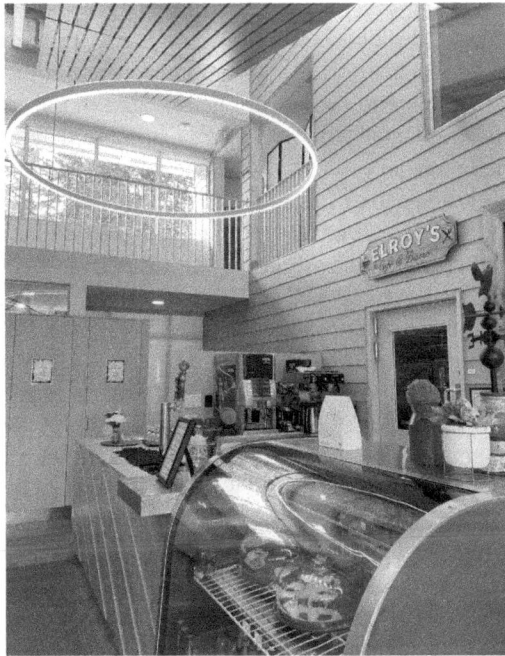

Figure 12.2b Cafe counter space in Langely Village

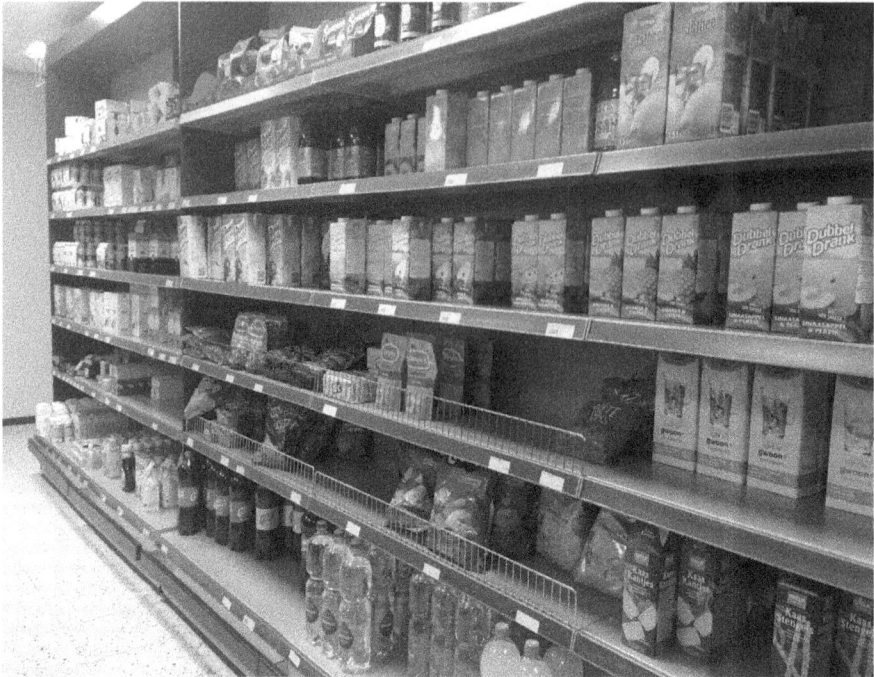

Figure 12.3a Products displayed in Hogeweyk grocery store

4) Cafe spaces

The size, function and interior design of the cafes were dramatically different. The cafe space at the Hogeweyk resembles the interior of a restaurant, as seen in most public spaces in the Netherlands. As seen in the image to the left in Figure 12.2 (a), the cafe counter space in the Hogeweyk resembles a typical Dutch cafe with a large size and function. The restaurant has a full-service kitchen, a menu and an extensive wine and beer menu. This space is open to residents and the general public and can be rented for private events.

In comparison, the cafe space at the Langley Village is much smaller and is similar to counter spaces seen in institutional settings such as libraries or hospitals in British Columbia. The cafe space does not have an extensive menu; however, like in the Hogeweyk, the residents and visitors can purchase coffee, beer, wine and snacks. As seen in Figure 12.2(b), behind the counter, the wall furnishing the 'Elroy's Café' sign is attached to a wall that resembles the outside of a building, providing a theatrical impression of the space. The combination of the sign and the inside wooden wall is designed to look like an outside wall, and the open space above the café does not resemble any common public space beyond the Village. Furthermore, above the cafe counter space, an open space with a metal railing is part of the staff-only area. This arrangement and layout give a sense of surveillance.

5) Grocery stores

Both sites have stores where residents can purchase grocery items: the Hogeweyk Super in the Hogeweyk and the General Store in the Langley Village. Similar to observations made in café

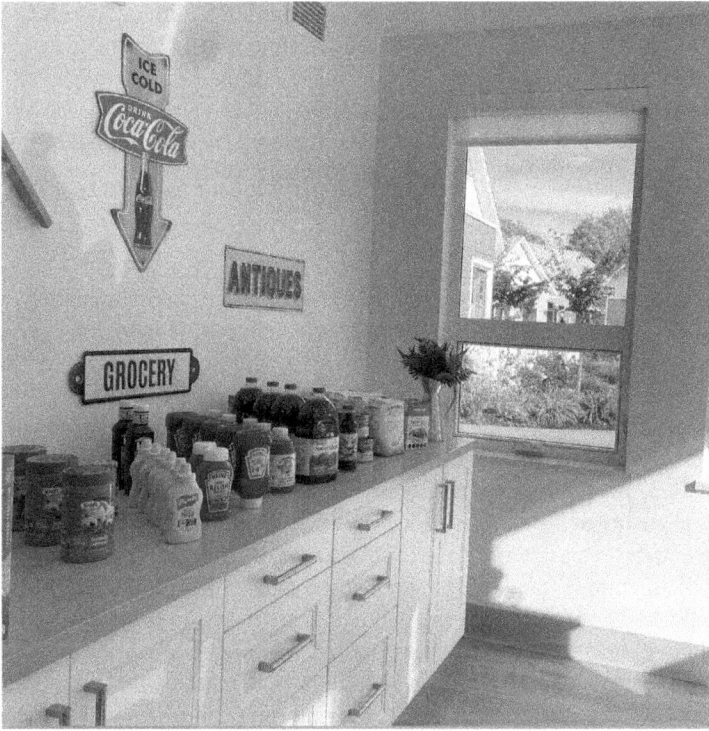

Figure 12.3b Products displayed in Langley Village grocer

spaces, the scale of the grocery store is much larger and typical of public space at the Hogeweyk compared to the Langley Village. Both sites have a counter space where residents can pay for products independently and interact with staff. The setup of the Dutch model includes features such as grocery carts and a moving conveyor belt as seen in a typical supermarket. The products in the Hogeweyk are displayed in an aisle format similar to a grocery store layout beyond the village (Figure 12.3a). The Langley Village grocer is smaller and has a similar layout to a British Columbia convenience store. There are no aisles and far fewer products in the Langley Village. The products are displayed on a counter space with a combination of decorative signage above (for cola, groceries and antiques) (Figure 12.3b).

General reflections

Dementia villages are an innovative dementia care intervention that has become a healthcare buzz trend in several countries. With design elements inspired by the hospitality industry, this care approach is a step away from the traditional institutional care environment. Although dementia villages are a secure environment, once inside, there is a sense of freedom, and without apparent barriers, it does not feel like a gated community. A dementia village approach allows for a safe environment where people with dementia can wander and live. The model supports the notion that if a secure environment is essential for safety, people with dementia must suffer as little as possible with measures in place to promote the feeling of freedom (Landeweer et al., 2021). However, the out-of-the-way locations of these two villages appear to keep people with dementia separated from normal society. This observation is similar to those of other critics who argue that dementia-specific villages are a form of segregation based on an illness where people are segregated in a place resembling a neighbourhood but with no access to communities (Graham, 2021; Hansen et al., 2021; Rahman & Swaffer, 2018; Steele et al., 2020). Integrating the dementia villages within more central areas of towns and cities, as seen in Denmark (Kielsgaard et al., 2021), would allow the village and the residents to be more integrated into a more realistic, diverse, mixed-generational society.

Design decisions

Both sites are designed to resemble a town or village. These 'micro societies' are said to be dementia-inclusive, where they contain a society in which people with dementia can fully participate (World Health Organization, 2021). However, within both villages, not all features of the built and social environments are common or 'normal' in society outside the village. For instance, there are few vehicles, no shops to buy clothing, and no bikes or children moving through the streets. Additionally, as described in this chapter and noted by other researchers (Chrysikou et al., 2018; Haeusermann, 2018; Huang et al., 2022; Lorey, 2019), these societies have theatrical elements or holiday resort features that do not resemble 'real' society. This type of design can be described as dementia deception and can cause some residents to become restless and agitated when they know they are staying in a fake environment (Huang et al., 2022). To avoid this, dementia village architects and designers need to take note of all details of surrounding neighbourhoods and reflect as many ordinary society references and public space features as possible to support the wellbeing of people with dementia (Chrysikou et al., 2018; Van Steenwinkel et al., 2016; Sturge et al., 2021). In addition, the designs within dementia villages should be dementia-friendly. A dementia-friendly design approach essentially means making design decisions that compensate for impaired cognition by promoting orientation, safety and intuitive usability (Kirch & Marquardt, 2021). For example, contrasting colour schemes on the walls and furniture to enable orientation, navigation and mobility (Marquardt et al., 2014). As described in this chapter, the design of the grocery store and layout of products at the 'Hogeweyk Super' (Figure 12.3a) is more 'familiar' compared to the Canadian store. However, the organisation of the products in Langley Village is considered dementia-friendly, where people with dementia prefer grocery store layouts with fewer products compared to shelves with many products (Brorsson et al., 2020). These observations present a design conflict between making spaces in dementia villages 'familiar' or dementia-friendly, where it can be challenging to do both. Community visioning activities, including people with dementia living in the community (Roberts & Shehadeh, 2021), could help guide the direction of these design decisions to ensure that such design features are appropriate and accessible.

Standardisation and evaluation

Comparing the two villages, there are noted similarities and differences. The main similarity is that both sites are purpose-built dementia villages with clustered housing for people with moderate to severe dementia. Differences were observed in the architecture and design of amenity spaces. These differences could be related to the culture, creativity and values of the design team and architect; however, other contributing factors could exist. Translating the Dutch model to other countries may be challenging with different styles of architecture, budgets, building regulations and healthcare systems. This translation can be further complicated without a standard definition describing what a dementia village is (Kielsgaard et al., 2021) or published design principles that describe and guide the design process. This lack of clarity is similar to other 'in-vogue' healthcare architecture phenomena, such as healing architecture (Simonsen et al., 2022) and home-like environments (Marquardt et al., 2014). Neither of these concepts has a clear definition or design principles, making it challenging to create these types of architecture as intended. Therefore, a standard definition of a dementia village is required, followed by design principles to guide the development of sites internationally. This toolset should be research-based, reflect lessons learnt and describe how regulations (e.g. building or welfare systems) have influenced the design of a dementia village in different countries.

Although it has been suggested that the dementia model has been 'tried and tested' (Haeusermann, 2018, p. 150), no published post-occupancy evaluations have tested how the dementia model works to improve the quality of life for people with dementia. Therefore, more evidence is needed to understand and evaluate how specific features of the built environment of a dementia village work in practice. The perspectives of all users, including people with dementia, should be captured through an operational evaluation. Such knowledge would result in common indicators to test how dementia villages support or hinder residents' quality of life. Furthermore, it should be noted that dementia villages are not the silver-bullet solution for a complicated problem. There are limited beds in dementia villages, the cost of care is not affordable for most people and often spaces are allocated to people at the later stage of dementia. For people with limited incomes or at the early stage of dementia, a dementia village is not a suitable option. Therefore, more evidence-based, equitable healthcare solutions for dementia care have to be identified.

Limitations

This chapter is based on one-day observations: a limited amount of time spent compared to other studies. For instance, in the Haeusermann (2018) study, the author lived in a dementia village for four months, while Peoples et al. (2020) conducted observations over 12 days in Denmark. Longer, more frequent observations would allow for a more systematic, detailed understanding of how specific environmental features supported residents' mobility or engagement. Additionally, consultations with user groups (e.g. residents, staff and family) could enrich and contextualise observations and assumptions (as described in the Peoples et al. (2020) study). Furthermore, interviews with the architect and design team would provide insight into the care vision and challenges faced in translating the philosophy of the village to another context.

Conclusion

As we continue to reimagine what dementia care looks like, the dementia village model holds much promise. The dementia village model is a step away from the typical institutional residential care model that several countries have enthusiastically adapted. However, there are divided opinions on dementia villages. Some believe the model is ideal for providing care, while others are more critical, stating that the secured world is fake and deceptive. Based on observations from two site tours, one in the Netherlands and one in Canada, there are similarities and differences. Impressions from the site tours brought up questions including what a dementia village is, how design decisions are made, and how the villages work to improve the quality of life. The future designs of these villages should be based on evidence-based design principles derived from evaluations, best practices and research. This toolset needs to be inclusive of the perspective of people with dementia to ensure that no design assumptions are made. This approach to design will result in evidence-based care models that support autonomy and a better quality of life for older adults and people with dementia.

References

Brorsson, A., Öhman, A., Lundberg, S., Cutchin, M. P., & Nygård, L. (2020). How accessible are grocery shops for people with dementia? A qualitative study using photo documentation and focus group interviews. *Dementia, 19*(6), 1872–1888.

Chrysikou, E., Tziraki, C., & Buhalis, D. (2018). Architectural hybrids for living across the lifespan: Lessons from dementia. *The Service Industries Journal, 38*(1–2), 4–26.

Fleming, R., & Purandare, N. (2010). Long-term care for people with dementia: Environmental design guidelines. *International Psychogeriatrics, 22*(7), 1084–1096.

Gauthier, S., Albert, M., Fox, N., Goedert, M., Kivipelto, M., Mestre-Ferrandiz, J., & Middleton, L. T. (2016). Why has therapy development for dementia failed in the last two decades? *Alzheimer's and Dementia, 12*(1), 60–64.

Geuna, A. (2020). Examining end-of-life care spaces as 21st century collective living types. In F. Berlingieri, & F. Zanotto (Eds.), *Comparison: Conference for artistic and architectural research. Book of proceedings* (Vol. 1, p. 399). LetteraVentidue Edizioni.

Gilbert, J., Ward, L., & Gwinner, K. (2019). Quality nursing care in dementia specific care units: A scoping review. *Dementia, 18*(6), 2140–2157.

Glass, A. P. (2014). Innovative seniors housing and care models: What we can learn from the Netherlands. *Seniors Housing and Care Journal, 22*(1), 74–81.

Graham, M. E. (2021). The securitisation of dementia: Socialities of securitisation on secure dementia care units. *Ageing and Society, 41*(2), 439–455.

Haeusermann, T. (2018). The dementia village: Between community and society. In F. Krause (Eds.) et. al., *Care in Healthcare: Reflections on Theory and Practice* , (pp. 135–167). Palgrave Macmillan.

Hansen, T. E., Præstegaard, J., Tjørnhøj-Thomsen, T., Andresen, M., & Nørgaard, B. (2021). Dementia-friendliness–A matter of knowledge, responsibility, dignity, and illusion. *Journal of Aging Studies, 59*, 100970.

The Hogeweyk. (2023, September 18). *The Hogeweyk® - normal life for people living with severe dementia*. https://hogeweyk.dementiavillage.com/

Huang, Y., Liu, H., & Cong, Y. (2022). Is deception defensible in dementia care? A care ethics perspective. *Nursing Ethics*. doi: 10.1177/09697330221092336.

Jenkins, C., & Smythe, A. (2013). Reflections on a visit to a dementia care village. *Nursing Older People, 25*(6), 14–9. doi: 10.7748/nop2013.07.25.6.14.e478.

Kielsgaard, K., Horghagen, S., Nielsen, D., & Kristensen, H. K. (2021). Moments of meaning: Enacted narratives of occupational engagement within a dementia town. *Journal of Occupational Science, 28*(4), 510–524.

Kirch, J., & Marquardt, G. (2021). Towards human-centred general hospitals: The potential of dementia-friendly design. *Architectural Science Review, 66*(44), 1–9. DOI:10.1080/00038628.2021.1933889

Landeweer, E. G. M., Frederiks, B. J. M., Vinckers, F., Janus, S., & Zuidema, S. U. (2021). *Open deuren voor PG?: Een exploratief ethisch onderzoek naar mogelijke alternatieven voor een gesloten deur in het kader van de implementatie van de Wet zorg en dwang*.UNO-UMCG. https://research.vumc.nl/ws/files/24522369/Onderzoeksrapport_Alternatieven_voor_een_gesloten_deur.pdf. https://research.vumc.nl/ws/files/24522369/Onderzoeksrapport_Alternatieven_voor_een_gesloten_deur.pdf

Livingston, G., Huntley, J., Sommerlad, A., Ames, D., Ballard, C., Banerjee, S., Brayne, C., Burns, A., Cohen-Mansfield, J., Cooper, C., Costafreda, S. G., Dias, A., Fox, N., Gitlin, L. N., Howard, R., Kales, H. C., Kivimäki, M., Larson, E. B., Ogunniyi, A., Orgeta, V., Ritchie, K., Rockwood, K., Sampson, E. L., Samus, Q., Schneider, L. S., Selbæk, G., Teri, L., & Mukadam, N. (2020). Dementia prevention, intervention, and care: 2020 report of the Lancet Commission. *The Lancet*. https://doi.org/10.1016/S0140-6736(20)30367-6

Lorey, P. (2019). Fake bus stops for persons with dementia? On truth and benevolent lies in public health. *Israel Journal of Health Policy Research, 8*(1), 1–7.

Marquardt, G., Bueter, K., & Motzek, T. (2014). Impact of the design of the built environment on people with dementia: An evidence-based review. *HERD: Health Environments Research and Design Journal, 8*(1), 127–157.

Morgan, R. C., Castro, J., Garcia, J. G., Gibson, B. T., Hall, S., Hauber, E., ... Yoder, H. M. (2019). There's no place like a Home-Or a nursing home that looks like home: A visit to de Hogeweyk. *Journal of Aging Law & Policy*, *10*, 143.

Nichols, E., Steinmetz, J. D., Vollset, S. E., Fukutaki, K., Chalek, J., Abd-Allah, F., ... Liu, X. (2022). Estimation of the global prevalence of dementia in 2019 and forecasted prevalence in 2050: An analysis for the Global Burden of Disease Study 2019. *The Lancet Public Health*, *7*(2), e105–e125.

Pedro, C., Duarte, M., Jorge, B., & Freitas, D. (2020). 440-Dementia villages: Rethinking dementia care. *International Psychogeriatrics*, *32*(Suppl. 1), 158–158.

Peoples, H., Pedersen, L. F., & Moestrup, L. (2020). Creating a meaningful everyday life: Perceptions of relatives of people with dementia and healthcare professionals in the context of a Danish dementia village. *Dementia*, *19*(7), 2314–2331.

Rahman, S., & Swaffer, K. (2018). Assets-based approaches and dementia-friendly communities. *Dementia*, *17*(2), 131–137.

Roberts, E., & Shehadeh, A. (2021). Community visioning for innovation in integrated dementia care: Stakeholder focus group outcomes. *Journal of Primary Care and Community Health*, *12*. doi:10.1177/21501327211042791

Simonsen, T., Sturge, J., & Duff, C. (2022). Healing architecture in healthcare: A scoping review. *HERD: Health Environments Research and Design Journal*. doi:10.1177/19375867211072513

Steele, L., Carr, R., Swaffer, K., Phillipson, L., & Fleming, R. (2020). Human rights and the confinement of people living with dementia in care homes. *Health and Human Rights*, *22*(1), 7.

Sturge, J., Nordin, S., Patil, D. S., Jones, A., Légaré, F., Elf, M., & Meijering, L. (2021). Features of the social and built environment that contribute to the well-being of people with dementia who live at home: A scoping review. *Health and Place*, *67*, 102483.

The Village. (2023, September 18). The Village Retirement Residence | Verve Senior Living. https://www.thevillagelangley.com/

Tierney, L., Doherty, K., Breen, J., & Courtney-Pratt, H. (2022). Community expectations of a village for people living with dementia. *Health & Social Care in the Community*. *30*(6), e5875-e5884.

Van Steenwinkel, I. V., Verstraeten, E., & Heylighen, A. (2016). Adjusting an older residential care facility to contemporary dementia care visions. In P. Langdon, J. Lazar, A. Heylighen, & H. Dong (Eds.), *Designing around people* (pp. 219–228). Cham: Springer International Publishing.

Verbeek, H., Van Rossum, E., Zwakhalen, S. M., Kempen, G. I., & Hamers, J. P. (2009). Small, homelike care environments for older people with dementia: A literature review. *International Psychogeriatrics*, *21*(2), 252–264.

Vernooij-Dassen, M., & Jeon, Y. H. (2016). Social health and dementia: The power of human capabilities. *International Psychogeriatrics*, *28*(5), 701–703.

Vernooij-Dassen, M., Verhey, F., & Lapid, M. (2020). The risks of social distancing for older adults: A call to balance. *International Psychogeriatrics*. https://doi.org/10.1017/S1041610220001350

Vinick, D. (2019). Dementia-friendly design: Hogeweyk and beyond. *British Journal of General Practice*, *69*(683), 300–300.

Wang, H., Li, T., Barbarino, P., Gauthier, S., Brodaty, H., Molinuevo, J. L., & Yu, X. (2020). Dementia care during COVID-19. *The Lancet*, *395*(10231), 1190–1191.

World Health Organization. (2021). *Towards a dementia-inclusive society: WHO toolkit for dementia-friendly initiatives (DFIs)*. World Health Organization.

13 Evaluation of technologies and products for psychosocial intervention and support for and with people living with dementia

Michael P. Craven

Introduction

This chapter concerns evaluation of products, services, or interventions, as they are also called throughout this section of the book, relating to health and well-being, with an emphasis on co-design. Co-design means inclusion of all user groups in a collaborative and joint design process. In a truly shared approach, this means 'designing with' rather than 'deciding for' people who will use the product. In the context of health and well-being it is important to involve people with lived experience of a health condition in the design process. This includes people living with dementia as a group of particular interest (Tsekleves & Keady, 2021).

Evaluation is a critical stage in design, both to assess whether the right thing is being developed and whether the resulting thing has been 'designed right', such that it fulfils its intended purpose and is acceptable to its users. It is therefore important that we think about what co-design means in the evaluation stage of design. This chapter will discuss various tools for evaluation and how they can be used in co-design or subsequent user elicitation.

Formative evaluation typically refers to assessments during the design process prior to final design and can be used to explore concepts and to test prototypes that will be further refined. The process is iterative such that design ideas and prototypes will be tested and changed multiple times. A variety of formative evaluation tools and methods such as personas and scenario-based design are available to help designers and researchers probe into the everyday experiences of persons living with a health condition and to also understand their relationships with others. Such methods, described in more detail later in this chapter, are well suited to co-design and can be readily applied in a group workshop format of public contributors and researchers.

Summative evaluation determines how well a final design or set of designs performs. This could use a comparative approach to assess one or more designs against each other, or to assess the design with reference to an established framework or performance benchmark. Summative evaluation can also be carried out with users in a workshop format or in one-to-one (person with condition or carer/supporter and researcher) or two-to-one (person, carer/supporter and researcher) interviews.

The attempt to measure psychosocial impact of technologies for people living with disabilities has resulted in a number of useful tools for their summative evaluation (Day et al., 2002; Scherer & Craddock, 2002). However, until recently, there were few tools available to specifically measure psychosocial wellbeing of persons with dementia, although a large number of quality-of-life (QoL) measures exist (Craven et al., 2014a). Better understanding of psychosocial factors should also help match individuals with appropriate technologies and also pre-empt issues that might lead to their abandonment. Furthermore, an appreciation of motivation and other individual factors is critical to the success of psychosocial interventions, and these can be explored using behavioural and predictive models.

DOI: 10.4324/9781003318262-17

The following sections introduce the 'Designing for people with Dementia' collaboration (MinD) and give examples of (both formative and summative) evaluation methods that were used and developed within it. The chapter then goes on to introduce the AIR model: a pragmatic model to consider the combined interactions of Activities, Internal World of the individual with dementia and Relationships with others, and the positive or negative influences on these. This model resulted from learning throughout the co-design and evaluation activities of MinD and can be used to steer similar activities in the future.

Tools for evaluation in co-design

In the 'Designing for people with dementia: designing for mindful self-empowerment and social engagement' (MinD) collaboration (funded by the European Union's Horizon 2020 Research and Innovation Staff Exchange, Marie Skłodowska-Curie Action – grant agreement No. 691001) a variety of methods were considered to support engagement with public contributors (participants with lived experience of dementia) in the co-design process. Some of these, such as personas and scenarios, are covered in some detail in the MinD Guidelines and Tools that were produced to explain and support their application (MinD, 2023). Personas and scenario techniques were mainly used in MinD to scope out design ideas but they also have a role in evaluation, since they provide a frame to think about the success or otherwise of the fulfilment of an activity in context of the person and their relationships.

Personas (Cooper et al., 2014) are user models that are based on real people, typically produced as composite archetypes which are then expressed as an individual. Personas have found good application in the context of dementia by researchers (Jais et al., 2018). In MinD, examples of personas were co-created from conversations with public contributors. These were fictional individuals who are named and described in enough detail to include the following four areas: biography, personality, health and social environment. Including a fictional person's life story gives expression to values, interests and habits, whereas outlining personality traits gives insight into attitudes and, for example, plausible reactions to having a diagnosis of dementia and how they deal with the change of identity that can accompany it. Knowing their health and care needs can suggest strategies to help solve or ameliorate problems through design. Providing information about social environment can help designers think about likely responses of an individual's social network to different situations, which can have a major impact on how a person experiences life with dementia. In the final MinD Persona Toolkit the four areas described above were supplemented with a set of individual needs to be addressed by design (MinD, 2023).

Scenario-based design (Carroll, 1995) is another design method where one aims to articulate situations that users face by breaking the whole down into its constituent tasks or steps. The rational for using scenarios in design with people with dementia is that they and carers often encounter difficulties in ordinary situations. Furthermore, it is not always easy to recognise these situations, to see what causes them and to find solutions for them. Mindful Scenario Task Analysis (MSTA), as used within MinD, drew on and synthesised scenario-based design and elements of hierarchical task-analysis (HTA) (Preece et al., 2002) with a specific focus on mindfulness.

To develop MSTA (MinD, 2023), a co-design workshop was initially held with people with lived experience of dementia and MinD researchers. After orientation to the goals of the workshop and an introduction to create a level playing field, a draft scenario framework conceived by the researchers was presented to small groups. It covered the various stages of preparing for, partaking in and looking back on difficult social situations, the details of which each group embellished from personal experiences. The MSTA grid was constructed as tasks broken down into mindful and non-mindful activities and included mind-states (both emotional and cognitive) as well as the activity at hand. It encouraged advanced planning and thinking about tactics and overall strategies to cope with the activity as it took place over time. A completed MTSA grid was built from the experiences of each group of workshop participants of real events.

Application and experience with using MTSA

One example scenario of a social situation was going to a party where the individual with dementia did not know everyone and was accompanied by a carer/supporter. As well as the period of the party, the task breakdown included preparation, travel to and from the venue, points of arrival and departure and post-event reflection. An accessible guide to scenario completion was developed. A further dimension was added to cover aspects of help or hinderances at the various stages.

Examples of mindful planning for the party occasion were: advance thinking about what outfit to wear, what to say, how to relax and to gain knowledge of who would be there. Mindful (and less mindful) states included worrying thoughts and reactions and physical sensations such as feeling nervous or suddenly needing the toilet. Strategies could include sitting near someone familiar and have a prearranged signal to one's carer to leave the party. Helps and hinderances could be time of day, specific difficulties such as heavy traffic that might cause distress en route. Table 13.1 shows the example of one MTSA grid completed from the group session, from the perspective of a carer taking their husband to a dance class.

To conclude the scenario-building co-design workshop, since this was considered to be quite novel in the context of dementia, the team wished to gain feedback from participants. Ten of the eleven participants (including carers/supporters and researchers) chose to respond and the overall message was that the session was informative and enjoyable as it included people with direct lived experience of dementia and resulted in significant collaboration, generosity, humanity and risk-taking, the latter point pertinent to researchers being out of their comfort zones as experts. The main criticisms were about the meeting room (computer presentation equipment used in the introduction and seating plan), minimal opportunity for preparation and lack of diversity in the group.

As such, these techniques found a purpose in the Activities, Internal World and Relationships (AIR) model described later in this chapter. But first we consider an example of formative evaluation.

Example of a formative evaluation

Let's meet up! was one of the MinD (2022) prototypes consisting of a screen-based system and software to enable social engagement that was aimed at empowering and giving confidence for people living with dementia to take part in social activities (Niedderer et al., 2020). The system was designed to encourage people with dementia to stay in touch with their loved ones and to remain physically active by arranging joint activities. Its function was to help initiate, plan and prepare for going out to perform the activity with another person. It was conceived as a user interface to an interactive 'map' of activities and participants with functions to visualise and mediate the social participation.

The need for such an application was discovered during earlier phases of the MinD programme co-design process. The programme had previously determined seven broad 'transition areas' of importance for mindful design in dementia:

Table 13.1 MSTA scenario-based design template for engaging in a social situation

Define and complete for each scenario	Preparation	On the way	While there	Going home	Afterwards
Activities including planning and reflection	Getting dressed and shaving	Driving to the venue	Remembering the dance steps And dancing	Discussing the achievement	Reflecting on the evening
Mindful (and less mindful) states	Thinking about being with people (Dizziness, anxiety)	Apologising for being cross about other drivers (Feeling nervous, uncertain)	Enjoying the entertainment (Feeling uncomfortable and embarrassed)	Sense of achievement (Mood lifted, feeling 'high')	Reasoning about the value of going (Feeling 'pressure' eased off)
Mindful strategies	Addressing excuses not to go Motivation to dress smartly Choosing the music to dance to in advance	Thinking about why we are going Addressing worries about being late	Finding people who make you feel comfortable Addressing feelings of inadequacy in front of dance teachers	Talking about what was most enjoyable Discussing listening to enjoyable music even if not able to have danced.	Discuss positives of having done something 'normal' Talking about people in the room
Things that help (or hinder)	Boosting confidence (Telling off/ criticism)	Distraction during the journey e.g. private jokes (Traffic may be too heavy)	Knowing that the activity is off fixed time (People who might judge)	Leaving later to avoid heavy traffic	('High' feeling wearing off)

1) Coming to terms with the diagnosis: acceptance, self-value and identity.
2) Feeling useful by helping others: sustaining self-value and emotions through self-realisation.
3) Self-realisation through purposeful activities: compensating limitations through new activities.
4) Coming to terms with emotions: defining and valuing yourself and in relation to others.
5) Importance of feelings arising from keeping relationships going: empathy in planning, decision-making and negotiation with carers, friends and family.
6) Maintaining social participation: negotiating and continuing relationships with carers, friends and family.
7) Negotiation and communication when planning activities.

For the *Let's Meet Up!* concept the designers were informed by transition areas 6 and 7 which indicated that it can be hard for people with dementia to keep relationships going, that friends and family may not always understand them that well and that participating in group activities may become more difficult. Other design considerations were related to cross-cutting

MinD themes: the importance of having a sense of continuation and familiarity which could be attained through attending the same regular activity events, with the same people, or using familiar things. The design brief sought to offer ways of encouraging motivation and confidence while offering new pastimes which might compensate for the necessary loss of some activities. It also asked for cognitive simplicity through a table or bulletin board interface and to have features that could help with reminders about arrangements.

The digital prototype was initially called the *Social Engagement Map* (SEM) and then later renamed *Let's Connect!* and finally *Let's Meet Up!*. The purpose of the application was to link an individual with dementia to a team of supporters. The team would be open to a variety of mutual activities and the software would manage communication about that activity to make it happen. Functions included arranging the schedule such as the date and time of cinema show-ings or swimming pool opening times and remembering to take the correct items e.g. ticket, towel. After completing earlier design iterations to decide which specific elements to include in the user interface, the application was mocked up as an interactive Portable Document Format (PDF) running on a personal computer.

The process of formative evaluation was to run a session with a group of volunteers with lived experience of dementia and other disabilities where the participants could try out the prototype, engage in group discussion and if possible complete an individual questionnaire with a researcher facilitating. A commonly used set-up for user experience (UX) testing in human–computer interaction (HCI) design was employed to test alternative forms of interaction which included use of a physical puck (tangible interface) of various sizes. One HCI technique, Wizard-of-Oz (Dahlbäck et al., 1993), was used to simulate user interaction of the puck device on a large TV screen by means of a human controlling the result of user selections on the inter-active PDF (see Figure 13.1).

It was found that participants in this session were enthusiastic about trying out the proto-type and were able to make recommendations about the unfamiliar interface. The outcome of the evaluation with 12 participants was that participants expressed, when prompted, different preferences for location of the interface in the home and opinions about the type and location of screen (laptop/tablet, table top or wall mounted). They mainly wished the device to be for personal use but to have it continually connected to supporters who would have some access the planner function. A majority wished for a degree of personalisation, had preference for and against or were ambivalent towards animation or other attention-grabbing functions. All partici-pants wished to have touch as one interface option with half also being accepting of either tan-gible, pen/stylus or mouse selection, with a mix of preferences for these. A majority expressed that having a tangible device was fun to use and encouraged social interaction (although others disagreed) and users identified a number of usability benefits (ease of seeing, manipulating and selecting choices), as well as the intended benefit of aiding memory.

Some concerns were the weight and possible disadvantage for a type of dementia (Lewy Bodies) that is accompanied by motor impairment and fear of screen damage. Most found the screen visual layout to be accessible and understandable, except for a criticism of the colour contrast. Half found the default number of objects on the screen to be about right, with some expressing too many or too few, but none required more help with decisions about which activities to choose. A few additional features were suggested including more names for all contact photos, more reminders, personalised reminders, emergency contacts and a detailed checklist of things to take and customisation of the activities list. Opinion was offered on the tangible design including change from a puck to a ring, or addition of a handle to make it easy to manipulate.

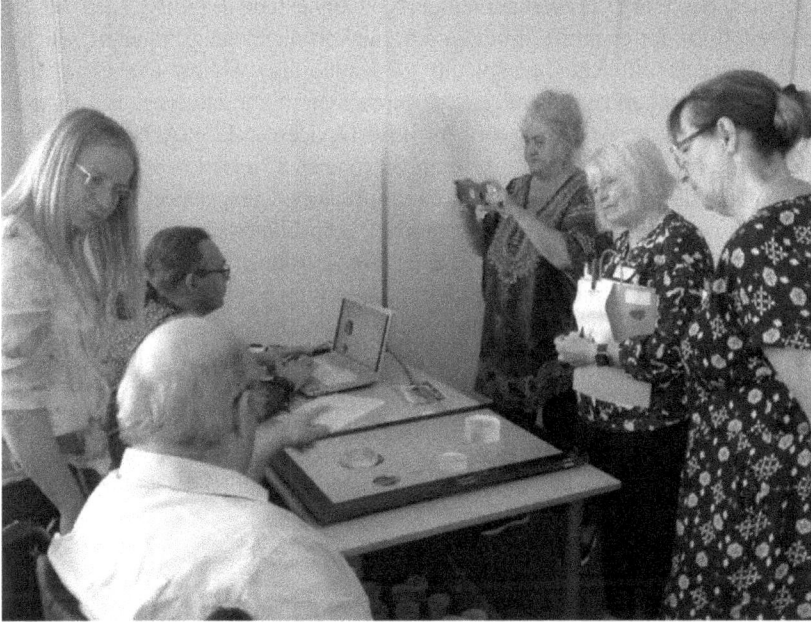

Figure 13.1 Wizard-of-Oz technique used to simulate user interaction with puck devices on a large TV screen

The above outline of results are not intended to be exhaustive but are presented to show the extent of feedback from a single workshop at an early stage of design that mainly shone light on usability issues and preferences. Subsequently, further user evaluations were conducted to explore the potential psychosocial impact of the design (Niedderer et al., 2020).

Summative evaluation tools

In the previous section we considered how tools for formative evaluation are particularly suited to co-design. Now we consider more traditional user evaluation methods that can be used for summative evaluation once a design has been developed and is approaching its final form. Most of these were not used to any great extent in the MinD programme but this section provides a brief review of tools and techniques that were considered potentially useful for evaluation, some of which are general to technologies, assistive technologies or health behaviours and others that are specifically concerned with psychosocial aspects of dementia.

Usability and user experience

A typical approach to evaluating the experiences of people with technologies once they have been designed is in terms of usability. The System Usability Scale (SUS, 2022) provides a quick tool for measuring usability, created in the 1980s and was originally intended to make comparisons of systems A and B e.g. products and services, including computer hardware, software, mobile devices, websites and applications. SUS questions cover five useful aspects of successful design including frequency of use, complexity, ease of use, level of support or learning that is needed to use it and consistency of design. The SUS is easy to apply but the results need careful interpretation and are not explicitly aligned to health and wellbeing products.

User experience (UE or UX) evaluation tools typically extend usability. The User Experience Questionnaire (UEQ), for example, provides a framework in six areas, three of which are 'classical usability' aspects (efficiency, perspicuity, dependability), two are user experience aspects (originality, stimulation) and an overall users' impression of attractiveness is measured.

Another tool, the Psychosocial Impact of Assistive Devices Scale (PIADS) was designed in the 1990s to help researchers explore the long-term acceptance or rejection of assistive technologies by users living with disabilities. It consists of three subscales: Competence, Adaptability and Self-esteem. PIADS is very much about how the individual's capabilities are changed by the introduction of an assistive technology and can be applied in a pre-post manner i.e. does the design improve (or not) the attributes listed in the subscales? In PIADS, there is no explicit aspect of social engagement covered in the sub-scale descriptors except for 'ability to participate'. Furthermore, some descriptors such as 'performance', 'quality of life' and 'wellbeing' are rather broad. Nor is the scale specifically intended for assessing the impact of technologies for memory problems or cognitive impairments. However, there are a good number of descriptors that add detail to the more basic or functional usability scale. As well as being suitable as a tool for summative evaluation it could help in discussions about the potential impact of the design on different dimensions during the design process.

Positive psychology measures

Stoner et al. (2017) created two new positive psychology outcome measures for research in dementia care. They had noted that positive psychology has largely been confined to the qualitative literature because of the lack of robust outcome measures. The two new scales were the Positive Psychology Outcome Measure (PPOM) and the Engagement and Independence in Dementia Questionnaire (EID-Q). Both are questionnaire based and are answered on a five-point interval scale (Not true at all, Rarely true, Sometimes true, Often true, True nearly all the time) and ask a person with dementia about the period of the last month. Questions are scored 0–4. There are two subscales for the 16-item PPOM: Hope (e.g. *I have a positive outlook on life*) and Resilience (e.g. *I am able to adapt to things*) with eight questions in each. The subscales can be summed to calculate hope scores and resilience scores as well as the total PPOM score. EID-Q has 26 items and 5 subscales: Activities of Daily Living (e.g. *I can look after myself as much as I need to)*, Decision-making (e.g., *I'm confident in making decisions*), Activity Engagement (e.g. *I can take part in groups/ activities with others*), Support (e.g. *My friends/ family care about me*) and Reciprocity (e.g. *I can help my friends/ family as much as I would like*) and responses can be similarly summed to provide a score in each subscale, as well as an overall score. These scales could readily be used to assess psychological changes seen by individuals who try out an assistive technology, as part of a summative evaluation.

Another scale worthy of mention is Sense of Coherence (SoC) developed by Antonevsky in the 1970s. SoC was used in the context of dementia in a mixed-method study by Alm and colleagues (Alm et al., 2015). SoC is measured by three dimensions: Meaningfulness, Manageability and Comprehensibility. Meaningfulness is the extent to which an individual believes that life makes sense emotionally and that one possesses the motivation and desire to cope with encountered stimuli. Comprehensibility is the extent to which an individual perceives life's challenges in a clear, ordered and structured manner, where an individual with strong comprehensibility will find logic in various external and internally encountered stimuli. Manageability means that an individual who perceives that the requisite resources to cope successfully with life's challenges are available and they will endure and not be overwhelmed. The study of Alm et al. formed part of a larger project where couples were interviewed about their experiences in long-term ongoing existing support groups as well as well as adult children of persons with dementia to find out what it means for them to have a parent with dementia. Analysis using SoC showed that having social connections and having support was identified as meaningful by all. It also showed that what made everyday life with dementia comprehensible was the ability to understand the disease or to be given tools to better understand how to care for a person with dementia. The study showed that feeling supported by others and normalising the disease made everyday life manageable, and children of the group felt relief in talking talk to others in the same situation and not feeling as though they were the only ones with a parent suffering from dementia. It is therefore seen that SoC has possible use in the evaluation of technologies that are designed to support relationships and developing mindful practices.

Behaviour change models

A different approach to evaluation with end users is to focus on behaviour change as is seen in the COM-B model proposed by Michie et al. (2011). The model targets three areas of importance in behaviour change:

- Capability – the individual's psychological and physical capacity to engage in an activity.
- Opportunity – factors which lie outside of the individual which make behavior possible, prompt it or present a barrier to it.
- Motivation – processes which energise and direct behaviour; both planned and habitual.

In this author's other work on cognitive assessment and training technologies, a qualitative analysis with thematic analysis using COM-B was supplemented with further data-driven codes (Harrington, 2022). It should be added that criticism of COM-B has also been made for its attempts to systematise clinical practice on the grounds of inability of this and other health psychology models to cope with patient variability (Ogden, 2016).

The theory of planned behaviour (Ajzen, 2011) is another common reference in the healthcare context, which is focussed on intentions that lead to behaviour, where attitude (beliefs) toward behaviour, subjective norm (beliefs about others' attitudes and beliefs) and 'perceived behavioural control' all affect intention. However, TPB has received criticism in recent years (Sniehotta et al., 2014) and this criticism highlights the lack of attention to unconscious influences on behaviour and the role of emotions, as well as its predictive validity.

The AIR model

Mutual and mindful capacity-building processes were introduced in the MinD programme through the duration of the partnership, enabling creative opportunities for people with dementia and their carers to think like designers and allowing designers to gain insight into user experience of dementia (individuals living with the condition and carers). Preceding these joint activities, an earlier exploratory workshop had brought people with lived experience of dementia and researchers together to think about design concepts relating to textiles as technologies. This was intended to help the programme prepare for a research visit to a MinD partner organisation which specialised in 'smart textiles' who were interested in applications in health, where we wished to provide input from people with dementia into the design thinking on potential products.

In this session, a miscellany of textiles, including clothes, fabrics, swatches and soft furnishings, were available for participants to touch, smell, drape, manipulate creatively before considering their attributes, their appeal and their applications within people's lived in worlds

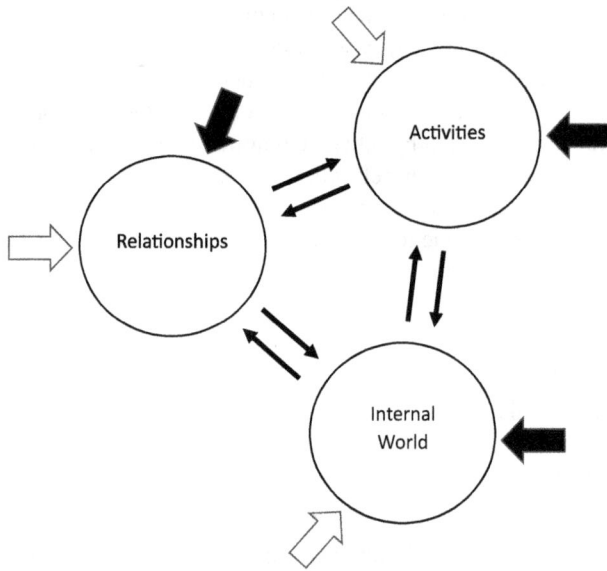

Figure 13.2 The AIR model with mutual interactions (thin arrows), negative external influencers (black arrows) and positive external influencers (white arrows)

(external and internal). The session revealed a rich language from users to describe attributes of clothing (tightness, warmth, colour, weight etc.), mindful attributes (feelings of comfort, security, being trapped; aesthetics of clashing or matching; status and dignity, fit to cultural and social etc.), actions performed (dressing, changing, washing, carrying etc.) and technological aspects (sensing, actuating and potential applications relating to smart functions). This led the researchers to think about how activities with clothing were influenced by individual cognitive and emotional factors.

Combining learning from this workshop with the experience of scenario-building, that had highlighted the importance of relationships in achieving tasks in the context of dementia, and discussions about impact of design on dementia in the wider consortium, led to a pragmatic model to consider the combined interactions of Activities, Internal World of the individual with dementia and Relationships with other, and the positive or negative influences on these; the AIR model (see Figure 13.2).

The three components of AIR are interrelated such that a lack of activities, or a less than ideal approach to them, can have detrimental effects on both the internal world and on the relationships of the person, whilst turmoil in the internal world can prevent someone participating in enjoyable activities and could harm relationships. There can be positive or negative influences on any and each of the three components, and they can therefore affect the whole system. A measure of success from design is enabling a new beneficial activity or maintaining an existing one, whilst improving relationships with people or environments, or enhancing the internal world. It is suggested that this model is valuable in three ways:

- *It is consistent with a mindful approach to design as facilitating experience.* It reminds us of the importance of bringing the internal and external worlds together and, as there is no specific dimension of time, it rests in the moment.

- *It informs co-design.* In designing with and for people with dementia, we can consider any or all of the three components. Design could focus on one component, such as the activity or activities, but in thinking about how the design may work we can take into account the likely impacts on relationships and on the internal world. Alternative designs can be targeted at changes to one or multiple components.
- *It informs evaluation.* This means working collaboratively to decide the suitability of prototype designs for people living with dementia and other actors. The three components of AIR give us a framework to assess if, how and why a design is effective. Conversely, it can suggest improvements to a design that are informed by users.

The MinD project used the AIR model to co-produce and evaluate two technologies/products; *Let's Meet Up!*, as described earlier, and *The Good Life Kit* (GLK), a compendium of two serious games together with a booklet of information, reflections and mindfulness exercises (MinD, 2023).

To support formative evaluation, a package of evaluation tools was produced that incorporated aspects of TAM, UX testing and also reflected the AIR themes to explore the potential for the technology to impact on those. In the context of the GLK evaluation tools were developed to capture not only the usability and experience of playing the set of board games and associated material at the prototype stage, but also facilitated reflection of the games' influence on players' inner selves and relationships with others.

One of the board games in GLK, *This is Me* (more recently renamed *All About Us*), was designed to support people diagnosed with dementia to increase wellbeing through mindful life-storytelling in a convivial setting (Niedderer et al., 2022). It was conceived to help people adopt a positive outlook on life using mindful questions to enable reflection and seeing new perspectives. The game consists of a game board, 66 question cards and a dice with six symbols as well as a set of counters (See Figure 13.3). The board shows a life-story path, divided into

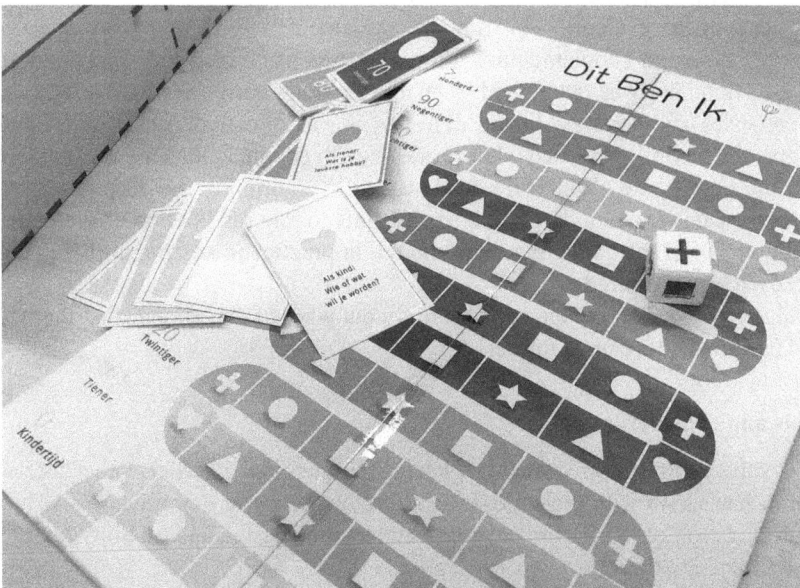

Figure 13.3 'This is Me' board game prototype during development (Dutch language version '*Dit Ben Ik*'). Photograph from Niedderer et al. (2022) https://creativecommons.org/licenses/by/4.0/

decades from childhood to 100+ years. A set of cards were designed to ask questions comprising of six categories (memories, activities, relationships, experiences, achievements, dreams) which were open-ended and phrased in the present tense to facilitate an in-the-moment experience. Selections on the board were made using a dice.

The *TIM* game was evaluated to understand whether people with dementia and carers were able and willing to use the game (adoption and usability) and what their experience was of using the game. We were interested in whether *TIM* enhanced wellbeing (emotional wellbeing, social engagement, agency) and experiences of reminiscence and mindfulness. These aspects are closely related to the Internal World aspect of the AIR model. We were also interested in seeing how the game affected mutual understanding between players that would align with the Relationships aspect of AIR. Further details of the game and the evaluation process are described in Niedderer et al. (2022).

A semi-structured questionnaire was developed by researchers from the MinD team, one of whom was the lead for the Public and Patient Involvement (PPI) group in the UK with whom the questionnaire was piloted before the final evaluation. The questionnaire was designed to elicit aspects of appreciation, usability and adoption of the game as well as potential impact. The questionnaire and user elicitation approach was broadly based on the principles of TAM (Davis, 1993) and employed categories of questions similar to those in the User Experience Questionnaire (UEQ, 2022) and to those of the AIR Model. The questionnaire comprised seven sections including personal information and prior experience with games; opinion about the aesthetics of the design; ease of use (ergonomic aspects of visualisation and handling); feelings about the process of playing and difficulties experienced; feelings experienced through/during the act of storytelling (regarding self and the benefit, importance or difficulties of sharing personal experiences and emotions); potential impact (how the game has helped, on the day, or may help players in general with socialising and sharing experiences, mutual appreciation and talking about the future); and further use (why, where and with whom people might play the game and whether they would recommend it to others).

Each section of the evaluation instrument consisted of two to four main questions, augmented by prompts and supplementary questions to gain more detail. The semi-structured interview questionnaire was developed to enable as much parity as possible across the four different countries and settings. In the delivery, it was effectively used as a conversation guide, to give the flexibility needed when working with people with dementia, and also taking account of the time frame of the different settings. In addition to the questions, a five-point 'smiley' emoji scale was included to ask participants to rate satisfaction of the main purpose of each section and of the game overall, although in practice it was found that the conversational approach was preferred.

The evaluation of *TIM* provided a means to try out ways of operationalising the AIR model, which will need to be developed further.

Other tools and considerations

Some tools suitable for group workshops have been mentioned earlier. Other techniques for evaluation in interviews with technologies and products are the Cognitive WalkThrough and the Think Aloud protocol which are covered in interaction design and usability texts (Preece et al., 2002; Barnum, 2020).

This chapter has mainly addressed evaluation that is suited to earlier stages of dementia. Evaluation methods need to adapt to address the changing nature of the dementia journey but there is a gap at later stages, which is also seen for QoL measures (Craven et al., 2014a). People in the late stages of dementia are often confined to a chair or bed and may experience sensory deprivation. Compassionate design for such vulnerable groups, as covered in Chapter 10 of this book, and associated techniques and products, aim to address this gap (Treadaway et al., 2018). Compassionate design in the context of dementia stresses personalised design to retain a person's sense of self and maintain their dignity; sensory design to keep in the present moment and not rely on past or future; and connecting design to encourage moments of high-quality connection with others. The associated *LAUGH* project used a number of evaluation tools including the new edition of the Pool Activity Level (PAL) tool, which added a focus on to the sensory level of functioning, and the Bradford Dementia Wellbeing Scale (Treadaway et al., 2020).

Since these are rather disconnected from co-design, this chapter has not attempted to cover in detail predictive techniques from Technology Adoption Modelling (TAM) (Davis, 1993) but these are now briefly mentioned. Chaurasia et al. (2016) employed the unified theory of acceptance and use of technology (UTAUT) to predict mobile technology adoption by people living with dementia using a variety of features to classify them as either likely adopters or likely non-adopters. This kind of model, whilst considering the importance of a wide range of factors (including access to internet resources, profile and capabilities of the individual, health status and genetic factors), could be considered to be quite impersonal and overly medical. However, whilst TAM approaches in general are somewhat pragmatic i.e. are not based on a theory such as one from health psychology, they include additional factors that could find use in the structuring of a user evaluation.

Implementation of healthcare interventions, whether they are products, services or combinations is another important area for evaluation of healthcare design. Until recently there were no set guidelines on how to increase the uptake of psychosocial interventions in practice. To address this, Streater et al. (2016) developed the Implementation Readiness (ImpRess) checklist for manualised interventions, that included criteria deemed useful in measuring readiness for implementation and applied it to trials of cognitive stimulation therapy in dementia. This checklist is currently being extended to cover implementation aspects of digital interventions. The Nonadoption, Abandonment and Challenges to the Scale-Up, Spread and Sustainability (NASSS) framework is also aimed at improving implementation of healthcare technology services (Greenhalgh et al., 2017).

Finally, a sometimes overlooked aspect of evaluation is that of non-functional requirements. Success of design project can be dominated by features that are not directly associated with the design such as available development and evaluation time, cost, or choice of platform. Consideration of non-functional requirements also brings into the technology evaluation process concepts that are present in psychosocial scales mentioned earlier, such as 'comprehensibility'. Non-functional factors may act to constrain the design process and limit implementation choices (Craven et al., 2014b). Evaluation of non-functional requirements can also extend to the 'involvementability' of co-production processes with end-users (Molinari-Ulate et al., 2022).

Acknowledgements

This chapter draws greatly from the MinD collaboration and as so represents the work of many others in addition to the author, as evidenced in the references, in particular the authors of Gosling et al. (2019) and Niedderer et al. (2020, 2022). Credit is due to all others of the MinD secondment participants and public contributors who worked tirelessly together from different countries on developing the design ideas, prototypes, guidelines and tools. The evaluation workpackage of MinD 'WP6: Implementation and User Testing' was led by colleagues at the University of Nottingham. *This is Me* has since been developed into a board game product, renamed *All About Us*, with additional thanks to Manchester Metropolitan University and Relish (London).

Reference list

Ajzen, I. (2011). The theory of planned behaviour: Reactions and reflections. *Psychology and Health, 26*(9), 1113–1127. https://doi.org/10.1080/08870446.2011.613995

Alm, A. K., Hagglund, P., Norbergh, K., & Hellzén, O. (2015). Sense of coherence in persons with dementia and their next of kin: A mixed-method study. *Open Journal of Nursing, 5*, 490–499. https://doi.org/10.4236/ojn.2015.55052

Barnum, C. M. (2020). *Usability testing essentials. ready, set test* (2nd ed.). Morgan Kaufmann, Elsevier Inc. https://doi.org/10.1016/C2018-0-01372-9.

Carroll, J. M. (1995). *Scenario based design: Envisioning work and technology in systems development.* John Wiley & Son.

Chaurasia, P., McClean, S. I., Nugent, C. D., Cleland, I., Zhang, S., Donnelly, M. P., Scotney, B. W., Sanders, C., Smith, K., Norton, M. C., & Tschanz, J. (2016, October). Modelling assistive technology adoption for people with dementia. *Journal of Biomedical Informatics, 63*, 235–248. https://doi.org/10.1016/j.jbi.2016.08.021

Cooper, A., Reimann, R., Cronin, D., & Noessel, C. (2014). *About face: The essentials of interaction design* (4th ed.). Wiley.

Craven, M. P., De Filippis, M. L., & Dening, T. (2014a). Quality of life tools to inform co-design in the development of assistive technologies for people with dementia and their carers. In L. Pecchia, L. L. Chen, C. Nugent, & J. Bravo (Eds.), *Ambient assisted living and daily activities. IWAAL 2014*. Lecture Notes in Computer Science (Vol. 8868). Springer. https://doi.org/10.1007/978-3-319-13105-4_57

Craven, M. P., Lang, A. R., & Martin, J. L. (2014b). Developing mhealth Apps with researchers: Multi-stakeholder design considerations. In A. Marcus (Ed.). *Design, user experience, and usability: User experience design for everyday life applications and services, lecture notes in computer science, Vol. 8519, DUXU 2014 / HCII 2014, Part III* (pp. 15–24). Springer. https://doi.org/10.1007/978-3-319-07635-5_2

Dahlbäck, N., Jönsson, A., & Ahrenberg, L. (1993, December). Wizard of Oz studies---Why and how. *Knowledge-Based Systems, 6*(4), 258–266. https://doi.org/10.1016/0950-7051(93)90017-N

Davis, F. D. (1993). User acceptance of information technology: System characteristics, user perceptions and behavioral impacts. *International Journal of Man-Machine Studies, 38*(3), 475–487. https://doi.org/10.1006/imms.1993.1022

Day, H., Jutai, J., & Campbell, K. A. (2002, February 15). Development of a scale to measure the psychosocial impact of assistive devices: Lessons learned and the road ahead. *Disability and Rehabilitation, 1–3*, 31–37. https://doi.org/10.1080/09638280110066343

Gosling, J., Craven, M. P., Dening, T., Coleston-Shields, D., Aberturas, A. G., Martín, S. G., & Abrilahij, A. (2019). The AIR model (Activities, Internal world, Relationships): A pragmatic framework for evaluating co-design. In K. Niedderer, G. Ludden, R. Cain, & C. Wölfel (Eds.), *International MinD conference 2019 designing with and for people with Dementia: Wellbeing, empowerment and happiness.* http://hdl.handle.net/2436/623319

Greenhalgh, T., Wherton, J., Papoutsi, C., Lynch, J., Hughes, G., A'Court, C., Hinder, S., Fahy, N., Procter, R., & Shaw, S. (2017). Beyond adoption: A new framework for theorizing and evaluating nonadoption, abandonment, and challenges to the scale-up, spread, and sustainability of health and care technologies. *Journal of Medical Internet Research, 19*(11), e367. https://doi.org/10.2196/jmir.8775

Harrington, K., Craven, M. P., Wilson, M. L., & Landowska, A. (2022). Perceptions of cognitive training games and assessment technologies for dementia: Acceptability study with patient and public involvement workshops. *JMIR Serious Games, 10*(2), e32489. https://doi.org/10.2196/32489

Jais, C., Hignett, S., Estupiñan, Z. T. G., & Hogervorst, E. (2018). Evidence based dementia personas: Human factors design for people living with dementia. In A. Polak-Sopinska, J. Krolikowski, & M.

Wrobel-Lachowska (Eds.), *Ergonomics for people with disabilities: Design for accessibility. Warsaw, Poland: Sciendo* (pp. 215–226). https://doi.org/10.2478/9783110617832-018

Michie, S., van Stralen, M. M., & West, R. (2011). The behaviour change wheel: A new method for characterising and designing behaviour change interventions. *Implementation Science*, 6(1), 42. https://doi.org/10.1186/1748-5908-6-42

Min, D. (2023). Designing for Dementia website. *Resources*. Retrieved May 13, 2023, from https://designingfordementia.eu/resources/

Molinari-Ulate, M., Woodcock, R., Smith, I., van der Roest, H. G., Franco-Martín, M. A., & Craven, M. P. (2022). Insights on conducting digital patient and public involvement in dementia research during the COVID-19 pandemic: Supporting the development of an "E-nabling digital co-production" framework. *Research Involvement and Engagement*, 8(1), 33. https://doi.org/10.1186/s40900-022-00371-9

Niedderer, K., Harrison, D., Gosling, J., Craven, M., Blackler, A., Losada, R., & Cid, T. (2020). Working with experts with experience: Charting co-production and co-design in the development of HCI-based design. In R. Brankaert, G. Kenning, et al. (Eds.), *HCI and design in the context of dementia. Human–computer interaction series*. Springer. https://doi.org/10.1007/978-3-030-32835-1_19

Niedderer, K., Holthoff-Detto, V., van Rompay, T. J. L., Karahanoğlu, A., Ludden, G. D. S., Almeida, A., Durán, R. L., Aguado, Y. B., Lim, J. N. W., Smith, T., Harrison, D., Craven, M. P., Gosling, J., Orton, L., & Tournier, I. (2022). This is Me: Evaluation of a boardgame to promote social engagement, wellbeing and agency in people with dementia through mindful life-storytelling. *Journal of Aging Studies*, 60, 100995. https://doi.org/10.1016/j.jaging.2021.100995

Ogden, J. (2016). Celebrating variability and a call to limit systematisation: The example of the behaviour change technique taxonomy and the behaviour change wheel. *Health Psychology Review*, 10(3), 245–250. https://doi.org/10.1080/17437199.2016.1190291

Preece, J., Rogers, Y., & Sharp, H. (2002). *Interaction design* (2nd ed.). John Wiley & Sons.

Scherer, M., & Craddock, G. (2022). Matching Person & Technology (MPT) assessment process. *Technology and Disability*, 14(3), 125–131. https://doi.org/10.3233/TAD-2002-14308

Sniehotta, F. F., Presseau, J., & Araújo-Soares, V. (2014). Time to retire the theory of planned behaviour. *Health Psychology Review*, 8(1), 1–7. https://doi.org/10.1080/17437199.2013.869710

Stoner, C. R., Orrell, M., Long, M., Csipke, E., & Spector, A. (2017). The development and preliminary psychometric properties of two positive psychology outcome measures for people with dementia: The PPOM and the EID-Q. *BMC Geriatrics*, 17(72), 1–11. https://doi.org/10.1186/s12877-017-0468-6

Streater, A., Spector, A., Aguirre, E., Stansfeld, J., & Orrell, M. (2016). ImpRess: An Implementation Readiness checklist developed using a systematic review of randomised controlled trials assessing cognitive stimulation for dementia. *BMC Medical Research Methodology*, 16(167). https://doi.org/10.1186/s12874-016-0268-2

System Usability Scale, SUS. Retrieved May 13, 2022, from https://www.usability.gov/how-to-and-tools/methods/system-usability-scale.html

Treadaway, C., Fennell, J., & Taylor, A. (2020, July 1–3). Compassionate Design: A methodology for advanced dementia. In K. Christer, C. Craig, & P. Chamberlain (Eds.), *Proceedings of the 6th European conference on Design4Health* (p. 667).

Treadaway, C., Taylor, A., & Fennell, J. (2018). Compassionate design for dementia care. *International Journal of Design Creativity and Innovation*, 7(3), 144–115. https://doi.org/10.1080/21650349.2018.1501280

Tsekleves, E., & Keady, J. (2021). *Design for people living with dementia. Interactions and innovations*. Routledge.

User Experience Questionnaire, UEQ. Retrieved May 13, 2022, from https://www.ueq-online.org/

14 Identifying and categorising mindfulness-based design interventions to support people with dementia and their wellbeing

Kristina Niedderer, Isabelle Tournier, Donna Maria Coleston-Shields and Tom Dening

Introduction and conceptual foundations

There is an increasing recognition that design can be helpful in supporting people living with dementia and their wellbeing, particularly for people with early to mid-stage dementia living in their own homes. Through its ubiquitous presence, design has a pivotal role in supporting people in their everyday lives. However, much of the focus is still on cognitive and functional support as well as safeguarding, which design can provide, whereas support for wellbeing remains under-researched (Ludden et al., 2019; Niedderer et al., 2021). By design, we include here design products as well as environments and any services and interactions related to them.

In this chapter, we make a case for the benefits of integrating mindfulness within design to promote wellbeing and develop a framework for distinguishing different categories of mindful design for wellbeing. To this end, we first introduce the key concepts and premises, including wellbeing, psychosocial interventions, design, mindfulness and their interconnections. We then discuss key examples of existing design and mindfulness interventions using concept analysis (Im, 2018). The discussion enables us to identify six distinct categories of mindful design and offers the criteria for distinguishing them. The framework is intended both as a guide for designers and to assist people with dementia, carers and care professionals in choosing appropriate design interventions. It further offers the theoretical basis for future empirical research to explore, refine and evaluate the proposed categories of mindful design for wellbeing.

The impact of dementia on wellbeing

Dementia is one of the main societal challenges of the 21st century. With currently no cure, the focus is on care to improve wellbeing and quality of life for people living with dementia. While much focus has been on the later stages of dementia and care-home provision, it is important to bear in mind that around two-thirds of people with dementia live in their own homes and that more support is needed for them (Clarkson et al., 2017).

Dementia is characterised by the progressive decline of cognitive functions, accompanied by changes in behavioural and emotional functions (Dening & Sandilyan, 2015), termed behavioural and psychological symptoms of dementia (Cerejeira et al., 2012). The latter affect 50% to 80% of people with dementia (Ballard et al., 2008), impact people's sense of wellbeing negatively (Ferring, 2015) and contribute to poor quality of life and early institutionalisation (Cerejeira et al., 2012). For example, people with dementia often struggle with 'self-identity, independence, control and status, activities, stigma, and how to view the future', especially following diagnosis (Low, 2018). In social contexts, they may also experience emotional and social challenges, including a lack of confidence, difficulties in relating to and empathising

DOI: 10.4324/9781003318262-18

with other people, disinhibited behaviour or social withdrawal, which can lead to a reduction in social engagement and its quality (Aldridge et al., 2017; Feast et al., 2016, p. 429).

However, social contact is vital to a person's wellbeing, to stimulating mental faculties and to maintaining emotional balance and quality of life (Fernández-Mayoralas et al., 2015; Mendes de Leon et al., 2003). This need has been recognised by the United Nations Convention on the Rights of Persons with Disabilities, including the right to protection of integrity, independent living and inclusion in the community (United Nations, 2006, Articles 17&19). Encouraging social engagement is therefore crucial for people with dementia. Alcove (2013, pp. 21–22) recommends psychosocial interventions as a priority in addressing psychosocial needs.[1] Johnston and Narayanasamy (2016) further highlight the role of psychosocial interventions in supporting people with dementia in social context.

Supporting wellbeing through psychosocial interventions

Today, there is an increasing number of psychosocial interventions for people living with dementia and cognitive decline (Chow, 2021; McDermott et al., 2019; Moniz-Cook et al., 2008; Guss et al., 2014). While some of them may be subsumed under the broader term of 'non-pharmacological interventions' (Whitlatch & Orsulic-Jeras, 2018), McDermott et al. (2019) point out that this negatively defined term does not describe what it covers and therefore is less useful than the term 'psychosocial intervention'. We follow McDermott et al. (2019, p. 393), adopting their definition of psychosocial interventions:

> as those physical, cognitive or social activities that may maintain or improve "functioning, interpersonal relationships and well-being in people with dementia.
>
> (Moniz-Cook et al., 2008)

In spite of this definition, few interventions focus on and define wellbeing as a whole. Rather, psychosocial interventions variously focus on a mixture of process, means and outcome-based measures, including cognitive, emotion-oriented, sensory and behaviour management (O'Neil et al., 2011); cognitive functioning and independence, reducing stress, anxiety or depression, supporting relationships and communication, maintaining quality of life (Guss et al., 2014, pp. 4–5). While some individual aspects of wellbeing are mentioned in these studies, such as social interaction or emotions, agency only appears in the form of independence, which is only one facet of agency. In this light, Oyebode and Parveen (2019) observe the need to develop psychosocial interventions that focus less on control of behaviours and more on wider aspects of life for people with dementia, especially to 'promote living well in the community post-diagnosis' (p. 8). Similar conclusions are drawn in the context of environmental design for dementia (Ludden et al., 2019). In addition, there is a lack of a clear rationale and theoretical underpinning to the development of psychosocial interventions, to support rigorous evaluation (Orgeta et al., 2022; Oyebode & Parveen, 2019).

Facets and importance of wellbeing

Discourses of wellbeing highlight the importance of subjective wellbeing for people with dementia (Kaufmann & Engel, 2016; Kitwood & Bredin, 1992). While wellbeing may be seen as a 'fluctuating subjective state' (Strohmaier & Camic, 2017), it comprises a number of tangible criteria, namely emotional wellbeing, social engagement and agency as distinguished by Niedderer et al. (2021) based on a review and synthesis of previous definitions and their criteria (Kaufmann & Engel, 2016; Kitwood & Bredin, 1992; Power, 2016; Strohmaier & Camic, 2017). The three

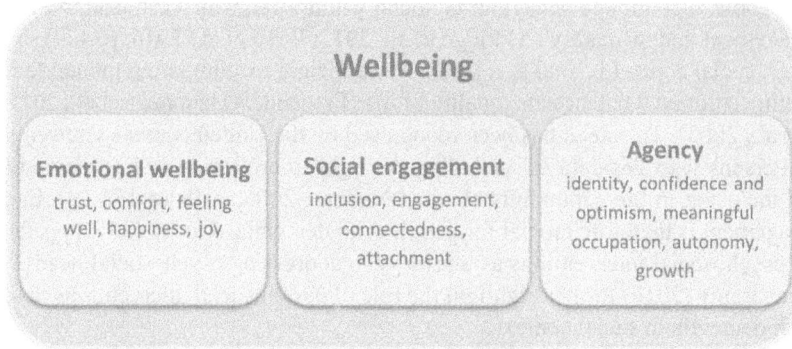

Figure 14.1 Facets of wellbeing, following Niedderer et al., 2021

aspects of wellbeing are strongly interlinked (see Figure 14.1). Emotional wellbeing is closely connected to the level and quality of a person's social engagement. Being socially connected and having caring others who empathise with the person's feelings, thoughts and behaviours can enhance
wellbeing (Aminzadeh et al., 2007; Fernández-Mayoralas et al., 2015) and has been shown to be
associated with more positive emotion expressions (Lee et al., 2017). Social inclusion can also add
a sense of agency or autonomy as an important determinant of wellbeing (Ryan & Deci, 2017).
Agency can be broadly defined as meaningful intentional action. Examples include learning, starting new activities or decision-making and can improve both confidence and optimism (Schlosser,
2015; Zeilig et al., 2019) and offer growth (Power, 2016).

Promoting wellbeing through mindfulness and design

Mindfulness is closely associated with promoting wellbeing. Meditation-based approaches to
mindfulness are now recognised in the dementia context. Other approaches, including cognitive
and design-based interventions, have been used in relation to ageing, mental health as well as areas
of everyday life. Mindfulness approaches, both meditation-based and cognitive, include elements
such as being in the present moment, non-judgemental acceptance of emotions and events (Kabat-
Zinn, 2003; Langer, 1989, 2010). Being in the present moment, and not having to rely on one's
memory, can help with relaxation and ameliorate stress and anxiety (Wells et al., 2013). Non-
judgemental acceptance of emotions and events, oneself and others, can also help with relaxation
and reflection on these can help engender new views and perspectives (Langer, 1989, 2010). Both
can provide useful support for people with dementia. One of the issues with mindfulness is that it
is often related to therapy and requires training, rather than being easily accessible in everyday life.

Design is a useful means for introducing mindfulness into everyday life because of its ubiq-
uity: design surrounds us everywhere, from clothing to housing, transport to communication.
Its utility and widespread use make design a powerful means to support people in everyday life.
When designed into everyday objects, mindfulness can become embedded through use in people's lives (Niedderer, 2014, 2017a). Design, in its broad sense, can be understood as 'courses
of action aimed at changing existing situations into preferred ones' (Simon, 1996, p. 111). Thus
understood, design includes the creation of objects, services, systems, architecture and the environment. Design interventions can offer support within therapy and care settings but also beyond
these in everyday life and social situations (Niedderer et al., 2017). They can support people with
dementia who still live at home to continue to live there better for longer (Niedderer et al., 2021).

Our approach

In light of the above discussion of the benefits of mindfulness and design, we propose that mindfulness-based design interventions may be a useful way to supporting people's wellbeing, especially within everyday and social contexts. We present the rationale and theoretical underpinning for developing mindfulness-based design interventions as a demonstration for others to follow. To this end, we explore the tenets of mindfulness and design-based interventions, and their interconnections, to derive a framework for how we can design for mindful wellbeing for people with dementia in everyday life.

Using mindfulness with people with dementia to foster wellbeing

Due to its assumed cognitive demands, mindfulness has mainly been applied with carers of people with dementia or with older adults, but not with people with dementia themselves. Because of its benefits relating to pain and stress reduction, and to mood improvement, specially adapted approaches are emerging to make mindfulness more accessible. The following discussion provides an overview of the concept of mindfulness before discussing its application with people with dementia.

Mindfulness for wellbeing

The literature on mindfulness is dominated by two major theoretical frameworks. The first defines mindfulness as 'awareness that emerges through paying attention on purpose, in the present moment, and non-judgmentally to the unfolding of experience moment by moment' (Kabat-Zinn, 2003, p. 145). Related to Buddhist meditative practices, applications include mindful meditation and stress reduction programmes, variously comprising formal meditation techniques, such as breathing exercises, body scan, sitting meditation, mindful hatha yoga and informal mindfulness techniques, such as mindful eating, to further 'stillness' or explore patterns of behaviour, thinking, feeling and action (Kabat-Zinn, 2003; Miller et al., 1995; Wells et al., 2013).

Associated with Langer's work on cognitive mindfulness and choice, the second approach presents mindfulness as the process of actively drawing novel distinctions by not relying on automatic categorisations (Langer, 1989). Mindfulness is nurtured by one's orientation to the present, alertness to distinctions, sensitivity to different contexts and openness to novelty (Djikic, 2014, p. 140).

Present-centred awareness, or awareness of the present moment, is a key aspect of both approaches. Bishop et al. (2004) explain that attentional skills (self-regulation), including sustained attention, switching and inhibition, enable staying in the present moment. Orientation to experience adds content, comprising

> an attitude of curiosity about where the mind wanders … [and] … the different objects within one's experience at any moment. All thoughts, feelings, and sensations that arise are … seen as relevant and … subject to observation.
>
> (p. 233)

This leads to a stance of acceptance, which allows being experientially open to the reality of the present moment, and which benefits emotional wellbeing by reducing cognitive overload as well as emotional distress. Meditation and related practices are the main medium of the first mindfulness approach. Cognitive mindfulness uses external stimulation, such as creative cognitive tasks (Alexander et al., 1989) or deliberate environment triggers, objects or situational settings (Langer,

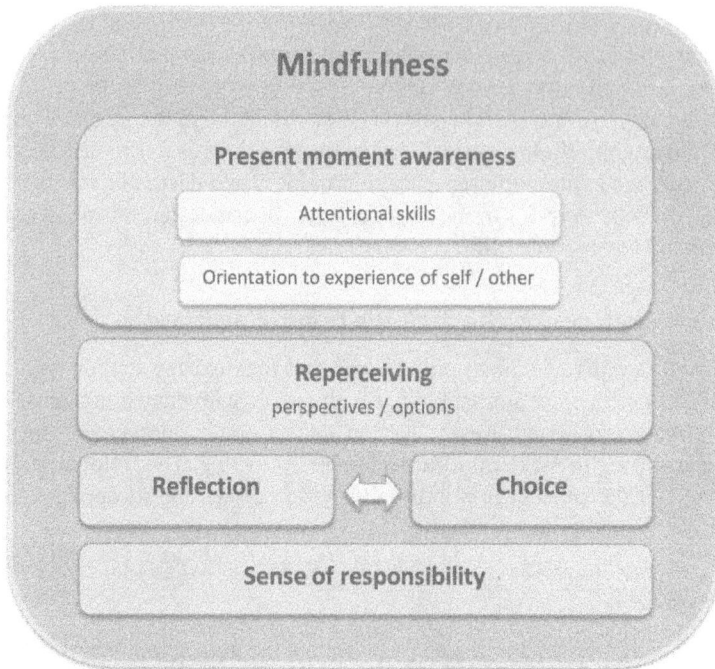

Figure 14.2 Key aspects of mindfulness

1989, pp. 82ff, 100ff), and is based on re-conceptualising self, one's situation or environment, associated choices and motivations. Mindfulness thus enables a shift in perspective, which Shapiro et al. (2006) term reperceiving, and which allows one to 'choose to reflect and self-regulate in ways that foster greater health and wellbeing' (p. 380). Choice and reflection allow taking responsibility for oneself and one's life, encouraging perceptions of self-realisation and self-empowerment that have a positive impact on wellbeing (Langer, 1989, pp. 82ff, 100ff).

This discussion reveals key aspects of mindfulness: awareness of the present moment, based on attentional skills and orientation to experience and relating to both self and/or others, enables reperceiving. Reperceiving, in turn offers new perspectives or options and hence choice, which requires reflection, and leads to a sense of responsibility (Figure 14.2).

Using mindfulness with people with dementia

Mindfulness appears to have benefits for people with dementia in several areas, though cognitive improvements have not yet been conclusively demonstrated. Applying mindfulness to dementia has been hampered by assumptions about the negative effects of cognitive impairment on people's ability to practice mindfulness. For the purposes of this chapter, we challenge these assumptions and have reviewed recent work on mindfulness with people with dementia.

We have conducted a meta-review of six integrative and narrative reviews on, or including, mindfulness approaches with people with mild cognitive impairment (MCI) and early to mid-stage dementia (EMD) (Anderson et al., 2017a, 2017b; Berkh et al., 2018; Burgener et al., 2015; Robertson, 2015; Russell-Williams et al., 2018). From these reviews, we have identified five relevant pilot studies (Clarke et al., 2017; Innes et al., 2014; Moss et al., 2012; Newberg et al.,

2010; Wells et al., 2013), two randomised controlled trials (Alexander et al., 1989; Quintana-Hernández et al., 2016) and one study on the ability of people with dementia to learn and participate in mindfulness meditation and training (Bousfield & Stott, 2019). All studies included were based on mindfulness meditation or mindfulness-based stress reduction training, except for one study on cognitive mindfulness training (Alexander et al., 1989), which instead used exercises for drawing cognitive distinctions through a combination of structured word-production and unstructured creative mental activity tasks.

Mindfulness practices require attentional and self-regulatory efforts progressively impaired in people with dementia. Using mindfulness-based approaches can therefore appear counterintuitive. However, progressive loss of memory and difficulties to project into the future tend to amplify the importance of the present moment for people with dementia (Power, 2011, p. xii). Bousfield and Stott (2019) found no significant difference in the ability to learn mindfulness techniques compared to people without cognitive decline. Rather, people with MCI using mindfulness-based stress reduction displayed a positive impact on regions of the brain negatively impacted by MCI and Alzheimer's disease because the training stimulates these regions of the brain (Wells et al., 2013).

In studies of mindfulness meditation involving people with MCI or EMD, Moss et al. (2012) observed improvements in mood, anxiety, tension and fatigue. Innes et al. (2014) found improvements in mood, stress, psychological wellbeing and quality of life. Using an adapted form of mindfulness-based stress reduction, Clarke et al. (2017) observed improvements in quality of life, but no changes in mood and anxiety. Quintana-Hernández et al. (2016) compared the effects of the mindfulness-based Alzheimer's stimulation programme on cognitive capacity with cognitive stimulation therapy and progressive muscle relaxation. They found that mindfulness-based Alzheimer's stimulation is as effective as cognitive stimulation therapy, and that it can slow cognitive impairment in persons with Alzheimer's disease. This confirms Alexander et al.'s (1989) earlier findings on the benefits of mindfulness meditation to cognition and longevity, while cognitive mindfulness therapy – predictably – offered less relaxation but had benefits in perceived control and word fluency, supporting perceptions of empowerment (p. 961).

In summary, the use of mindfulness practices with people with dementia suggests that there are psychological and behavioural benefits and cognitive and neuroprotective effects for the brain. While mindfulness meditation helps with cognition, emotions, wellbeing and quality of life, cognitive mindfulness therapy can support a sense of control and empowerment. Even though mindfulness approaches do require cognitive processes that are affected by dementia, nonetheless, tailored programmes, support from caregivers and external tools and reminders can make mindfulness training feasible and enjoyable for participants (Clarke et al., 2017). One limitation of the studies described here is that the participant samples may be relatively limited and may not reflect the full diversity of societies. With a focus on Anglophone countries, the applicability of the findings elsewhere will need further research. Nevertheless, it is of interest that different mindfulness approaches seem to have contrasting effects.

Using design to embed mindfulness in everyday life

This section considers how design can embed mindfulness in people's lives to support wellbeing. We first discuss how mindful design works. We then discuss selected examples with regard to the identified aspects of mindfulness as well as wellbeing.

Designing mindfulness

The idea of mindfulness in design was first proposed by Niedderer in 2007, and then gradually refined (2014, 2017a, 2017b). Niedderer proposed that (aspects of) mindfulness can be

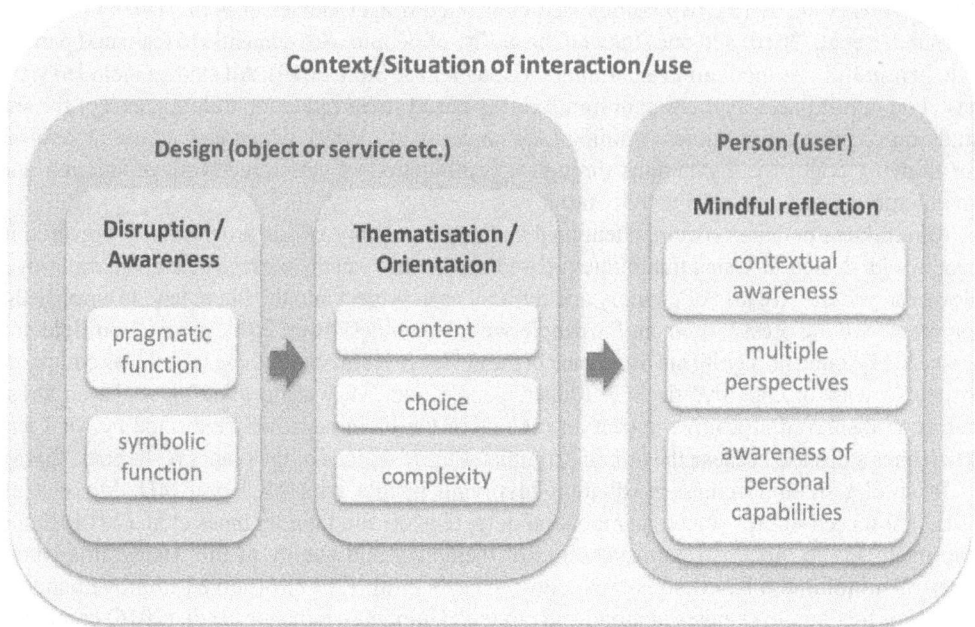

Figure 14.3 Mindful design mechanisms, adapted from Niedderer (2017b)

embedded within objects and through objects in people's lives, drawing on the mindful aspects of awareness, orientation and reflection. Using an object's function, either relating to its practical or symbolic use, to disrupt a user's action helps to draw their attention to it. Orienting the user's attention to the potential consequences of their actions and offering choices for completing the action by offering relevant content and related action choices (thematisation) offers reperceiving and reflection on the different potential actions or perspectives (Figure 14.3). For example, health features on smartwatches can prompt awareness of our state of health and promote activities, such as standing up or breathing mindfully, by buzzing the wearer to raise attention and displaying a banner asking them to breathe deeply or stand up for a minute.

The key here is that we can embed content and choice into the object. In meditation-based mindfulness exercises, content is provided through orientation to experience by focusing on breathing, the body, imagery, mantras, or similar. Design offers the option of externalising this focus to provide relevant content. In addition, the object's ability to afford different actions provides the user with a choice and thus requires reflection and a sense of responsibility for the choice made. In the following examples, we discuss different ways in which this can work.

Considering the different examples of mindful design

Still very new, a small but increasing number of studies demonstrates how mindfulness thinking and practice can be embedded within and through design interventions. One of the difficulties is finding these examples. Generally, many of these studies or design examples have not been tested in such a way as to be included in any peer-reviewed academic papers. In fact, many are not tested at all but simply released as commercial products and evidence, therefore, remains anecdotal although there is now an emerging literature on smart devices and apps, which can include various aspects of mindfulness (e.g. Hwang et al., 2021) as well as on coloring (e.g. Jakobsson Støre & Jakobsson, 2022).

Finding relevant products can be even more challenging because of the broad use of the term 'design'. In many cases, mindfulness is not mentioned explicitly even though interventions or products can be shown to incorporate aspects of mindfulness. In other instances, mindfulness is used loosely in the context of commercial designing as a means for designers to become more creative or perhaps to design more responsibly (e.g. IDEO[2]). For these reasons, the examples we provide here are not systematic but eclectic and purposive, and we offer the following analysis and discussion in the hope that it will lead to a clearer, extended and more evidence-based practice of mindful design in the sense in which it has been developed by Niedderer (2014, 2017a, 2017b). In the following, we discuss the selected examples in terms of their approach to mindfulness and potential impact on wellbeing. We have identified six types of approaches relating to the way they engender or promote mindfulness.

1) *Initiating mindfulness practices*

In everyday life, it is not always easy to remember one's mindfulness practices. Design interventions, in the form of fitness trackers, smart watches, or phone apps, can act as prompts to raise awareness of this need (Hwang et al., 2021; Saganowski et al., 2020). A basic example of this application is the health feature of many smartwatches, such as the Apple watch, which can be set to prompt the user at regular times (e.g. every hour) to breathe more deeply. Thus, it creates awareness of health and exercise needs and gives the user a choice for them to take (or not take) the suggested action. This application draws on a combination of cognitive and meditation-based approaches, using the first to initiate the second. It can thus promote a general sense of wellbeing (comfort, feeling well) associated with breathing (or alternative) exercises performed. In addition, the choice of completing the exercise might add a sense of agency and satisfaction.

2) *Guiding mindfulness practices*

Extending the first approach, there are various design interventions to guide mindfulness training or exercise instead of an in-person trainer. Foremost, these come in the format of books or apps (e.g. Chaskalson, 2014; Hwang et al., 2021; Kabat-Zinn, 2013; Saganowski et al., 2020), or physical mindfulness cards (e.g. 'Mindfulness Cards' by Rohan Gunatillake or '31 Day Mindfulness Challenge' by Sharon Jeffreys). The kind of mindfulness training or exercise these designs offer varies and can include, for example, mindfulness-based cognitive therapy or stress reduction training, mediation, or mindful reflection during the day. Generally, there is little evaluation of the performance, but one app, which offers thought distancing training, was evaluated by Chittaro and Vianello (2014), who found that such design interventions can significantly surpass the effectiveness of traditional mindfulness training.

In both the first and second sets of examples, the interventions take on the function of the traditional trainer, both as prompts and guidance, allowing access to mindfulness exercises anywhere and anytime, integrating them within daily life. The aspect of wellbeing achieved, depends on the mindfulness exercise chosen, but generally, effects have been found to relate to a reduction in stress, anxiety and depression, and an increase in life satisfaction and quality of life (e.g. Hwang et al., 2021).

3) *Supporting mindfulness practices*

Another design approach focuses on supporting formal mindfulness practices. The design example by Thieme et al. (2013) aims to support the practice of mindful breathing in a therapeutic context related to mental health. This design is an interactive orb, which can be held during exercise. It visualises the person's heartbeat through a gentle light pulsing in time with it. It has been developed and evaluated with regard to promoting mindful awareness of the relationship of breathing exercise and heart rate during therapy sessions to help with relaxation. A related approach, in an informal context, is provided through wearables, which can offer similar interactive sensory feedback (Saganowski et al., 2020) and are closely linked to approach 2.

4) *Triggering mindful experiences through nature-based stimuli*

In interventions relating to environment design, nature-based imagery has been used in mindfulness practices to trigger meditative states through effortless attention ('soft fascination') as a sense of being away from worries and routines without relying on effortful cognitive processes (Kaplan & Kaplan, 1989, 2011). Stimuli including daylighting, natural sounds and natural landscapes have been found to improve sleep quality, reduce anxiety and increase wellbeing (Ozdemir & Akdemir, 2009; Whear et al., 2014).

5) *Using meditative activities to promote mindful experiences*

For some time now, there has been a rise in arts or craft-based activities claiming to promote a mindful experience. Colouring books, especially those with Mandala motifs, where outlines are provided ready to be coloured in, currently appear to be one of the most popular activities. Research suggests that colouring, whether mindfulness-related or not, can help reduce anxiety and promote wellbeing based on the principle of 'flow', or focused activity (e.g. Mantzios et al., 2022; Singh, 2018; Jakobsson Støre & Jakobsson, 2022).

6) *Including cognitive mindfulness in everyday social activities*

While the five examples above predominantly rely on meditation-based mindfulness approaches, the last example considers the use of cognitive mindfulness based on Langer's work (1989, 2010). The *This is Me* game,[3] which was developed and evaluated with people with dementia, is a life-storytelling board game that offers players a series of mindful-reflective questions relating to experiences and aspirational activities for each decade of life (Niedderer et al., 2021). Langer (1989) has shown that being in the present moment and developing new perspectives can improve physical and mental wellbeing in relation to ageing. According to Langer, one way of putting oneself into the present moment is by putting one's mind into the present, such as by speaking in the present tense, even if speaking about the past (pp. 100–113). Following Langer's experiments on using supportive prompts to put one's mind into the present moment, all question cards are phrased in the present tense. In addition, the players can decide how to answer the cards and the game can be played flexibly, offering aspects of choice and reflection. During the evaluation, players of the game demonstrated mindful instances of 'in the moment' enjoyment as well as acceptance of experiences, both good and bad. The game fostered experiences relating to all three aspects of wellbeing: emotional wellbeing, social engagement and agency. While we have focused here on the example of the game, some of the mindfulness cards mentioned above also offer exercises based on cognitive mindfulness.

Discussion: establishing a framework for categorising mindful design interventions

The above discussion of examples has highlighted six different categories of mindful design interventions, which we summarise with a definition in Table 14.1.

Table 14.1 Six mindful design categories and their definitions

	Category	Definition
1.	**Design for initiating mindfulness practices**	Design for raising awareness ('prompt') to initiate mindfulness practices, usually in everyday life context.
2.	**Design for guiding mindfulness practices**	Design for delivering mindfulness meditation or training in everyday or therapeutic, contexts.
3.	**Design for supporting mindfulness practices**	Design for supporting mindfulness practice in therapeutic, or everyday, contexts.
4.	**Nature-based design for triggering mindful experiences**	(Multi)sensory design of mindfulness-state-supporting environments, within or without therapeutic context.
5.	**Activity-based design for triggering mindful flow**	Designs to promote 'mindful flow' through creative or sensory activities, with or without mindfulness instructions.
6.	**Designing cognitive mindfulness for everyday**	Design for embedding mindful mindset and choices in everyday (social) contexts through cognitive mechanisms.

Reflecting on these categories, categories 1 to 3 are closely interrelated in that they encompass a prompt, guidance for, and feedback on mindful practice. The starting point is the prompt accompanied by a directive for what action to practice, whereas guidance provides specific detail on how to practice and feedback offers further help to improve one's practice. This work includes both meditation and cognitive-based approaches and is largely focused on mental and physical wellbeing, especially emotional wellbeing. Studies of mindfulness practices have to date largely focused on emotional wellbeing, but further work is needed, for example in extending this research to the context of dementia.

Categories 4 and 5 are based on less formal approaches to mindfulness in that they seek to promote a meditative state, albeit in two different ways: nature-based designs seek to induce this state through sensory immersion, whereas activity-based designs seek to do so through immersion in some, usually repetitive, arts and craft activity. Category 4 has a sound theoretical underpinning, but both categories would benefit from further research or translation into design interventions. Finally, category 6 explicitly relates to cognitive mindfulness. In line with prior research (Alexander et al., 1989; Niedderer et al., 2021), it is more strongly focused on agency and social engagement and has been evaluated in the dementia context. There, is much scope for innovation to explore the breadth of possible applications through design.

In summary, the emergence of these different approaches is promising, but there is a need for more detailed and systematic research. We hope that the distinction of these different categories of mindful design will support understanding of, and further research into novel design options. In turn, this will engender both the development of new products and their evaluation, and this will subsequently lead to more choice and better interventions.

Conclusion: designing for mindful wellbeing

This chapter has brought together and reviewed challenges concerning subjective wellbeing, self-empowerment and social engagement for people with dementia; the application of mindfulness with people with dementia; and different mindful design approaches. In doing so, it has elicited the key criteria for six mindful design approaches as a framework for the application of mindful design interventions in the dementia context.

The framework aims to enable a better understanding of how to design and choose mindful design. The framework's purpose thus is twofold: it can benefit designers as a guide for understanding and creating mindful design solutions with and for people with dementia; and it can assist users, including people with dementia, formal and informal carers and care professionals in understanding and choosing appropriate (types of) design interventions in relation to desired outcomes to support them in everyday/social life or relevant therapies.

A limitation is that there are few existing examples of mindful design being applied within the dementia context. The framework is therefore developed theoretically based on the discussion of mindfulness practices with people with dementia and of mindful design examples in other contexts to demonstrate the potential and benefits. The strength of the framework is that it will enable others to develop, test against and populate the framework with examples from clinical, dementia care and design practice, which – we hope – over time will lead to the refinement and development of the framework and its categories.

Acknowledgements

This article has been developed as part of the MinD project, and we want to thank all colleagues, who have supported us in the development of this chapter.

The MinD project has received funding from the European Union's Horizon 2020 research and innovation programme under the Marie Skłodowska-Curie grant agreement No 691001. This document reflects only the authors' view and the Research Executive Agency is not responsible for any use that may be made of the information it contains. Further information on the MinD project is available here: www.designingfordementia.eu

Notes

1 For the purposes of this paper, we use the term psychosocial to include psychological, behavioural and social issues and needs. The inclusion of the behavioural aspect in the term 'psychosocial' acknowledges the use of behavioural interventions as part of psychosocial studies (e.g. Burgio and Fisher, 2000) and the application of psychosocial interventions to behavioural issues (Alcove, 2013), thus emphasising psychosocial aspects over bio-psychosocial ones as distinguished by Stenner (Stenner, 2017, p. 2).
2 https://www.ideo.com/blog/5-ways-mindfulness-can-make-you-a-better-designer [accessed 5 May 2022]
3 Commercially available under the name *All About Us*, produced by Relish.

References

Alcove. (2013). *The European joint action on dementia: Synthesis report 2013*. Retrieved November 23, 2019, from https://www.alcove-project.eu/images/pdf/ALCOVE_SYNTHESIS_REPORT_VF.pdf
Aldridge, H., Fisher, P., & Laidlaw, K. (2017). Experiences of shame for people with dementia: An interpretative phenomenological analysis. *Dementia*. https://doi.org/10.1177/1471301217732430
Alexander, C. N., Chandler, H. M., Langer, E. J., Newman, R. I., & Davies, J. L. (1989). Transcendental meditation, mindfulness and longevity: An experimental study with the elderly. *Journal of Personality and Social Development, 57*(6), 950–964.
Aminzadeh, F., Byszewski, A., Molnar, F. J., & Eisner, M. (2007). Emotional impact of dementia diagnosis: Exploring persons with dementia and caregivers' perspectives. *Aging and Mental Health, 11*(3), 281–290. https://doi.org/10.1080/13607860600963695
Anderson, J. G., Lopez, R. P., Rose, K. M., & Specht, J. K. (2017b). Nonpharmacological strategies for patients with early-stage dementia or mild cognitive impairment: A 10-year update. *Research in Gerontological Nursing, 10*(1), 5–11.

Anderson, J. G., Rogers, C. E., Bossen, A., Testad, I., & Rose, K. M. (2017a). Mind–body therapies in individuals with dementia: An integrative review. *Research in Gerontological Nursing, 10*(6), 288–296.

Ballard, C., Day, S., Sharp, S., Wing, G., & Sorensen, S. (2008). Neuropsychiatric symptoms in dementia: Importance and treatment considerations. *International Review of Psychiatry.* https://doi.org/10.1080/09540260802099968

Berkh, L., Warmenhoven, F., van Os, J., & van Boxtel, M. (2018). Mindfulness training for people with dementia and their caregivers: Rationale, current research, and future directions. *Frontiers in Psychology.* https://doi.org/10.3389/fpsyg.2018.00982

Bishop, S. R., Lau, M., Shapiro, S., Carlson, L., Anderson, N. D., Carmody, J., Susan Abbey, S., Speca, M., Velting, D., & Devins, G. (2004). Mindfulness: A proposed operational definition. *Clinical Psychology, 11*(3), 230–241.

Bousfield, C., & Stott, J. (2019). Impact of dementia on mindful attention: A cross-sectional comparison of people with dementia and those without. *Mindfulness, 10*(2), 279–287.

Burgener, S. C., Jao, Y. L., Anderson, J. G., & Bossen, A. L. (2015). Mechanism of action for nonpharmacological therapies for individuals with dementia: Implications for practice and research. *Research in Gerontological Nursing.* https://doi.org/10.3928/19404921-20150429-02

Burgio, L. D., & Fisher, S. E. (2000). Application of psychosocial interventions for treating behavioral and psychological symptoms of dementia. *International Psychogeriatrics, 12*(Suppl. I), 351–358.

Cerejeira, J., Lagarto, L., & Mukaetova-Ladinska, E. B. (2012). Behavioral and psychological symptoms of dementia. *Frontiers in Neurology.* https://doi.org/10.3389/fneur.2012.00073

Chaskalson, M. (2014). *Mindfulness in eight weeks.* Harper Thorsons.

Chittaro, L., & Vianello, A. (2014). Computer-supported mindfulness: Evaluation of a mobile thought distancing application on naive meditators. *International Journal of Human-Computer Studies, 72*(3), 337–348.

Chow, G., Gan, J. K. E., Chan, J. K. Y., Wu, X. V., & Klainin-Yobas, P. (2021). Effectiveness of psychosocial interventions among older adults with mild cognitive impairment: A systematic review and meta-analysis. *Aging and Mental Health, 25*(11), 1986–1997. https://doi.org/10.1080/13607863.2020.1839861

Clarke, A. C., Chan, J. M. Y., Stott, J., Royan, L., & Spector, A. (2017). An adapted mindfulness intervention for people with dementia in care homes: Feasibility pilot study. *International Journal of Geriatry and Psychiatry, 32*, e123–e131.

Clarkson, P., Hughes, J., Xie, C., Larbey, M., Roe, B., Giebel, C. M., Jolley, D., Challis, D., & Members of the HoSt-D (Home Support in Dementia) Programme Management Group. (2017). Overview of systematic reviews: Effective home support in dementia care, components and impacts-Stage 1, psychosocial interventions for dementia. *Journal of Advanced Nursing, 73*(12), 2845–2863. https://doi.org/10.1111/jan.13362

de Leon, M., Glass, C. F. T. A., & Berkman, L. F. (2003). Social engagement and disability in a community population of older adults: The New Haven EPESE. *American Journal of Epidemiology, 157*(7), 633–642.

Dening, T., & Sandilyan, M. B. (2015). Dementia: Definitions and types. *Nursing Standard, 29*(37), 37–42.

Djikic, M. (2014). Art of mindfulness: Integrating eastern and western approaches. In A. Ie., C. T. Ngnoumen & E. J. Langer (Eds.), *The Wiley Blackwell Handbook of Mindfulness* (pp. 139-148). John Wiley & Sons, Ltd.

Feast, A., Orrell, M., Charlesworth, G., Melunsky, N., Poland, F., & Moniz-Cook, E. (2016). Behavioural and psychological symptoms in dementia and the challenges for family carers: Systematic review. *British Journal of Psychiatry.* https://doi.org/10.1192/bjp.bp.114.153684

Fernández-Mayoralas, G., Rojo-Pérez, F., Martínez-Martín, P., Prieto-Flores, M.-E., Rodríguez-Blázquez, C., Martín-García, S., Rojo-Abuín, J.-M., & Forjaz, M.-J. (2015). Active ageing and quality of life: Factors associated with participation in leisure activities among institutionalized older adults, with and without dementia. *Aging and Mental Health, 19*(11), 1031–1041. https://doi.org/10.1080/13607863.2014.996734

Ferring, D. (2015). Alzheimer's disease: Behavioral and social aspects. In J. D. Wright (Ed.), *International encyclopedia of the social & behavioral sciences* (Vol. 1, pp. 584–590). Elsevier.

Guss, R., Middleton, J., Beanland, T., Slade, L., Moniz-Cook, E., Watts, S., & Bone, A. (2014). *A guide to psychosocial interventions in early stages of dementia*. The British Psychological Society.

Hwang, W. J., Ha, J. S., & Kim, M. J. (2021). Research trends on mobile mental health application for general population: A scoping review. *International Journal of Environmental Research and Public Health*, *18*(5), 2459. https://doi.org/10.3390/ijerph18052459

Im, E. O. (2018). Theory development strategies for middle-range theories. *Advances in Nursing Science*, *41*(3), 275–292. https://doi.org/10.1097/ANS.0000000000000215

Innes, K. E., Selfe, T. K., Khalsa, D. S., & Kandati, S. (2014). Effects of meditation versus music listening on perceived stress, mood, sleep, and quality of life in adults with early memory loss: A pilot randomized controlled trial. *Journal of Alzheimer's Disease*, *52*(4), 1277–1298.

Jakobsson Støre, S., & Jakobsson, N. (2022). The effect of mandala coloring on state anxiety: A systematic review and meta-analysis. *Art Therapy*. https://doi.org/10.1080/07421656.2021.2003144

Johnston, B., & Narayanasamy, M. (2016). Exploring psychosocial interventions for people with dementia that enhance personhood and relate to legacy-An integrative review. *BMC Geriatrics*. https://doi.org/10.1186/s12877-016-0250-1

Kabat-Zinn, J. (2003). Mindfulness-based interventions in context: Past, present, and future. *Clinical Psychology: Science and Practice*, *10*(2), 144–156.

Kabat-Zinn, J. (2013). *Full catastrophe living. Using the wisdom of your body and mind to face stress, pain, and Illness* (Rev. ed.). Random House Publishing. ISBN: 9780345539724.

Kaplan, R., & Kaplan, S. (1989). *The experience of nature: A psychological perspective*. Cambridge University Press.

Kaplan, R., & Kaplan, S. (2011). Well-being, reasonableness, and the natural environment. *Applied Psychology: Health and Well-Being*, *3*(3), 304–321.

Kaufmann, E. G., & Engel, S. A. (2016). Dementia and well-being: A conceptual framework based on tom Kitwood's model of needs. *Dementia*, *15*(4), 774–788. https://doi.org/10.1177/1471301214539690

Kitwood, T., & Bredin, K. (1992). Towards a theory of dementia care: Personhood and well-being. *Ageing and Society*, *12*(3), 269–287. https://doi.org/10.1017/s0144686x0000502x

Langer, E. J. (1989). *Mindfulness*. Da Capo Press.

Langer, E. J. (2010). *Counterclockwise*. Hodder & Stoughton.

Lee, K. H., Boltz, M., Lee, H., & Algase, D. L. (2017). Does social interaction matter psychological well-being in persons with dementia? *American Journal of Alzheimer's Disease and Other Dementias*, *32*(4), 207–212. https://doi.org/10.1177/1533317517704301

Low, L.-F., Swaffer, K., McGrath, M., & Brodaty, H. (2018). Do people with early stage dementia experience prescribed disengagement®? A systematic review of qualitative studies. *International Psychogeriatrics*, *30*(6), 807–831. https://doi.org/10.1017/s1041610217001545

Ludden, G. D. S., van Rompay, T. J. L., Niedderer, K., & Tournier, I. (2019). Environmental design for dementia care - Towards more meaningful experiences through design. *Maturitas*, *128*, 10–16. https://doi.org/10.1016/j.maturitas.2019.06.011

Mantzios, M., Tariq, A., Altaf, M., & Giannou, K. (2022). Loving-kindness colouring and loving-kindness meditation: Exploring the effectiveness of non-meditative and meditative practices on state mindfulness and anxiety. *Journal of Creativity in Mental Health*, *17*(3), 305–312. https://doi.org/10.1080/15401383.2021.1884159

McDermott, O., Charlesworth, G., Hogervorst, E., Stoner, C., Moniz-Cook, E., Spector, A., Csipke, E., & Orrell, M. (2019). Psychosocial interventions for people with dementia: A synthesis of systematic reviews. *Aging and Mental Health*, *23*(4), 393–403. https://doi.org/10.1080/13607863.2017.1423031

Miller, J. J., Fletcher, K., & Kabat-Zinn, J. (1995). Three-year follow-up and clinical implications of a mindfulness meditation-based stress reduction intervention in the treatment of anxiety disorders. *General Hospital Psychiatry*, *17*(3), 192–200.

Moniz-Cook, E., Vernooij-Dassen, M., Woods, R., Verhey, F., Chattat, R., De Vugt, M., Mountain, G., O'connell, M., Harrison, J., Vasse, E., Dröes, R. M., Orrell, M., & For The Interdem* Group. (2008). A European consensus on outcome measures for psychosocial intervention research in dementia care. *Aging and Mental Health*, *12*(1), 14–29. https://doi.org/10.1080/13607860801919850

Moss, A. S., Wintering, N., Roggenkamp, H., Khalsa, D. S., Waldman, M. R., Monti, D., & Newberg, A. B. (2012). Effects of an 8-week meditation program on mood and anxiety in patients with memory loss. *Journal of Alternative and Complementary Medicine.* https://doi.org/10.1089/acm.2011.0051

Newberg, A. B., Wintering, N., Khalsa, D. S., Roggenkamp, H., & Waldman, M. R. (2010). Meditation effects on cognitive function and cerebral blood flow in subjects with memory loss: A preliminary study. *Journal of Alzheimer's Disease.* https://doi.org/10.3233/jad-2010-1391

Niedderer, K. (2007). Designing mindful interaction: The category of the performative object. *Design Issues, 23*(1), 3–17.

Niedderer, K. (2014). Mediating mindful social interactions through design. In A. Ie., C. T. Ngnoumen & E. Langer (Eds.), *The Wiley Blackwell Handbook of Mindfulness* (Vol. 1, pp. 345–366). John Wiley & Sons, Ltd. https://doi.org/10.1002/9781118294895.ch19

Niedderer, K. (2017a). Facilitating behaviour change through mindful design. In K. Niedderer, S. Clune, & G. Ludden (Eds.), *Design for behaviour change* (pp. 104–115). Routledge.

Niedderer, K. (2017b). Promoting sustainability through mindful design. In J. Chapman (Ed.), *The Routledge handbook of sustainable product design* (pp. 527–539). Routledge. https://doi.org/10.4324/9781315693309

Niedderer, K., Clune, S., & Ludden, G. (Eds.). (2017). *Design for behaviour change: Theories and practices of designing for change*. Routledge.

Niedderer, K., Holthoff-Detto, V., van Rompay, T. J. L., Karahanoğlu, A., Ludden, G. D. S., Almeida, R., Losada Durán, R., Bueno Aguado, Y., Lim, J. N. W., Smith, T., Harrison, D., Craven, M. P., Gosling, J., Orton, L., & Tournier, I. (2021). This is Me: Evaluation of a board game to promote social engagement, wellbeing and agency in people with dementia through mindful life-storytelling. *Journal of Aging Studies, 60.* https://doi.org/10.1016/j.jaging.2021.100995

O'Neil, M. E., Freeman, M., Christensen, V., Telerant, R., Addleman, A., & Kansagara, D. (2011). *A systematic evidence review of non-pharmacological interventions for behavioral symptoms of dementia.* Department of Veterans Affairs.

Orgeta, V., Palpatzis, E., See, Y. N., Tuijt, R., Verdaguer, E. S., & Leung, P. (2022). Development of a psychological intervention to promote meaningful activity in people living with mild dementia: An intervention mapping approach. *Gerontologist, 62*(4), 629–641. https://doi.org/10.1093/geront/gnab047

Oyebode, J. R., & Parveen, S. (2019). Psychosocial interventions for people with dementia: An overview and commentary on recent developments. *Dementia, 18*(1), 8–35.

Ozdemir, L., & Akdemir, N. (2009). Effects of multisensory stimulation on cognition, depression and anxiety levels of mildly-affected Alzheimer's patients. *Journal of the Neurological Sciences.* https://doi.org/10.1016/j.jns.2009.02.367

Power, G. A. (2011). Foreword. In H. Lee & T. Adams (Eds.), *Creative approaches in dementia care* (pp. x–xiii). Palgrave Macmillan.

Power, G. A. (2016, November 30). *Dementia beyond disease: Enhancing well-being* (Rev. ed.). Health Professions Press.

Quintana-Hernández, D. J., Miró-Barrachina, M. T., Ibáñez-Fernández, I. J., Pino, A. S., Quintana-Montesdeoca, M. P., Rodríguez-de Vera, B., Morales-Casanova, D., Pérez-Vieitez Mdel, C., Rodríguez-García, J., & Bravo-Caraduje, N. (2016). Mindfulness in the maintenance of cognitive capacities in Alzheimer's disease: A randomized clinical trial. *Journal of Alzheimer's Disease, 50*(1), 217–232.

Robertson, G. (2015). Spirituality and ageing – The role of mindfulness in supporting people with dementia to live well. *Working with Older People.* https://doi.org/10.1108/WWOP-11-2014-0038

Russell-Williams, J., Jaroudi, W., Perich, T., Hoscheidt, S., El Haj, M., & Moustafa, A. A. (2018). Mindfulness and meditation: Treating cognitive impairment and reducing stress in dementia. *Reviews in the Neurosciences.* https://doi.org/10.1515/revneuro-2017-0066

Ryan, R. M., & Deci, E. L. (2017). *Self-determination theory: Basic psychological needs in motivation, development, and wellness.* Guilford Publishing.

Saganowski, S., Kazienko, P., Dziezyc, M., Jakimow, P., Komoszynska, J., Michalska, W., Dutkowiak, A., Polak, A., Dziadek, A., & Ujma, M. (2020.). Consumer wearables and affective computing for wellbeing support. In *MobiQuitous 2020 - 17th EAI international conference on mobile and ubiquitous systems: Computing, networking and services (MobiQuitous '20)* (pp. 482–487). Association for Computing Machinery. https://doi.org/10.1145/3448891.3450332

Schlosser, M. (2015). Agency. In *The Stanford encyclopedia of philosophy*. Stanford University. Retrieved January 11 , 2021, from https://plato.stanford.edu/archives/win2019/entries/agency/

Shapiro, S. L., Carlson, L. E., Astin, J. A., & Freedman, B. (2006). Mechanisms of mindfulness. *Journal of Clinical Psychology*. https://doi.org/10.1002/jclp.20237

Simon, H. (1996). *The sciences of the artificial* (3rd ed.). MIT.

Singh, N. (2018). *Does colouring promote mindfulness and enhance wellbeing? A randomised controlled trial* (PhD Thesis). University of Surrey.

Stenner, P. (2017). *Liminality and experience. A transdisciplinary approach to the psychosocial*. Palgrave Macmillan.

Strohmaier, S., & Camic, P. (2017, November 24). *Conceptualising what we mean by 'wellbeing' in the dementias*. Royal Society for Public Health conference 'Powerful Partners: Advancing Dementia Care through the Arts & Sciences. Retrieved April 8, 2021, from https://repository.canterbury.ac.uk/item/88v33/conceptualising-what-we-mean-by-wellbeing-in-the-dementias

Thieme, A., Wallace, J., Johnson, P., McCarthy, J., Lindley, S., Wright, P., Olivier, P., & Meyer, T. (2013). Design to promote mindfulness practice and sense of self for vulnerable women in secure hospital services. In Proceedings of the SIGCHI Conference on Human Factors in Computing Systems (CHI '13). Association for Computing Machinery, New York, NY, USA, pp. 2647–2656. https://doi.org/10.1145/2470654.2481366.

United Nations. (2006). *Convention on the rights of persons with disabilities*. Retrieved October 31, 2023, from https://www.ohchr.org/en/instruments-mechanisms/instruments/convention-rights-persons-disabilities

Wells, R. E., Yeh, G. Y., Kerr, C. E., Wolkin, J., Davis, R. B., Tan, Y. Spaeth, R., Wall, R. B., Walsh, J., Kaptchuk, T. J., Press, D., Phillips, R. S., & Kong, J. (2013). Meditation's impact on default mode network and hippocampus in mild cognitive impairment: A pilot study. *Neuroscience Letters*. https://doi.org/10.1016/j.neulet.2013.10.001

Whear, R., Coon, J. T., Bethel, A., Abbott, R., Stein, K., & Garside, R. (2014). What is the impact of using outdoor spaces such as gardens on the physical and mental wellbeing of those with dementia? A systematic review of quantitative and qualitative evidence. *Journal of the American Medical Directors Association*. https://doi.org/10.1016/j.jamda.2014.05.013

Whitlatch, C. J., & Orsulic-Jeras, S. (2018). Meeting the informational, educational, and psychosocial support needs of persons living with dementia and their family caregivers. *Gerontologist*. https://doi.org/10.1093/geront/gnx162

Zeilig, H., Tischler, V., van der Byl Williams, M., West, J., & Strohmaier, S. (2019). Co-creativity, wellbeing and agency: A case study analysis of a co-creative arts group for people with dementia. *Journal of Aging Studies*, *49*, 16–24. https://doi.org/10.1016/j.jaging.2019.03.002

15 Mindful design for designers

The dimensions of socio-cognitive mindfulness and correlating the Mindful Design Evaluation Scale and visual cards for expert use

Michaelle Bosse and Christian Wölfel

Motivation

Human-technology interaction and user behaviour have changed substantially over the past few decades due to digital transformation (Yasav, 2015). The problem is no longer a lack of information, but the coordination of this amount of information almost simultaneously (Endsley, 2001). This new human behaviour of constantly communicating and being informed digitally has led the world population to a different kind of problem: a massive movement towards mental health problems such as addictions and concentration problems (Alhassan et al., 2018; Parasuraman et al., 2017; Mutchler et al., 2011; Cha & Seo, 2018).

Another side of the digital transformation brings to light the difficulties of adapting the development of high-tech household and industrial devices to human cognitive factors of attention, learning and information processing. The inability of these devices to cater to these human factors has led to a lack of acceptance, adoption and uncertainty among many people (e.g. Lewis, 2000).

The human capacity to process information is limited (Schaub, 2008). During conscious information processing, not as many stimuli can be processed as would be necessary to fully understand situations, potential actions and their consequences (Spieß, 2002). When people take in information with alertness, their attention focuses on specific objects, processes and thoughts. Their attention can be directed voluntarily (by interests) or stimulated involuntarily (passively) (Davies et al., 2000). At some point, adjusting human attention and cognition to the amount of information available becomes impossible with consequences for emotional balance and psychological wellbeing. Feeling overwhelmed and lost in this whirlwind of external and internal needs has become a significant health issue worldwide (e.g. Shanafelt et al., 2015; Rama Devi & Nagini, 2014).

How can design help to address digital-transformation-related issues of stress and cognitive overload?

To address the issues of stress and distraction that are further promoted by the digital transformation, studies on mindfulness have increasingly focused on the Western research field of psychology for cognitive enhancement since the 1990s (Kabat-Zinn, 1990; Langer, 2000). Researchers and practitioners of mindfulness have identified mindfulness interventions from Buddhist philosophy that date back over 2500 years (Hanh, 1975; Kabat-Zinn, 1990).

Two predominant streams of mindfulness research and practice can be found in the literature: meditative mindfulness (Kabat-Zinn, 2003) and socio-cognitive mindfulness (Djikic, 2014; Langer, 1992; Yeganeh & Kolb, 2009). One part defines mindfulness as 'the awareness that emerges through paying attention on purpose, in the present moment, and non-judgmentally to the unfolding of experience moment by moment' (Kabat-Zinn, 2003, p. 145).

DOI: 10.4324/9781003318262-19

This approach refers to Buddhist meditation practices and considers mindfulness as a positive influence on attention that would increase during the process of maintaining meditation as a daily practice (Gunaratana, 2012; Hanh, 1987; Kabat-Zinn, 2003; Williams et al., 2011). Both strands of literature refer to the commitment to the notion of being in the present moment. However, the socio-cognitive strand presents mindfulness as the process of actively making new distinctions by not relying on automatic categorisations (Le et al., 2014). Proponents of this concept explain that mindfulness is actualised by maintaining orientation to the present, alertness to differences, sensitivity to different contexts, openness to novelty and creativity (Langer, 1992).

The qualities and benefits of the meditative path have been explored and practised more widely than the socio-cognitive one. However, the socio-cognitive approach is more applicable to the design process, as it can be promoted by consciously made design decisions. The dimensions of socio-cognitive mindfulness can be implemented in design processes and methods. Furthermore, the socio-cognitive stream has more potential to incorporate mindfulness into people's everyday lives by provoking, for example, awareness during product use by design. Following this stream, mindfulness can be embedded in design and neither the designers nor the users need to meditate according to the ancient Buddhist technique to reach their state of awareness; something that we can hardly expect everyone to do in order to counter the stress and cognitive overload daily life brings us. We argue here that we go for the alternative approach that helps developers and designers evaluate to what extent their design proposals elicit mindfulness in the context of product interaction.

Mindfulness is a broad field with enormous potential for psychological treatment of people who need to improve cognitive factors such as attention, psychological wellbeing and emotional self-regulation. Studies based on mindfulness show its benefits in treating psychiatric patients and those who want to improve their cognitive performance. Based on these findings, studies on appropriate measures of the mindfulness state have increased. Self-assessment of mindfulness and other methods for operationalising and measuring clinical use are mostly based on an Eastern Buddhist perspective that has been developed and validated (Pirson et al., 2012).

Studies of mindfulness have been conducted in the fields of psychology and neurobiology for emotion regulation, cognitive enhancement and therapeutic meditation, as well as stress reduction, chronic pain, depression, improved memory and attention in children in school and enhanced performance in sports. However, in the design domain, mindfulness has received growing attention only more recently (e.g. performative objects for mindfulness, Niedderer, 2014; mindful design interventions for mental health, Thieme et al., 2013; Niedderer et al., 2020; meditative mindfulness as a collaborative creative process, Rosenberg, 2015; digital products and services for meditative mindfulness, Gunatillake, 2016; increase empathy and awareness, change behaviour, Rojas et al., 2016, 2017).

The design approach based on socio-cognitive mindfulness is referred to as mindful design (e.g. Niedderer, 2007, 2014, 2017; see Chapter 14 of this book). The concept of mindful design was introduced by Niedderer (2007) to describe how design artefacts can promote and enhance mindful awareness of physical and social actions. Niedderer also notes that mindful design can be associated with behavioural change, expanding the understanding of social-cognitive mindfulness by changing the expected functions of artefact use.

The mindful design approach is of significant importance for socio-cognitive awareness, self-empowerment, originality in design, subjective wellbeing and subsequent behaviour change of users. According to literature, mindful design can take effect through meditation and being aware in a socio-cognitive way. As a result, mindful design can potentially deliver:

- Cognitive improvements for concentration and maintaining focus on the present activity, orientation and improvement of memory (Langer, 2000, 2014).
- Awareness at the present, identifying new opportunities, promoting people to creativity and novelty (ibid.).
- Consequently improved psychosocial and subjective wellbeing (e.g. relaxation, mood, emotion, self-regulation, self-determination, self-confidence.
- Contribution to behaviour change (Lockton, 2010, 2012) through engagement, reflection and awareness with self and others.

To enable the mindful design approach, it is necessary to support designers in developing design solutions that improve cognitive abilities, self-regulation and subjective wellbeing for user groups who can benefit from it.

Designers are experts in human–artifact interaction in general, and their main task is to develop and anticipate design solutions. They learn and practice various approaches, methods and tools. In this context, most designers have limited knowledge and expertise in terms of mindfulness and mindful design. Conversely, most experts in mindfulness have no training and expertise in designing and anticipating design solutions. This necessitates either interdisciplinary collaboration or methodological support for one or the other discipline. In the field of mindful design, we suggest that, if possible, interdisciplinary collaboration or methodological guidance and support on mindfulness for designers are appropriate approaches. Depending on projects, organisational constraints and team dynamics, interdisciplinary collaboration is not always feasible. Therefore, there is a need for systematic methods that assist designers in designing and evaluating the mindfulness of their design proposals well before high-fidelity prototyping and user tests can be conducted. The next sections will elaborate on how we propose this can be accomplished.

Criteria-based evaluation of design proposals

The implementation of design criteria is essential for systematic design processes. It guides designers and decision-makers and limits their design space for a clear and focused project pursuit. For Baxter (1995), clearly formulated design specifications and criteria are essential to guide the design teams and remind them of the projects' priorities throughout the whole process. These criteria are defined at the beginning of the design process where the most important project information and requirements are condensed into a design brief. It serves then as a self-assessment reference that allows designers to evaluate user needs, production specifications or market expectations during development. The more clearly and detailed these criteria are described, the better they can achieve the project goals.

A project must consider a number of specifications, most of these given explicitly in the design brief; some need to be derived in the early stages of the design process. These specifications can provide requirements on the technical limitations of the project, such as in terms of production, industry, materials, costs and form and are defined as objective aspects. There are also more subjective aspects for project development, such as positive user experience, psychological needs fulfilment or consumer preferences and expectations, which can be further subcategorised and prioritised depending on the project requirements.

There is an agreement that in interdisciplinary product development processes, design criteria should be measurable and described quantitatively if possible, e.g., measured on a scale to prioritise and categorise the different criteria in the same process. On the one hand, the lack of defined criteria for the project can lead to a vague or unsuccessful outcome, and on the other hand, too much restriction of the project pursuit due to the specific design criteria list can reduce creativity and innovative aspects for the product.

A tool for the systematic promotion and evaluation of mindful design proposals can steer a product design process by structuring design goals and eventually help designers do an expert evaluation of concepts or apply self-assessments in user research.

While there are evaluation scales on mindfulness, most of these are self-assessment scales from the field of psychology and have not been developed or validated to be used in product design evaluation. However, influential research on user-experience design and evaluation has demonstrated the successful and well-accepted transfer of evaluation approaches and scales from psychology to user-experience design. One such example is the fundamental and now widely accepted transfer of the Needs Scale for user-experience design. This approach and scale are based on the human psychological needs theories and scales of Sheldon and colleagues (2001), which have later been adapted and transferred to a user experience design approach and corresponding design and evaluation methods (Hassenzahl et al., 2010). Sheldon et al. (2001) suggest ten needs as a source of positive experiences – in the context of 'satisfying events'. Seven, respectively eight of which were identified as significant for human–technology interaction, hence for design. Hassenzahl et al. (2010; Partala & Kallinen, 2012), developed and validated design and evaluation methods (visual cards and standardised questionnaires) for these. Other similar approaches and methods that partly combine design prompts (most often in the form of visual cards) and standardised evaluation scales are Interaction Vocabulary (Diefenbach et al., 2013), AttrakDiff 2.0 (Hassenzahl et al., 2003) or the CUE model and MeCUE 2.0 (Thüring & Mahlke, 2007; Minge & Thüring, 2018), all of which deal with specific aspects or qualities of human–technology interaction. These tools were developed to be used in a user-centred design process, to provide a positive experience for users and to provide guidance and evaluation for designers to see if the products developed meet the needs of their target groups. Each of the above tools has a specific goal that is pursued during the design process. These tools join the ranks with other visual design tools that help in the design (synthesis) phases that also serve as, or have counterparts for, evaluation phases.

The above examples of transfer from psychology to design approaches and evaluation methods all deal with human-centred aspects of human–technology interaction. More specifically, those are focused on non-instrumental qualities of human–technology interaction. Attention to these non-instrumental qualities is considered to be essential for systematic experience design (Thüring & Mahlke, 2007). In this regard, mindful design is a specific form of experience design, as it focuses on socio-cognitive factors rather than instrumental qualities such as function, reliability or usability of products. Accordingly, it can be assumed that psychological models and scales on mindfulness can be potentially transferred to design in order to allow for systematic mindful design and respective evaluation.

The assessment of mindfulness

With the increased application of mindfulness-based interventions, the accurate measurement of both the general tendency to be mindful (a trait) and the individual level of mindfulness at a given time (a state) has become a significant clinical and research issue (Medvedev et al., 2017). Researchers in the field of psychology have discussed the differences between state and trait characteristics over the years. A temporary emotional change creates the state. It is defined as an emotional response to internal and external factors that produce physical, behavioural, cognitive and psychological changes. Depending on the level of arousal, frustration, subjective perception and context, it can determine the duration and intensity of the emotion felt (Galor, 2012).

On the other hand, 'trait' is a more permanent facet of the personality, implying a more permanent and stable level of feeling. Traits describe an individual's personality characteristics that are constant over time, for example, whether the person is very anxious, shy or angry. These personality characteristics (traits), in combination with various situational factors, lead to different emotional states, including extraversion, self-esteem, perfectionism and impulsivity. While some forms of therapy or behaviour modification can influence traits, they generally do not change without concerted effort (Spielberger & Sydeman, 1994).

For Ackerman (2017), the state of mindfulness refers to a temporary state of awareness that an individual feels by observing their thoughts and feelings and being able to stay in the present moment even when distractions arise. Moreover, the mindfulness trait is characterised by the ability to achieve this state more frequently and to maintain focus on the present for a longer period of time.

Several self-report tools were developed to capture a general tendency towards mindfulness in daily life and have shown promising psychometric properties. Furthermore, a number of mindfulness self-report assessment scales have been developed and applied in research in order to evaluate the impact of mindfulness-based interventions. These vary in underlying concepts (meditative vs. socio-cognitive mindfulness), scope (state vs. trait, short-term vs. long-term assessment) and lengths, and accordingly they consist of a variety of scale items that cannot easily be recombined and transferred to mindful design. These scales include:

- the Mindfulness/Mindlessness Scale, MMS, Bodner and Langer (2001) and
- the Langer Mindfulness Scale, LMS (Pirson et al., 2012), a progression of the MMS

that provide a long-term assessment (of tendency, trait) of socio-cognitive mindfulness;

- Mindful Attention Awareness Scale, MAAS (Brown & Ryan, 2003),
- the Five-Facet Mindfulness Questionnaire, FFMQ (Baer et al., 2006),
- the Kentucky Inventory of Mindfulness Skills, KIMS, (Baer et al., 2004),
- the Freiburg Mindfulness Inventory, FMI (Walach et al., 2006) and
- the Cognitive and Affective Mindfulness Scale Revised, CAM-R (Feldman et al., 2007)

that provide a long-term assessment (of tendency, trait) of meditative mindfulness; and

- the Philadelphia Mindfulness Scale, PHLMS (Cardatiotto et al., 2008),
- the State Mindfulness Scale , SMS (Tanay & Bernstein, 2013),
- the Toronto Mindfulness Scale, TMS (Lau et al., 2006) and
- the Comprehensive Inventory of Mindfulness Experiences, CHIME (Bergomi et al., 2014, cf. Sliwinski et al., 2017),

that provide short-term assessment (of level, state) of meditative mindfulness.

A closer look shows that, furthermore the scales all have some constructs in common, but still also differ not just slightly. The differences in their scope, content and structure suggest that there is no consensus among researchers as to how mindfulness is conceptualised as a multifaceted construct, and if so, how these facets are defined and operationalised (Baer et al., 2008).

Among the self-assessment scales, only one has been used for design evaluation through the classification of interactive technologies: the CHIME. In their study, Sliwinski et al. (2017) presented interactive technology approaches to improve mindfulness and discussed their implications for games, smartphone apps and computer software. However, CHIME relates to meditative mindfulness. It also covers specific mindfulness dimensions and constructs that might not cover the whole spectrum. Our aim was to be able to assess socio-cognitive mindfulness in the most valid and reliable way possible in the context of design processes. We hence analysed the scales to derive a comprehensive set of constructs that can potentially be operationalised for an assessment of how design proposals can promote the mindfulness of users. An overview of the comparison of the mindfulness self-report assessment scales is shown in the matrix in Figure 15.1. It is subdivided by core characteristics and measured constructs. The constructs operationalised in the different scales are structured differently. Accordingly, there are some overlaps and inconsistencies across the scales. Restructuring was necessary. We give some examples below.

Curiosity is a part of novelty-seeking, which describes this mechanism in a very similar way. Curiosity within TMS was measured with the following construct: 'I was curious about what I might learn about myself by paying attention to how I react to certain thoughts, feelings, or sensations' and novelty-seeking in LMS with 'I try to think of new ways to do things.' However,

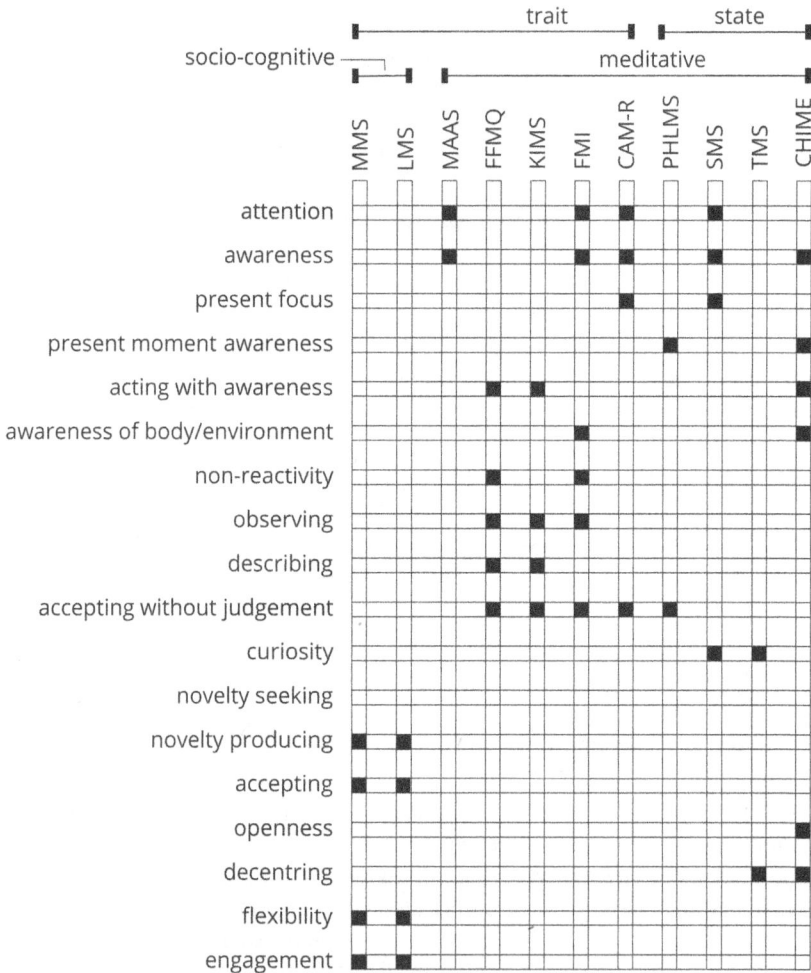

Figure 15.1 Overview of primary self-report assessments, categorised and analysed by underlying constructs

self-report TMSs have different measurement objectives. In the TMS measure, mindfulness is considered a state; in the LMS, it is considered a trait. The mechanism of mindful awareness is addressed in eight out of ten annotated self-assessments. Moreover, the other two statements also contain a description of awareness, for example, in TMS: 'I was aware of my thoughts and feelings without over-identifying with them,' or (MMS): 'I am rarely aware of changes'. This fact led to the decision to retain awareness as a socio-cognitive mindfulness mechanism for design products, even though this property is not explicit in the socio-cognitive self-assessment itself.

Attention has the same value as awareness for application in the design of products. However, attention was combined with another dimension of mindfulness, 'observing' (CHIME) or 'acting with awareness' (FFMQ). As the explanation of the dimension 'curiosity' shows, CHIME does not have the same measurement objectives. The focus is on measuring mindfulness through meditation, unlike the socio-cognitive assessment LMS.

It can be concluded that mindfulness assessment is practised by means of self-report scales that vary in form, but more importantly, in terms of underlying constructs that are being measured. However, they not only provide approaches to the structuring of dimensions of mindfulness but also provide assessment tools to measure mindfulness that have already been empirically validated for use in psychometric evaluations of interventions. As the transfer, implementation and validation of psychometric scales in user-experience design have shown in the past, it could be possible to adapt and transfer these mindfulness assessment methods to design. Hence, we will pursue our aim to develop a mindfulness evaluation tool for design based on the self-report scales reported above.

Development of the Mindful Design Evaluation Scale

The psychometric self-assessment for measuring socio-cognitive mindfulness was selected and adapted to the context of product development to measure the extent to which cognitive mindfulness of users can be promoted by interacting with mindful products. Considering that the self-assessment scales are all already methodologically evaluated, the development of this evaluation tool is divided into three steps:

- Phase 1 – What constructs and respective statements can be selected to provide a measure of mindfulness level in the context of design?
- Phase 2 – Are the statements valid, easy to understand and applicable to user-product interaction? Can they be answered quickly?
- Phase 3 – Can a newly arranged assessment scale be validated as a reliable means of expert assessment on how (many) design proposals promote mindfulness of users?

Phase 1 – Selection of Constructs and statements (scale Items)

The constructs (e.g. 'Attention') and respective statements (e.g. 'I find it difficult to stay focused on what's happening in the present' (MAAS, Brown & Ryan, 2003) of the self-assessment scales have been analysed and selected to be applied in the mindful design assessment scale.

Of the targets selected for a mindful design evaluation, two of the questionnaires consider socio-cognitive mindfulness mechanisms: the Mindfulness/Mindlessness Scale (MMS) of Bodner and Langer (2001) and the Langer Mindfulness Scale (LMS) of Pirson et al. (2012). The KIMS, FFMQ, CAMS-R, PHLMS and MAAS questionnaires were considered primarily because they address the mechanisms of attention and awareness necessary for a mindful state of mind. Of the latter, MAAS has been identified as appropriate to be partially adopted.

Based on a detailed analysis, two self-report questionnaires are identified to be suitable for applying the mindfulness dimension to the design process: the LMS and MAAS. Both self-reports are based on human psychological traits and long-term measurements and complement each other in their dimensions of novelty-seeking, novelty-producing and engagement from LMS and the dimensions of awareness and attention from the MAAS scale, which is also probably the most widely used scale to date. The MAAS is a reliable and validated self-report and can be used in combination with other self-reports (Brown & Ryan, 2003). Although the LMS is the only self-report that addresses socio-cognitive mindfulness principles, the dimensions of awareness and attention were frequently mentioned in all other self-reports except the MMS/LMS. Awareness and attention are the result of mindful interaction and can be measured without the need for meditation practice. According to Brown and Ryan (2003), this self-report aims to reliably measure inter- and intrapersonal variations in an individual's mindfulness, establish its relationships to other relevant psychological constructs and demonstrate its relevance to a variety of forms of psychological wellbeing.

The scale items were selected and organised in relation to the following dimensions: Novelty-Seeking and Novelty-Producing, Engagement, Awareness and Attention, which are essential to achieving the socio-cognitive state of mindfulness.

Phase 2 – Reliability, comprehensibility and applicability

The items taken from self-assessment scales have been altered as little as possible in order to allow for implementation in expert assessments. The selection and reformulation of the statement were refined based on constructs, homogeneity, general statements, easy understandability and whether they can be answered in relation to interacting with products.

The scale is introduced to the assessors by an instruction to rate the items based on anticipated product interaction. The scale to assess the mindfulness of products or design proposals ranges from 'reduce' to 'increase', depending on how the interaction between user and product is anticipated to influence the user's state of mindfulness. The 27 items are rated on uneven five-step metric scales that allow for neutral answers on the midpoint. This way, all items can be answered even if no impact is being reported. Figure 15.2 shows a mindful design evaluation sheet based on the described scale that addresses the constructs of Attention, Engagement, Novelty-Seeking, Novelty-Producing, Flexibility and Awareness in the moment of user interaction.

Phase 3 – Reliability assessment

The items have been transferred from empirically validated scales. The transfer and recombination, but also the changed field of application (human–technology interaction), as well as the change from self-assessment to expert assessment (including the necessary small changes of formulations), result in the need for an empirical reliability proof of the newly arranged scale.

This step was carried out to test the reliability of the developed questionnaire. Assessment sessions were conducted with five experts in the fields of design and psychology, including three designers and two mindfulness specialists (psychologists). One group, the designers, is familiar with the product development process and the decisions made during the design process based on non-countable aspects, such as creative, psychological dimension and subjective design criteria. The other group, the psychologists, is familiar with t cognitive qualities that people should have in order to achieve the state of mindfulness.

	Imagine _____, interacting with "_____", at the given scenario. Interacting with the product….	Reduce			Increase		Points
		2	1	0	-1	2	
1	He/she avoids thought provoking conversations.	O	O	O	O	O	
2	He/she is rarely aware of changes.	O	O	O	O	O	
3	He/she seldom notice what other people are up to.	O	O	O	O	O	
4	He/she is rarely alert to new developments.	O	O	O	O	O	
		-2	-1	0	1	2	
5	He/she is very curious.	O	O	O	O	O	
6	He/she likes to investigate things.	O	O	O	O	O	
7	He/she tries to think of new ways of doing things.	O	O	O	O	O	
8	He/she likes to be challenged intellectually.	O	O	O	O	O	
9	He/she likes to figure out how things work.	O	O	O	O	O	
10	He/she generates few novel ideas.	O	O	O	O	O	
11	He/she makes many novel contributions.	O	O	O	O	O	
12	He/she is very creative.	O	O	O	O	O	
13	He/she finds it easy to create new and effective ideas.	O	O	O	O	O	
		2	1	0	-1	-2	
14	He/she is not an original thinker.	O	O	O	O	O	
15	He/she finds it difficult to stay focused on what's happening in the present.	O	O	O	O	O	
16	He/she breaks or spills things because of carelessness, not paying attention, or thinking of something else.	O	O	O	O	O	
17	He/she tends not to notice feelings of physical tension or discomfort until they really grab his/her attention.	O	O	O	O	O	
18	It seems he/she is „running on automatic ", without much awareness of what he/she's doing.	O	O	O	O	O	
19	He/she finds himself/herself preoccupied with the future or the past.	O	O	O	O	O	
20	He/she finds himself/herself doing things without paying attention.	O	O	O	O	O	
21	He/she tends to walk quickly to get where he/she's going without paying attention to what he/she's experience along the way.	O	O	O	O	O	
22	When he/she does things, his/her mind wanders off and he/she's easily distracted.	O	O	O	O	O	
23	He/she doesn't pay attention to what he/she's doing because he/she's daydreaming, worrying, or otherwise distracted.	O	O	O	O	O	
24	He/she's easily distracted.	O	O	O	O	O	
25	He/she finds it difficult to stay focused on what's happening in the present.	O	O	O	O	O	
26	He/she rushes through activities without being really attentive to them.	O	O	O	O	O	
27	He/she does jobs or tasks automatically without being aware of what he/she's doing.	O	O	O	O	O	
	TOTAL						

Figure 15.2 Mindful design evaluation scale. Attention = AT, Engagement = E, Novelty Seeking = NS, Novelty Producing = NP, Awareness = AA

A number of different mindful design proposals have all been assessed by the experts based on the 27-item scale. The aim was to test if the assessments conducted by the experts are reliable, i.e. objectively measured. If this is the case, all different design proposals should be given the same scores by all different experts and the items contribute to the constructs as expected (e.g. all questions related to 'attention' statistically contribute to the respective construct).

Inter-rater reliability has been statistically tested as the degree of agreement between raters. It indicates how homogeneous or consistent the jurors' ratings are. The intra-class correlation coefficient was used as the reliability test in this study because there were more than two raters in a continuous assessment. Cronbach's alpha is a measure used to assess the reliability or internal consistency of a set of scale or test items (i.e. constructs).

In the statistical test, the Spearman correlation between psychologists' responses and the designer's responses is 0.648, indicating a positive relationship between the variables, while Cronbach's Alpha has a questionable internal consistency of 0.686. Consequently, it can be concluded that based on the 27-item scale, designers and psychologists do not rate the design proposals equally, hence the results cannot be considered being reliable in this setting.

However, when looking at the designer's responses only, the Spearman correlation between them is 0.804. The relationship between the variables of the underlying constructs is also positive, with Cronbach's Alpha showing excellent internal consistency of 0.824. This means that the designers have almost the same understanding when using the Mindful Design Evaluation Scale to evaluate the design proposals. Accordingly, the scale can be considered reliable in early design stages if used by design experts exclusively.

Visual mindful design cards as prompts and qualitative evaluation means in early design phases

The results of the theoretical analysis of (socio-cognitive) mindfulness and mindful design have been the basis for the described development of the standardised evaluation scale. However, it can also serve as a basis for guiding tools that support the design (synthesis) phase. In coherence with the working and reasoning styles of designers, respective design tools are available in visual forms that correlate with the constructs underlying the Mindful Design Evaluation Scale (cf. references to Interaction Vocabulary Cards, Diefenbach et al., 2013 or Needs Cards, Hassenzahl et al., 2010 and other visual cards related to assessment scales as described further above). The criteria and dimensions of mindfulness in human-product interactions can be presented and hence inform, inspire and trigger design activities and decisions. Furthermore, such visual cards can serve as explanatory or educational aids. Last but not least, they can be used as prompts in non-standardised qualitative assessments of design proposals. In any application, they can support the focus, comprehensiveness and clarity of the understanding of mindful design.

Figure 15.3 shows mindful design visual cards that have been derived from the constructs underlying the Mindful Design Evaluation Scale. The design and instructions on the cards were made to be simple and easy to follow. They can be used in the definition and evaluation phases and help to adhere to the mindful design criteria during design and learning processes

Discussion

Both visual cards as well as the Mindful Design Evaluation Scale have been developed and validated in educational settings and in the context of designing product-service-systems for people with dementia. However, while mindful design approach yields a particular potential to contribute to social wellbeing for people with dementia, it is not restricted to cognitive impairment

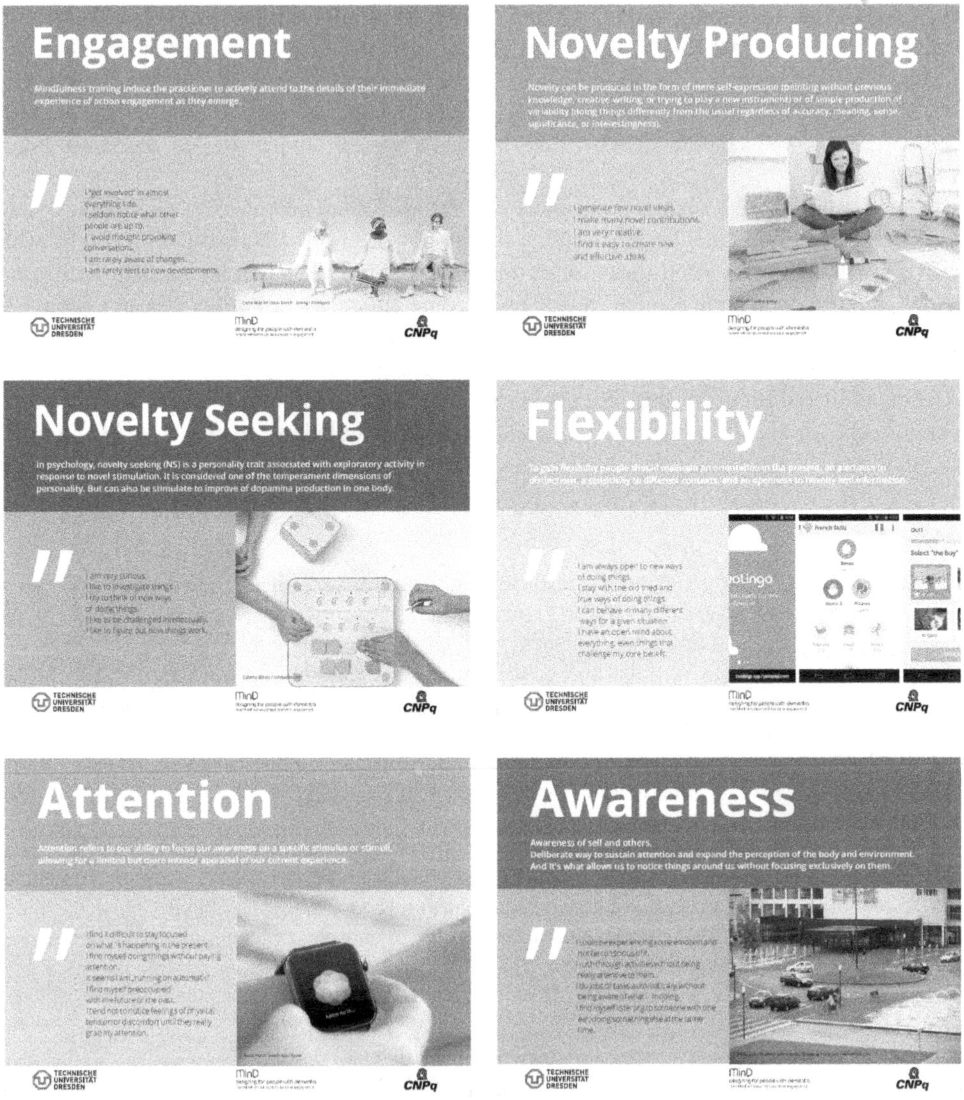

Figure 15.3 a–f Mindful design visual cards. Design and evaluation prompts based on the underlying constructs of the Mindful Design Evaluation Scale

problems. As mindfulness can contribute to positive experiences and wellbeing in a much wider range of contexts, mindful design also can. The presented design and evaluation methods can serve as support for mindful design. However, their impact in different fields of design and in different contexts needs further investigation.

The Mindful Design Evaluation Scale has been developed and tested as a means for expert assessments of design proposals in early stages of design processes. Specific challenges of such early stages are incomplete and fuzzy representations of the design outcomes. Design experts can deal with it; it is part of their daily work. Accordingly, they are experts in anticipating future interactions between users and final design solutions. They are, however, not experts in psychological underpinnings and correlating constructs of mindfulness. The provided Mindful Design Evaluation Scale fills this gap and allows for valid and reliable assessments if conducted by design experts. The scale does not, however, provide reliable results if applied by non-design experts such as psychologists who might be better experts in mindfulness but have a less aligned understanding of what final solutions typical (fuzzy) design proposals might evolve into.

In later stages of the design process, more concrete and more complete representations of the design solutions are available; high-fidelity prototypes or pre-production models might eventually be available. Based on these, other evaluation approaches can be applied that do not rely on the described competences in design outcome anticipation. Further research would be necessary in order to test if the Mindful Design Evaluation Scale can then be used in expert assessments conducted by non-designers. Furthermore, the instruction and item formulations could be re-altered to ego-perspective again in order to implement the scale in self-assessments in empirical user research. Again, validity and reliability would have to be proven by empirical investigations.

References

Ackerman, C. (2017). 11 mindfulness questionnaires, scales & assessments for measuring. *Positive Psychology*. Retrieved September 20, 2017, from https://positivepsychologyprogram.com/mindfulness-questionnaires-scales-assessments-awareness/#challenges-measuring-mindfulness

Alhassan, A. A., Alqadhib, E. M., Taha, N. W., Alahmari, R. A., Salam, M., & Almutairi, A. F. (2018). The relationship between addiction to smartphone usage and depression among adults: A cross sectional study. *BMC Psychiatry*, *18*(1), 1–8.

Baer, R. A., Smith, G. T., & Allen, K. B. (2004). Assessment of mindfulness by self-report: The Kentucky inventory of mindfulness skills. *Assessment 11*(3), 191–206. https://doi.org/10.1177/1073191104268029

Baer, R. A., Smith, G. T., Hopkins, J., Krietemeyer, J., & Toney, L. (2006). Using self-report assessment methods to explore facets of mindfulness. *Assessment*, *13*(1), 27–45. doi:/10.1177/1073191105283504

Baer, R. A., Smith, G. T., Lykins, E., Button, D., Krietemeyer, J., Sauer, S., et al. (2008). Construct validity of the five facet mindfulness questionnaire in meditating and nonmeditating samples. *Assessment*, *15*(3), 329–342. https://doi.org/10.1177/1073191107313003

Baxter, M. (1995). *Product design. Practical methods for the systematic development of new products*. CRC press.

Bergomi, C., Tschacher, W., & Kupper, Z. (2014). Konstruktion und erste Validierung eines Fragebogens zur umfassenden Erfassung von Achtsamkeit: Der comprehensive inventory of mindfulness experiences (CHIME). *.Diagnostica*, 60, 111-125.

Bodner, T. E., & Langer, E. J. (2001, June). *Individual differences in mindfulness: The mindfulness/mindlessness scale*. Poster presented at the 13th annual American Psychological Society Convention, Toronto, Ontario, Canada.

Brown, K. W., & Ryan, R. M. (2003). The benefits of being present: Mindfulness and its role in psychological well-being. *Journal of Personality and Social Psychology*84(4), 822–848.

Cardaciotto, L., Herbert, J. D., Forman, E. M., Moitra, E., & Farrow, V. (2008). The assessment of present-moment awareness and acceptance: The Philadelphia mindfulness scale. *Assessment*, *15*(2), 204–223. https://doi.org/10.1177/1073191107311467

Cha, S. S., & Seo, B. K. (2018). Smartphone use and smartphone addiction in middle school students in Korea: Prevalence, social networking service, and game use. *Health Psychology Open*, *5*(1). https://doi.org/2055102918755046

Davies, D. R., Matthews, G., Stammers, R. B., & Westerman, S. J. (2000). *Human performance: Cognition, stress and individual differences*. Psychology Press.

Diefenbach, S., Lenz, E., & Hassenzahl, M. (2013). An interaction vocabulary. describing the how of interaction. In *CHI'13 extended abstracts on human factors in computing systems* (pp. 607–612).

Djikic, M. (2014). Art of mindfulness: Integrating eastern and western approaches art of mindfulness: Integrating eastern and western approaches. In A. Ie., C. T. Ngnoumen & E. J. Langer (Eds.), Whiley *Blackwell Handbook of Mindfulness.* (Vol. 1, pp. 139–148). John Wiley & Sons, Ltd.

Endsley, M. R. (2001). Designing for situation awareness in complex system. In *Proceedings of the second international workshop on symbiosis of human, artifacts and environment.*

Feldman, G., Hayes, A., Kumar, S., Greeson, J., & Laurenceau, J.-P. (2007). Mindfulness and emotion regulation: The development and initial validation of the cognitive and affective mindfulness scale-revised (CAMS-R). *International Journal of Psychopathology and Behavioral Assessment 29, 177-190.*

Galor, S. (2012). *Clarifying states and traits.* https://drsharongalor.wordpress.com/2012/07/09/clarifyingstates-and-traits/, checked on 11/12/2017

Gunaratana, H. (2012). *The four foundations of mindfulness in plain English: Wisdom publications.*Simon and Schuster.

Gunatillake, R. (2016). *Designing mindfulness — How to make technology which takes care of the people who use it.* https://medium.com/@rohan_21awake/designing-mindfulness-how-to-make-technology-which-takes-care-of-the-people-who-use-it-8a6aaf76dea3

Hanh, T. N. (1975). The Miracles of Mindfulness..*An Introduction to the Practice of meditation.* Beacon Press.

Hanh, T. N. (1987). *Old path white clouds: Walking in the footsteps of the Buddha.* Parallax Press.

Hassenzahl, M., Burmester, M., & Koller, F. (2003). AttrakDiff: Ein Fragebogen zur Messung wahrgenommener hedonischer und[MS1] pragmatischer Qualität. *Mensch & Computer 2003: Interaktion in Bewegung*, 187–196.

Hassenzahl, M. (Ed.). (2008, September 2–5). User experience (UX): Towards an experiential perspective on product quality. IHM, '08. *Metz - France.*

Hassenzahl, M., Diefenbach, S., & Göritz, A. (2010). Needs, affect, and interactive products–Facets of user experience. *Interacting with Computers, 22*(5), 353–362.

Kabat-Zinn, J. (1990). *Full catastrophe living: Using the wisdom of your mind to face stress, pain and illness.* Dell.

Ie, A., Ngnoumen, C. T., & Langer, E. J. (Eds.). (2014). *The Wiley Blackwell Handbook of Mindfulness. Wiley Blackwell.* John Wiley & Sons, Ltd.

Kabat-Zinn, J. (2003). Mindfulness-based interventions in context. Past, present, and future. *Clinical Psychology: Science and Practice, 10*(2), 144–156. https://doi.org/10.1093/clipsy.bpg016

Langer, E. J. (1992). Matters of mind. Mindfulness/mindlessness in perspective. *Consciousness and Cognition, 1*(3), 289–305. https://doi.org/10.1016/1053-8100(92)90066-J

Langer, E. J. (2000). Mindful learning. *Current Directions in Psychological Science, 9*(6), 220–223.

Langer, E. J. (2014). Mindfulness forward and back. In A. Ie, C. T. Ngnoumen & E. Langer (Eds.), *The Wiley Blackwell Handbook of Mindfulness* (Vol. 1, pp. 7–20). John Wiley & Sons, Ltd.

Lau, M. A., Bishop, S. R., Segal, Z. V., Buis, T., Anderson, N. D., Carlson, L., et al. (2006). The Toronto mindfulness scale: Development and validation. *Journal of Clinical Psychology, 62*(12), 1445–1467. https://doi.org/10.1002/jclp.20326

Lewis, M. M. (2000). *The new thing: A Silicon Valley story.* WW Norton & Company.

Lockton, D. (2012). *Posiwid and determinism in design for behaviour change.* http://bura.brunel.ac.uk/bitstream/2438/6394/2/SSRN-id2033231.pdf

Lockton, D., Hårrison, D., & Stanton, N. A. (2010). The design with intent method: A design tool for influencing user behaviour. *Applied Ergonomics, 41*(3), 382–392. https://doi.org/10.1016/j.apergo.2009.09.001

Medvedev, O. N., Krägeloh, C. U., Narayanan, A., & Siegert, R. J. (2017). Measuring mindfulness: Applying generalizability theory to distinguish between state and trait. *Mindfulness, 8*(4), 1036–1046. https://doi.org/10.1007/s12671-017-0679-0

Minge, M., & Thüring, M. (2018, July 15–20). *The meCUE questionnaire (2.0): Meeting five basic requirements for lean and standardized UX assessment. Design, User Experience, and Usability.*

Theory and into Practice. 7th International Conference, DUXU 2018, Held as Part of HCI International 2018, Proceedings, Part I 7. Springer International Publishing, Las Vegas, NV, pp. 451–469.

Mutchler, L. A., Shim, J. P., & Ormond, D. (2011). Exploratory study on users' behavior: Smartphone usage. In Niedderer, K. (Ed.), *AMCIS 2011 proceedings - all submissions*. John Wiley & Sons, Ltd.

Niedderer, K. (2007). Designing mindful interaction: The category of performative object. *Design Issues*, *23*(1), 3–17.

Niedderer, K. (2014). Mediating mindful social interactions through design. In A. Ie, C. T. Ngnoumen & E. J. Langer (Eds.), *The Wiley Blackwell Handbook of Mindfulness*. (pp. 345-366). John Wiley & Sons, Ltd.

Niedderer, K. (2017). Facilitating behaviour change through mindful design. In K. Niedderer, S. Clune and G. (Eds.) *Design for behaviour change* (pp. 104–115). Routledge.

Niedderer, K., Tournier, I., Coleston-Shields, D. M., Craven, M., Gosling, J., Garde, J., & Griffioen, I. (2020). *Designing with and for people with dementia: Developing a mindful interdisciplinary co-design methodology*. Proceeding of 7th International Congress of the International Association of Societies of Design Research (IASDR).

Parasuraman, S., Sam, A. T., Yee, S. W. K., Chuon, B. L. C., & Ren, L. Y. (2017). Smartphone usage and increased risk of mobile phone addiction: A concurrent study. *International Journal of Pharmaceutical Investigation*, *7*(3), 125.

Partala, T., & Kallinen, A. (2012). Understanding the most satisfying and unsatisfying user experiences: Emotions, psychological needs, and context. *Interacting with Computers*, *24*(1), 25–34.

Pirson, M., Langer, E. J., Bodner, T., & Zilcha, S. (2012). The development and validation of the langer mindfulness scale - Enabling a socio-cognitive perspective of mindfulness in organizational contexts. *SSRN Journal*. https://doi.org/10.2139/ssrn.2158921

Rama Devi, V., & Nagini, A. (2014). Work-life balance and burnout as predictors of job satisfaction in private banking sector. In *Skyline Business Journal 9*(1), 50-53.

Rojas, F., English, S., Young, R., & Spencer, N. (2015). Making Mindfulness explicit in Design Education. In R. Vande & I. Digranes (Eds.), *Erik Bohemia Learnx design proceedings of the 3rd international conference for design education researchers*. Aalto University Press.

Rojas, F., English, S., Young, R., & Spencer, N. (Eds.). (2017). A design-relevant mindfulness device. *The Design Journal*, *20*(sup1), S767-S780..

Rosenberg, D. (2015). *Transformational design: A mindful practice for experience-driven design* (PhD. MA). Massachusetts Institute of Technology. Architecture: Design and Computation.

Schaub, H. (2008). Wahrnehmung, Aufmerksamkeit und situation awareness (SA). With assistance of Petra Badke-Schaub. In G. Hofinger & K. Lauche (Eds.), *Human factors* (pp. 59–76). Springer.

Shanafelt, T. D., Hasan, O., Dyrbye, L. N., Sinsky, C., Satele, D., Sloan, J., & West, C. P. (2015, December). Changes in burnout and satisfaction with work-life balance in physicians and the general US working population between 2011 and 2014. In *Mayo clinic proceedings* (Vol. 90, No. 12, pp. 1600–1613). Elsevier.

Sheldon, K. M., Elliot, A. J., Kim, Y., & Kasser, T. (2001). What is satisfying about satisfying events? Testing 10 candidate psychological needs. *Journal of Personality and Social Psychology*, *80*(2), 325.

Sliwinski, J., & Katsikitis, M. , Jones, C. M. (2017): A Review of Interactive Technologies as Support Tools for the Cultivation of Mindfulness. *Mindfulness*, *8*, 1150–1159.

Spieß, R. (2002). *Unbewusste Informationsverarbeitung. Forschungsansätze, Ergebnisse und methodische Probleme*. Verlag Dr. Kovač.

Spielberger, C. D., & Sydeman, S. J. (1994). State-Trait Anxiety Inventory and stale-trait ånger expression inventory. In M. E. Maruish (Ed.), *The use of psychological tests for treatment planning and outcome assessment* (pp. 292–232). Erlbaum.

Tanay, G., & Bernstein, A. (2013). State Mindfulness Scale (SMS): Development and initial validation. *Psychological Assessment*, *25*(4), 1286–1299. https://doi.org/10.1037/a0034044.

Thieme, A., Wallace, J., Johnson, P., McCarthy, J., Lindley, S., Wright, P., & Meyer, T. D. (2013, April). Design to promote mindfulness practice and sense of self for vulnerable women in secure hospital services. In *Proceedings of the SIGCHI conference on human factors in computing systems* (pp. 2647–2656).

Thüring, M., & Mahlke, S. (2007). Usability, aesthetics and emotions in human–technology interaction. *International Journal of Psychology*, *42*(4), 253–264.

Walach, H., Buchheld, N., Buttenmuller, V., Kleinknecht, N., & Schmidt, S. (2006). Measuring mindfulness: The Freiburg mindfulness inventory (FMI). *Personality and Individual Differences*, *40*(8), 1543–1555. https://doi.org/10.1016/j.paid.2005.11.025

Williams, J. M. G., & Kabat-Zinn, J. (2011). Mindfulness: Diverse perspectives on its meaning, origins, and multiple applications at the intersection of science and dharma introduction. *Contemporary Buddhism*, *12*(1), 1–18. https://doi.org/10.1080/14639947.2011.564811

Yasav, S. (2015). The impact of digital technology on consumer purchase behavior. *The Journal of Financial Perspectives: FinTech*, *3*(3).

Yeganeh, B., & Kolb, D. (2009). Mindfulness and experiential learning. *OD Practitioner*, *41*(3), 8–14.

16 Compassionate technology, value-based design for (e-)mental health

Geke Ludden, Matthijs Noordzij, Benedetta Lusi,
Charlotte van Lotringen and Randy Klaassen

Introduction

For decades, ICT has been put forward as a crucial tool to realise a more self-management and prevention-focused, economically viable mental healthcare. Furthermore, technology is assumed to open up fundamentally new paths of treatment by technology-mediated mechanisms, such as enhanced adaptability and personalisation through personal sensing (Mohr et al., 2017). These opportunities are reflected in the rise of digital technologies that are developed for the mental healthcare context. Although internet-delivered therapy is the most widespread use of digital technology in mental healthcare (Kemp et al., 2020), we also see more innovative developments in this field exploring the use of mobile applications, chatbots using artificial intelligence, virtual reality applications and serious games. Pilots aimed at introducing existing (off-the-shelf) technology from other areas in mental healthcare are ongoing. For example, there is significant interest in introducing wearable technology and virtual technology in mental healthcare. Wearable technology can, for example, be used to make people with mental illnesses, clients of mental healthcare services, more aware of changes in their body that reflect their emotional status (Derks et al., 2019; Van Doorn et al., 2022). Virtual technology offers opportunities to do therapeutic exercises, for example, to overcome trauma or fear (Kothgassner et al., 2019). Yet, the digital transition which these technologies promise has not taken place to the extent or pace envisioned. Clients show low adherence to the technology-mediated options. Many professionals show persistent hesitation in prescribing 'e-mental health' options and lack digital skills to confidently explain and adapt the existing options (Feijt et al., 2018). The societal readiness level of current technology for mental health is low, and often mostly a direct translation of components of existing face-to-face therapies. ICT in mental healthcare seems to be perceived by mental health professionals as a cold and inferior option, that mostly can be ignored in favour of the more human-friendly 'warm' and currently more effective face-to-face options.

However, studies have found that blended therapy can be as effective as face-to-face therapy (Hedman-Lagerlöf et al., 2023), though seemingly most effective if some form of guidance is present (see also Scholten & Granic, 2019) who discuss this specifically for youth). By making better use of the many new possibilities recent developments in technology offer, we might be able to work towards more sustainable mental health care. This chapter presents the results of the *Compassionate Technology* project run at the University of Twente with partners in mental healthcare (Dimence) and e-mental health tools (Minddistrict) to illustrate such possibilities. This project contends that the framing of mental health technology by many policymakers, designers and software developers is inappropriate. Whereas the focus of these stakeholders is on the usability and economic benefits of technology, the focus of the client and the professional is on human connection and alleviating mental suffering and increasing wellbeing. We propose,

DOI: 10.4324/9781003318262-20

therefore, that designing technology with pivotal human values and new ways of dividing tasks between people and technology can lead to societal readiness of technology and thus enable the transition towards sustainable mental health(care).

An essential value in mental health care is compassion: awareness of suffering, tolerating difficult feelings in the face of suffering and acting or being motivated to alleviate suffering. Compassion is both an attitude or sensitivity to suffering and wellbeing and taking the expedient action to improve the human condition (Strauss et al., 2016). This combination of both sensing and acting makes it a more comprehensive and useful concept to link to technology (which often both senses and acts) than, for example empathy or intimacy, which mainly have to do with the sensing aspects of interaction.

In the following, we will elaborate on the nature of compassion, reviewing current definitions and explaining the different roles of compassion in designing the digital transition in mental healthcare. To situate our work and views on compassion in the field, the chapter will continue to discuss how compassion is viewed in design research, and it will demonstrate how applying a designing for values approach (Smits et al., 2019), in which values of all stakeholders are taken into account, can support designing for this particularly important value in mental healthcare. This process will be illustrated through a case study showing how compassion can be embedded in design. This includes a discussion of the necessity to continuously (re-)evaluate the development of technology for mental health to enable a sustainable future of mental healthcare.

Compassion: a discussion of its definitions and roles

Compassion has been described by philosophers and in many religions as an indication of virtue in human beings. Compassion is widely recognised as being orientated towards reducing suffering (Strauss et al., 2016). Compassion can not only be directed toward ourselves (often referred to as self-compassion (Neff, 2012) and our loved ones, but also towards strangers and ultimately, to all humankind (Elices et al., 2017). It has also been described as an important value for organisations (see e.g. Cameron, 2017) and as an especially important value in healthcare (Shea & Lionis, 2017). This latter chapter aims to discuss the importance of compassionate care within healthcare settings, especially during times of austerity and for vulnerable individuals. It also addresses factors that may promote or hinder compassion and how compassion can be sustained long-term. In mental healthcare specifically, it was found that showing and training in compassion supports trust and directly deals with the high levels of shame and self-criticism that can be prevalent in mental illness (Gilbert, 2009). Strauss et al. (2016) provide an extensive review of existing definitions of compassion, and the ways in which it can be measured. They derive a new procedural definition of compassion as an interpersonal, cognitive, affective and behavioral *process* divided into five steps:

1) Recognising suffering; 2) understanding the universality of suffering in human experience; 3) feeling empathy for the person suffering and connecting with the distress (emotional resonance); 4) tolerating uncomfortable feelings aroused in response to the suffering person (e.g. distress, anger, fear) while remaining open to and accepting of the person suffering; and 5) motivation to act/acting to alleviate suffering. (Strauss et al., 2016, p. 6).

This definition is particularly relevant here, and we utilise it in the course of the work reported later on in this chapter.

Research on the link between compassion and technology for mental health care is still scarce. An exception is a recent scoping review (Kemp et al., 2020). This review aimed to identify which digital technologies are being used by patients and health professionals in the delivery of mental health care. Additionally, it investigated facilitators and barriers for the use of digital

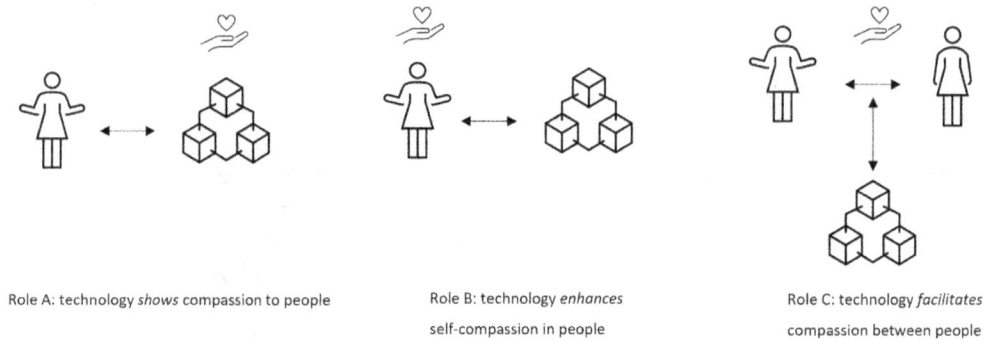

Role A: technology *shows* compassion to people

Role B: technology *enhances* self-compassion in people

Role C: technology *facilitates* compassion between people

Figure 16.1 The three ways in which technology can contribute to compassion

technology in the delivery of compassion in mental healthcare. Kemp et al. (2020) found that, when employed appropriately, digital technologies can facilitate and strengthen compassion and meaningful human connections in mental healthcare. In a review for the *Compassionate Technology* project, Van Lotringen et al. (2023) found three main ways in which technology can contribute to compassion in mental healthcare: by showing compassion to people (the technology itself is perceived as compassionate), by enhancing self-compassion in people and by facilitating compassion between people. Figure 16.1 shows these roles of technology in the interaction with people (clients and care professionals). A better understanding of the different roles and exactly which role would be best suitable for a particular situation can support developers of technology in embedding compassion within design. So far, many efforts to design for compassion in mental healthcare have focused on role B in Figure 16.1: technology that enhances self-compassion in people. For example, Ascone et al. (Ascone et al., 2020) draw from compassion-focused imagery exercises (Gilbert, 2010) to develop an immersive VR experience for individuals with occasional paranoid thoughts. The study then assesses levels of self-compassion in people, as well as emotion and paranoia by means of questionnaires. Conversely, Zhu et al. (Zhu et al., 2022) have designed a system to alleviate compassion fatigue in therapists. The intervention, tested in China during COVID-19, senses emotional fatigue in therapists during their sessions, and allows them to alleviate it through multisensory meditation. Although the paper mentions self-compassion as a proposed solution to compassion fatigue, the link between this theoretical underpinning and the embedding of self-compassion in design is less explicit.

While acknowledging compassion as an important value in mental healthcare, it is important to realise that compassion is seen as a phasic value: it only explicitly manifests at times of suffering, and in organisations, it has optimal effects when coupled with other values (Cameron, 2017). Similarly, in design for values (Friedman & Hendry, 2019), the focus is rarely on just one value. Below, we will elaborate on value-sensitive design approaches and how they may embed design for compassion.

Design for values and design for compassion

We refer to the word 'value' as what a person, or a group of people, consider important in life. Friedman and Hendry (2019) describe value-sensitive design (VSD) as a theoretically grounded approach that investigates the role of values in the design process. VSD allows designers to address ethical questions of responsibility. This is especially important when introducing new technologies where new or unexpected values may emerge. The approach consists of three phases. The first phase, 'conceptual investigations', aims at identifying and ordering all values at stake in a given context. The second phase, 'empirical investigations', studies the ideas of stakeholders about these values. The third phase, 'technical investigations', focuses on existing technologies and their embodied values. After thorough study of all value-related aspects of a typical context, the design of a new product or service can start. VSD has been applied in a wide range of domains, including nano pharmacy, transportation services and privacy in information technology. Since VSD as a basic methodology doesn't provide much direction as to how to embed a value in the design of a new product or service, this is part of ongoing research in the field. Later methodologies observe and identify values throughout the design process. Smits et al. (2022) developed Values that Matter (VtM), a method for designers to iterate on what values can be recognised in the design in its context, at any point of the creation and implementation process. In both VtM and VSD, the authors recommend that designers identify the values at stake in innovation processes and concretize the chosen ones in the final design. Smits et al.'s (2022) case of the design of a device for continuous monitoring of physiological signals in a hospital setting shows how complicated the VSD process can be. Typically, a designer or design team needs to choose which values to focus on during the design process, and how these can actually be implemented in the design and/or emerge from the interaction. Especially the implementation of values is not well described in the literature so far and this chapter aims to make a contribution here. Based on the above methodologies, looking specifically at designing for compassion, it is necessary to explain how such a value can be embedded in design or how a design can facilitate the emergence of this value.

As discussed above, in the domain of (mental) healthcare, compassion has been described by many authors as an important value for designers to have and to work with. For example, Goguen (2005) argues that compassion supports both better analysis and better ethics in design. Similar to what we see in the VtM method, Goguen advocates value discovery methods such as interviews combined with an iterative design process, leading to a value-centred design approach. Compassion and empathy as related concept have also been described as qualities that designers should use to connect to the people they are designing for and their needs. In this regard, Seshadri et al. (2014) offer a framework for fostering design thinking during the design process, a skill they describe as important to teach students who will design for people in complex and sensitive situations. Likewise, connecting to a vulnerable group of people, compassionate design was introduced as a method to design for dementia care in the context of developing analogue designs (Treadaway et al., 2018, see also Chapter 10 in this book). This method consists of three elements (sensory properties, connecting and personalisation) that centre around a focus on loving kindness for the individual. Compassionate design is rooted in positive psychology and builds on positive design methodology (Desmet & Pohlmeyer, 2013).

While the methods described above can help in understanding how to deal with the value of compassion in design, both in the process as well as in understanding the importance of the value in its context and outcome, the question of how design can promote the experience of compassion is still a challenging one. Can we embed the experience of compassion in design and can people experience a design as compassionate? In a study on multisensory aspects of compassion, we identified different aspects of compassion, both to investigate the multifaceted value that is compassion and to facilitate its embedding in design by breaking it down. We brainstormed with experts in mental healthcare to understand how we could translate the different aspects of compassion into *expressions of compassion*. This led to four different expressions of compassion, the development of which we present below by going through the procedural definition of compassion proposed by Strauss et al. (2016). This definition is particularly interesting from the point of view of design, as it includes different phases of the compassionate interaction and different aspects of compassion. 'Recognise suffering' is connected to being serious, heartfelt and sincere, qualities required to acknowledge someone else's suffering to ourselves and to the other. The second step, 'understanding the universality of suffering', is related to being vulnerable and humble, as it allows us to see the bigger picture and shrink ourselves in comparison to another (K. Neff, 2003). The third step, empathy, was not translated into an expression because it is about resonating with emotions in the moment. In the fourth step, courage is linked to the ability to stay with and bear difficult feelings that accompany suffering (Gilbert et al., 2017). Finally, the fifth step is connected to being authoritative, required to act with confidence and empathy based on all the previous four elements. Sincere, humble, courageous and authoritative describe the balance of both the empathic, kind, warm, open-minded caring aspect and the stronger, assertive one. In a course on multisensory design, students worked with this breakdown of compassion and embedded elements of compassion in their designs. The complete process is described in a paper (Lusi et al., 2022). In this chapter, we elaborate on one of the students' designs as an example of how such values can be used to create compassionate design, and how the compassionate design of technology can be embedded in a therapy process.

Embedding compassionate technology in therapy

In the previous sections, we have outlined how a design for values approach, focused on the value of compassion, can offer a way forward for better design of e-mental health and for embedding technology in mental healthcare. Eventually, this could (and should) lead to a more seamless integration of technology in mental healthcare with the aim to empower clients and to lower the barrier to accessing necessary care, and as a result, to lower the burden on the care system. In this section, we examine if and how following a compassionate design approach could lead to new technology that allows for more (self-)compassion and addresses the issue of introducing existing (off-the-shelf) technology in mental healthcare settings. To do so, we discuss a case study of a new technology-based application, the Balancial, that was designed to support clients and therapists in the process of cognitive behavioral therapy. The case study utilised a design for values approach, working with relevant stakeholders during the iterative design process.

Cognitive behavioural therapy (CBT) is a widely used and evidence-based method in psychotherapy used to restructure thinking and improve people's thoughts (e.g. feelings of worthlessness in clinical depression). Generally, CBT involves three separate stages. First, during the assessment stage, the behaviours, thoughts and feelings are explored to see how they may be contributing to people's psychological distress and wellbeing. Then, an intervention stage will follow, where the problematic behaviours or thoughts are targeted through an intervention. The third and last stage is about evaluating thoughts, feelings and behaviours that have occurred during the intervention and whether things have improved in the post-intervention stage (Teater, 2010). Balancial was envisaged as a therapeutic intervention that clients would use in their home environment to support self-compassion outside of the actual therapy sessions. Focusing on the sensory qualities and what a compassionate experience could mean for a product supporting self-compassion led to the understanding that such a product should make use of the sense of touch and be experienced as 'recognising suffering', the first step in the Strauss' definition of compassion. This means it should be experienced as serious, heartfelt and sincere; this translated into a design that showed both positive and negative sides of life in an honest and open way. Balancial therefore consisted of a weighing scale with blocks (physical elements) combined with a mobile application (see Figures 16.2 and 16.3). The blocks represent events, emotions, thoughts and other sorts of input provided by the user. The user puts the blocks on the surface, either on the 'positive' or 'negative' side, depending

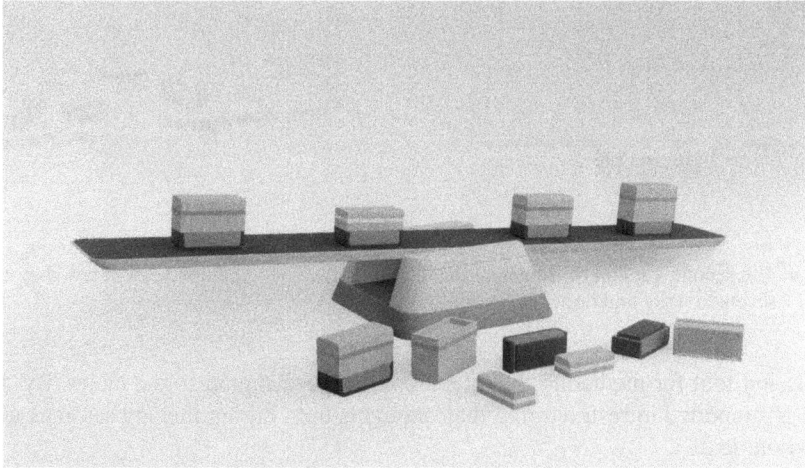

Figure 16.2 The first version of Balancial that could be used by clients at home as a planning and reflection tool is a weighing scale with blocks

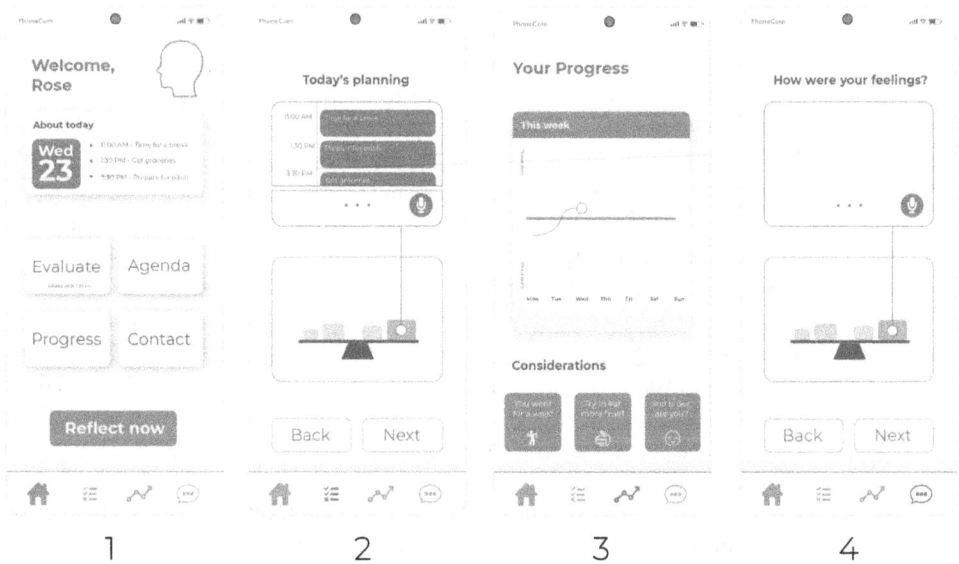

Figure 16.3 Screenshots of the mobile application, which supports the use of the physical part of Balancial to plan the activities of the day and reflect on them

on their emotional meanings. Balancial will then show the emotional balance of the day. The weight of the blocks indicates the mental/emotional impact the day's events had on the user. Either in the morning or evening, the user can give explicit value to each block by using the mobile application. Once the blocks are in place on the scale, the application can recognise their positions and translate this to an overview on the screen. By clicking on a block, a note or message can be attached to each block. Balancial can help a client evaluate their thoughts, emotions and events of the day and put them into perspective. It further serves as a reminder

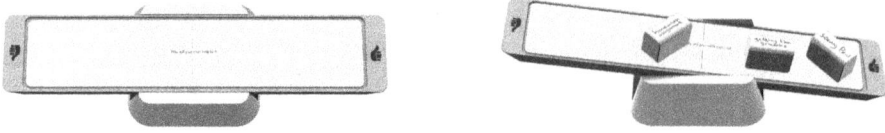

Figure 16.4 The second version of Balancial that could be used in a therapy session and that used paper
sheets to write and draw on

and discussion tool for mediating the interaction between therapist and client. By doing so,
the client is supported in restructuring their thoughts both during therapy sessions and in the
home environment.

Balancial was evaluated in conversation with five psychologists and therapists. In these interviews, a visualisation of a therapeutic journey, including the use of Balancial, was used. The
questions asked centred around positive and negative aspects of the design, compassion as a
value and the general workflow and specific features of Balancial. The outcomes of these interviews reflected some of the issues that started our Compassionate Technology project. The therapists saw difficulties in implementing new tools as well as benefits. The physical element of
Balancial was appreciated, and it was suggested that physically placing weights on the Balancial
could provoke more of an actual, tangible experience to enable or aid moments of reflection.
However, the digital element of Balancial was less appreciated. Interviewees suggested that too
many digital tools were already available and that Balancial could also be a low-tech solution
used by therapists and clients together. Further discussions centred around how the use of balance would be experienced (maybe not always compassionate) and how clients and therapists
would give meaning to different blocks.

Based on these insights, a re-design of Balancial was created that, instead of making use of a
mobile application, used a paper sheet to draw and write on (Figure 16.4). The blocks now also
have an area to write on, making it easier to remember what they represent and allowing their
use during a therapy session, where the client and therapist could 'build', as it were, the balance
in life. After a therapy session, the client could take the paper sheet home as a reminder of what
was discussed. During the next session client and therapist could reflect on the week using the
balance that was created on the paper sheet, replacing the blocks.

Being a student project, the study was relatively short and had limited involvement of stakeholders because, due to ethical concerns, we could not involve clients at this stage. Nevertheless,
the process of creating Balancial does show how different aspects of designing for compassion
may be used and combined. Starting from a better understanding of the (multisensory) experience of compassion (role A in Figure 16.1: product showing compassion) and supporting self-
compassion through its functionalities (role B in Figure 16.1), evaluation prompted us to move
to strengthening compassion within the interaction between therapist and client in the second
version (role C in Figure 16.1).

To facilitate compassion between therapist and client, Balancial uses characteristics that
seem common for compassionate technology. Firstly, the design concept uses the embodied
metaphor of a scale: when discussing the weights, the client can externalise their emotions
and thoughts to a tangible object (Hurtienne et al., 2007). This allows both client and therapist
to visualise and reshape the client's challenges on the scale to work towards their wellbeing.

Furthermore, the physical manipulation of the weights allows for off-loading of cognitive processes, which contributes to effective problem-solving (Manches & O'Malley, 2012). Finally, the weights become personalised elements, thus empowering the client to tailor the intervention to their own needs and wants, as well as supporting the therapist in choosing the best therapeutic path for the client. As opposed to role B (focused on self-compassion), facilitating compassion between people (role C) means designing for a shared experience that involves at least two people. This might include role-taking and team-based activities or even gamified elements. Importantly, the intervention space must create such a dynamic that allows for both individuals to feel with one another, while encouraging them to find meaningful ways to work towards the wellbeing of the individual suffering.

In some examples of compassionate technology, the system senses, represents and enables interactions (Van Lotringen, 2023). However, in the case of Balancial, the system does not sense the client's feelings; it is the client who inputs the information by assigning the meaning to the weights. The system then has the function of representing them and facilitating the interactions between client and therapist. When the client brings the Balancial's paper sheet home, the intervention will also allow for self-reflection.

Discussion

In this chapter, we have discussed how we can design for a value that is particularly important in mental healthcare: compassion. We have discussed different approaches to designing for compassion in the mental healthcare setting, where multiple stakeholders play a role. Integrating technology in such a setting is complex and requires a sensitive and iterative approach to design, as demonstrated through our case study. In addition to the development of value-based designs, it is also important to evaluate these to see if indeed the solutions that arise from this approach are successful, both in terms of acceptability and uptake, as well as in increasing wellbeing for the people using them.

The Compassionate Technology project adopts the view that designing technology with a pivotal human value and new ways of dividing tasks between people and technology can help promote the transition to sustainable mental health(care). So far, there is limited evidence as to the effects of following a design-for-values approach focused on the value of compassion. Compassion has been used as a theoretical grounding in design, but the mental health (technological) interventions that resulted from the design process are seldomly evaluated for compassion. Some studies have evaluated whether a technological intervention increased self-compassion in people (e.g. Falconer et al., 2016; Ascone et al., 2020; Huberty et al., 2019). However, they have not evaluated – to our knowledge – whether the technology itself is compassionate or has a compassionate role. This raises the question of what it means to design compassionate technology.

Currently, no evaluation tool exists to evaluate technology use in mental healthcare on compassion. To be able to evaluate whether our efforts to design for compassion are also experienced as compassionate, we are currently developing a new scale (van Lotringen et al., forthcoming). This scale is being developed based on literature on compassion and existing compassion measures, conversations with experts on compassion and scale development, combined with qualitative and quantitative input from professionals and clients in mental health care. Thus, we aim to make the process of compassion in the use of technology in mental health care visible and measurable, from both the professional and client perspective. The scale will have a regular version, for example, to evaluate a series of sessions in which an intervention was used, and a short version. The short version could be used to provide a repeated measure, for instance, for each interaction with an intervention. Evaluating e-mental health tools on their contribution to a compassionate process could help to draw comparisons between interventions and inform future design decisions.

Despite the current lack of evaluations of technology on compassion, we do know that putting compassion as a central value in organisations leads to organisations that are better in both subjective and objective outcomes (Cameron, 2017). Going beyond organisations in healthcare, for technology or design firms that are active in the (mental) healthcare domain, it is probably also a good idea to start emphasising the value of compassion in the organisation itself and to adopt designing for compassion approaches throughout their activities.

The case study described in this chapter has shown two ways to design for compassion: by focusing on the (sensory) experience and by better understanding what happens in the interaction between people and technology. Only through such thoroughly described case studies, and evaluation of design processes and outcomes, can we gain a better understanding of what the best practices to embed values – in this case compassion – in design. Should compassion be embedded in the technology, in the intervention (the system that technology is part of), or is it better to let compassion only come from within the human in a human–technology interaction? This multifaceted question is particularly relevant for designers and intervention developers that employ VSD, who wish to embed compassion in their designs.

Acknowledgements

This chapter describes work done in the project 'designing compassionate technology with high societal readiness levels for mental healthcare' (with project number 403.19.229) of the research programme Transitions and Behavior, which is financed by the Dutch Research Council (NWO), Minddistrict B.V. and Dimence Groep. The funding sources were not involved in the writing of this manuscript or the decision to submit it for publication. We would like to thank all the talented students from the University of Twente, who participated in the Multisensory Design course 2020–2021. Special thanks to Casper Hazebroek for allowing us to include the work on the Balancial project and its visuals in this chapter.

References

Ascone, L., Ney, K., Mostajeran, F., Steinicke, F., Moritz, S., Gallinat, J., & Kühn, S. (2020). *Virtual reality for individuals with occasional paranoid thoughts*. Extended Abstracts of the 2020 CHI Conference on Human Factors in Computing Systems (CHI EA '20). Association for Computing Machinery, New York, NY, 1–8. https://doi-org.ezproxy2.utwente.nl/10.1145/3334480.3382918

Cameron, K. S. (2017). *Organizational compassion* (E. M. Seppälä, E. Simon-Thomas, S. L. Brown, M. C. Worline, C. D. Cameron, & J. R. Doty, Eds., Vol. 1). Oxford University Press. https://doi.org/10.1093/oxfordhb/9780190464684.013.30

Derks, Y. P., Klaassen, R., Westerhof, G. J., Bohlmeijer, E. T., & Noordzij, M. L. (2019). Development of an ambulatory biofeedback app to enhance emotional awareness in patients with borderline personality disorder: Multicycle usability testing study. *JMIR mHealth and uHealth*, 7(10), e13479. https://doi.org/10.2196/13479

Desmet, P. M. A., & Pohlmeyer, A. E. (2013). Positive design: An introduction to design for subjective well-being. *International Journal of Design*, 7(3), 5–19.

Elices, M., Carmona, C., Pascual, J. C., Feliu-Soler, A., Martin-Blanco, A., & Soler, J. (2017). Compassion and self-compassion: Construct and measurement. *Mindfulness and Compassion*, 2(1), 34–40. https://doi.org/10.1016/j.mincom.2016.11.003

Falconer, C. J., Rovira, A., King, J. A., Gilbert, P., Antley, A., Fearon, P., Ralph, N., Slater, M., & Brewin, C. R. (2015). Embodying self-compassion within virtual reality and its effects on patients with depression. *BJPsych Open*, *2*(1), 74–80. https://doi.org/10.1192/bjpo.bp.115.002147, PubMed: 27703757, PubMed Central: PMC4995586.

Feijt, M. A., de Kort, Y. A., Bongers, I. M., & IJsselsteijn, W. A. (2018). Perceived drivers and barriers to the adoption of eMental health by psychologists: The construction of the levels of adoption of eMental health model. *Journal of Medical Internet Research*, *20*(4), e153. https://doi.org/10.2196/jmir.9485

Friedman, B., & Hendry, D. F. (2019). *Value sensitive design: Shaping technology with moral imagination.* The MIT Press.

Gilbert, P. (2009). Introducing compassion-focused therapy. *Advances in Psychiatric Treatment*, *15*(3), 199–208. https://doi.org/10.1192/apt.bp.107.005264

Gilbert, P. (2010). *Compassion focused therapy: Distinctive features.* Routledge.

Gilbert, P., Catarino, F., Duarte, C., Matos, M., Kolts, R., Stubbs, J., Ceresatto, L., Duarte, J., Pinto-Gouveia, J., & Basran, J. (2017). The development of compassionate engagement and action scales for self and others. *Journal of Compassionate Health Care*, *4*(1), 4. https://doi.org/10.1186/s40639-017-0033-3

Goguen, J. A. (2005). Semiotics, compassion and value-centered design. In K. Liu (Ed.), *Virtual, distributed and flexible organisations* (pp. 3–14). Kluwer Academic Publishers. https://doi.org/10.1007/1-4020-2162-3_1

Hedman-Lagerlöf, E., Carlbring, P., Svärdman, F., Riper, H., Cuijpers, P., & Andersson, G. (2023). Therapist-supported Internet-based cognitive behaviour therapy yields similar effects as face-to-face therapy for psychiatric and somatic disorders: An updated systematic review and meta-analysis. *World Psychiatry*, *22*(2), 305–314. https://doi.org/10.1002/wps.21088

Huberty, J., Green, J., Glissmann, C., Larkey, L., Puzia, M., & Lee, C. (2019). Efficacy of the mindfulness meditation mobile app "calm" to reduce stress among college students: Randomized controlled trial. *JMIR mHealth and uHealth*, *25*(6), e14273. https://doi.org/10.2196/14273, PubMed: 31237569, PubMed Central: PMC6614998.

Hurtienne, J., & Israel, J. (2007). *Image schemas and their metaphorical extensions: Intuitive patterns for tangible interaction. TEI'07.* 1st International Conference on Tangible and Embedded Interaction, 127–134. doi:10.1145/1226969.1226996

Kemp, J., Zhang, T., Inglis, F., Wiljer, D., Sockalingam, S., Crawford, A., Lo, B., Charow, R., Munnery, M., Singh Takhar, S., & Strudwick, G. (2020). Delivery of compassionate mental health care in a digital technology–driven age: Scoping review. *Journal of Medical Internet Research*, *22*(3), e16263. https://doi.org/10.2196/16263

Kothgassner, O. D., Goreis, A., Kafka, J. X., Van Eickels, R. L., Plener, P. L., & Felnhofer, A. (2019). Virtual reality exposure therapy for posttraumatic stress disorder (PTSD): A meta-analysis. *European Journal of Psychotraumatology*, *10*(1), 1654782. https://doi.org/10.1080/20008198.2019.1654782

Lusi, B., Ludden, G., Klaassen, R., van Lotringen, C., & Noordzij, M. (2022, June 16). *Embodiments of compassion in caring and non-caring products: Exploring design for values with a multisensory approach.* DRS. https://doi.org/10.21606/drs.2022.288

Manches, A., & O'Malley, C. (2012). Tangibles for learning: A representational analysis of physical manipulation. *Personal and Ubiquitous Computing*, *16*(4), 405–419. https://doi.org/10.1007/s00779-011-0406-0

Mohr, D. C., Zhang, M., & Schueller, S. M. (2017). Personal sensing: Understanding mental health using ubiquitous sensors and machine learning. *Annual Review of Clinical Psychology*, *13*(1), 23–47. https://doi.org/10.1146/annurev-clinpsy-032816-044949

Neff, K. D. (2003). Self-compassion: An alternative conceptualization of a healthy attitude toward oneself. *Self and Identity*, *2*(2), 85–101. https://doi.org/10.1080/15298860309032

Neff, K. D. (2012). The science of self-compassion. In C. Germer & R. Siegel*Compassion and wisdom in psychotherapy.*(pp. 79-92). New York: Guilford Press.

Scholten, H., & Granic, I. (2019). Use of the principles of design thinking to address limitations of digital mental health interventions for youth: Viewpoint. *Journal of Medical Internet Research*, *21*(1), e11528. https://doi.org/10.2196/11528

Seshadri, P., Reid, T., & Booth, J. (2014). A framework for fostering compassionate design thinking during the design process. *ASEE Annual Conference & Exposition Proceedings*, *2014*, 24.51.1–24.51.20. https://doi.org/10.18260/1-2--19943

Shea, S., & Lionis, C. (2017). *The call for compassion in health care* (E. M. Seppälä, et al. Eds., Vol. 1). Oxford University Press. https://doi.org/10.1093/oxfordhb/9780190464684.013.32

Smits, M., Bredie, B., Van Goor, H., & Verbeek, P. P. C. C. (2019). Values that matter: Mediation theory and design for values. In *Proceedings of the academy of design innovation management conference*.

Smits, M., Ludden, G., Peters, R., Bredie, S. J. H., van Goor, H., & Verbeek, P.-P. (2022). Values that matter: A new method to design and assess moral mediation of technology. *Design Issues*, *38*(1), 39–54. https://doi.org/10.1162/desi_a_00669

Strauss, C., Lever Taylor, B., Gu, J., Kuyken, W., Baer, R., Jones, F., & Cavanagh, K. (2016). What is compassion and how can we measure it? A review of definitions and measures. *Clinical Psychology Review*, *47*, 15–27. https://doi.org/10.1016/j.cpr.2016.05.004

Teater, B. (2010). Cognitive behavioral therapy. In M. Davies (Ed.), *The Blackwell companion to social work* (4th ed.). Wiley-Blackwell[MS1].

Treadaway, C., Fennell, J., Prytherch, D., Kenning, G., Prior, A., & Walters, A. (2018). *Compassionate design: How to design for advanced dementia – A toolkit for designers*. Cardiff Metropolitan University.

Van Doorn, M., Nijhuis, L. A., Monsanto, A., Van Amelsvoort, T., Popma, A., Jaspers, M. W. M., Noordzij, M. L., Öry, F. G., Alvarez-Jimenez, M., & Nieman, D. H. (2022). Usability, feasibility, and effect of a biocueing intervention in addition to a moderated digital social therapy-platform in young people with emerging mental health problems: A mixed-method approach. *Frontiers in Psychiatry*, *13*, 871813. https://doi.org/10.3389/fpsyt.2022.871813

Van Lotringen, C., Lusi, B., Westerhof, G. J., Ludden, G. D. S., Kip, H., Kelders, S. M., & Noordzij, M. L. (2023). The role of compassionate technology in blended and digital mental health interventions: Systematic scoping review. *JMIR Mental Health*, *10*, e42403.

van Lotringen, C., ten Klooster, P., Austin, J., Westerhof, G. J., Kelders, S. M., Lusi, B., & Noordzij, M. L. (forthcoming). Using Q-sort methodology to develop a compassionate technology evaluation scale with stakeholders in mental health care.

Zhu, Y., Zhu, D., & Liu, W. (2022). *Do not to be a trash can for other people's bad emotions compassion fatigue solutions for psychological counselors*. The Ninth International Symposium of Chinese CHI (Chinese CHI 2021). Association for Computing Machinery, New York, NY, 83–91. https://doi-org .ezproxy2.utwente.nl/10.1145/3490355.3490364

17 We want to play too

Co-design of a public intergenerational play space and service for improved mental health for older adults in the Australian Capital Territory

Jordan Mckibbin, Fanke Peng and Cathy Hope

Introduction

In Western cultures, age segregation of older adults and children is widespread, occurring institutionally, culturally and spatially (Hagestad & Uhlenberg, 2005). Age segregation appears in institutions such as schools and where age is an explicit or implicit criterion for participation (Hagestad & Uhlenberg, 2006). Cultural age segregation occurs in language and cultural artefacts such as music, fashion and food, with these cultural differences exacerbated by marketing that targets specific age demographics (Hagestad & Uhlenberg, 2005; Rogoff et al., 2010). Spatial age segregation occurs when people of different ages are not facilitated to occupy the same spaces, as is evident in housing and neighbourhood play and recreation spaces. The impacts of such age segregation are limited opportunities for culturally sanctioned and meaningful engagement between young and old outside of familial interactions, and possible intergenerational misunderstandings and conflicts. Age segregation as a barrier to intergenerational engagement can, in turn, lead to poorer mental health outcomes for older adults by contributing to ageism and social disconnectedness and isolation (Hagestad & Uhlenberg, 2006).

The issues and impacts of age segregation are exacerbated by the fact that the population worldwide is ageing as people live longer. The World Health Organisation (WHO) predicts that the proportion of people aged 60+ will double by 2050, and the number of people aged 80+ will triple in this same period (WHO, 2022). This exponential growth in the number of older adults is 'poised to become one of the most significant social transformations of the twenty-first century' affecting all sectors of society, including 'family structures and intergenerational ties' (United Nations, n.d.).

While increased longevity provides opportunities for older adults to enjoy an extended quality of life and ongoing contributions to the community, these opportunities are deeply interconnected with older adult health (United Nations n.d.) According to the United Nations, physical and social environments have significant impacts on older adults' health across the lifespan, either affecting health directly, 'or through barriers or incentives that affect opportunities, decisions, and health behaviour' (United Nations, n.d.).

This chapter outlines the first stage of a design project in Canberra, in the Australian Capital Territory (ACT), Australia in 2021, which seeks to contribute to the provision of better physical and social environments for older adults to improve mental and physical health outcomes by informing the design of the first intergenerational play space in the ACT. This design project is important because the ACT's projected ageing population growth mirrors those worldwide: in 2019, the ACT 65+ population was 12.5%, but this is expected to rise to 21% by 2053 (ACT Health, 2016; Community Services, 2019).

DOI: 10.4324/9781003318262-21

The site for the proposed dedicated intergenerational play space is Macnamara Park in the 40-year greenfield urban development of Ginninderry in the northwest of the ACT. Ginninderry will house approximately 30,000 residents in 11,500 dwellings, with around 1,800 dwellings and 4,600 residents currently in residence there. Ginnderry is notably more culturally diverse than the rest of the ACT, with over 65% of Ginninderry's current residents with both parents born overseas, compared with ACT average at 37% (Australian Bureau of Statistics, 2021). The development of Ginninderry aims to exemplify 'world's best practice in its design, 'construction and long-term liveability, and seeks to achieve this through a set of broad-ranging principles including 'collaborating with research and education institutions to drive innovation' and 'designing neighbourhoods that support and encourage community interactions through imaginative, functional and enjoyable public spaces' (Ginninderry Project Vision, 2021).

A multidisciplinary team facilitated by researchers from the University of Canberra in design, the built environment, play and health partnered with the Ginninderry design and community engagement team to answer the question: how do you design a successful intergenerational play space for older adult users? The research team undertook an interdisciplinary literature review and developed a co-design workshop for older adults. The design process then led to the use of service design to co-create an intergenerational programme to facilitate the use of the intergenerational play space. The focus in the first phase of this project is on understanding the needs of older adults (65+ in this project) because the needs of children (0–12 in this project) from play spaces and play elements are comparatively well known and fulfilled in public space (Mitchell et al., 2007).

This project seeks to address what Kaplan et al. (2007) refer to as a historical 'lack of attention to how the physical environment plays a role in promoting or inhibiting intergenerational engagement' (p. 81). This 'lack of attention' in the literature is reflected in the absence of purpose-built intergenerational play environments in the ACT, and the paucity of such play spaces in Australia and the world.

What is play?

To define intergenerational play, it is important to understand the characteristics of play. Play is a subjective experience that we engage in voluntarily, is self-directed, intrinsically motivated, guided by rules that allow creativity and imagination and that generates some form of positive affect (Davis et al., 2011; Eberle, 2014; Sicart, 2014; Gray, 2017). While play is mostly associated with childhood, people engage in play and are playful across the lifespan, including older adults (Goldmintz & Schaefer, 2007; Yarnal & Qian, 2011; Cosco, 2017).

One important characteristic of play is that it is multi-faceted. Examples of the spectrum of play include physical, cognitive, social, creative, imaginative, exploratory, sensory and nature play (Hughes, 2002; Shackell et al., 2008; Whitebread et al., 2012; City of Ballarat, 2017; Borzenkova, 2021). The multi-faceted nature of play offers people many and diverse modes of engaging in play culturally, physically, socially and cognitively (Henricks, 2006).

What is intergenerational play?

Intergenerational play is play that involves interaction, cooperation and possible mutual influence between generations (Villar, 2007). It differs from multigenerational play because while multigenerational play implies shared activity among generations, it does not necessarily involve interaction or influence across the generations (Cushing et al., 2022). Key to intergenerational play, then, is its 'relational' quality (Kaplan et al., 2007).

Agate et al. (2018) outlined a framework for exploring the experience of intergenerational play for older adults with their grandchildren. This framework consists of motivations, functions, constraints, negotiation/affordances and mechanisms. Motivations for older adults include the priority of engaging with family, a desire to help, and the many benefits sought from intergenerational play for both grandparent and grandchild. These benefits in this framework are referred to as functions, and include 'having fun, bonding, expressing love and interest in the other, making memories, getting to know each other and teaching lessons' (Agate et al, 2018, p. 405). Perceived constraints are physical, geographical and behavioural and act as barriers to engagement in mutual play. Negotiation involves navigating these constraints, such as changing roles when engaged in play – a finding supported by Davis et al. (2011) – and identifying activities in which grandparent and grandchild can play together. Affordances include everything from leisure affordances, such as staying healthy to ensure grandparents can engage in play, to utilised affordances like technology, board games and chairs to facilitate active or passive engagement in play. Finally, mechanisms are the 'components of the process through which grandparent and grandchild played together' (p410) and include focused time, talking and listening and interactive activities.

Kaplan et al. (2020) proposed the multi-dimensional conceptual approach to intergenerational play known as intergenerational contact zones (ICZ). These zones 'serve as spatial focal points for different generations to meet, interact, build relationships (e.g. trust and friendships), and, if desired, work together to address issues of local concern'. ICZs extend design beyond considerations of the physical properties of a space to incorporate how people use and perceive that space. Alongside the physical are temporal, psychological, sociocultural, political, institutional and ethical contact zones, which provide a more holistic view of intergenerational engagement and the many zones in which this engagement can be constrained or enabled.

Barriers to intergenerational play and impacts on older adults' mental health

While studies show that people play across the lifespan, the amount of time we play and the way that we play changes as we grow older (Burr et al., 2019). This change and decline in play as we age may, in part, be attributed to the socio-cultural view that play is childish and that adults should be productive with their time (Van Vleet & Feeney, 2015).

The view that play is for childhood is reinforced by the built environment in Australia, where there are exponentially fewer dedicated public spaces for play as we grow older. In the ACT, for example, there are 512 play spaces, 434 of which are designed for children aged 0–7 (Transport Canberra and City Services, 2018). There are notably fewer play spaces designed for teenagers (11 destination play spaces and 5 skate parks), and currently none designed for older adults in the ACT, such as those found in China, the USA and Europe designed for exclusive or primary use by older adults (Link, 2017; Levinger et al., 2018).

The perceived social stigma of playing for older adults and the age segregation of play spaces create barriers for older adults in visiting play spaces and engaging in play in those spaces. In a study by Mitchell et al. (2007), there was a unanimous perception from older adult participants that playgrounds are meant for children, and thus use of the equipment by adults would be negatively received. Older adults also do not feel welcome in public spaces where children play because of societal perceptions of 'stranger danger'. Further, there are physical safety concerns about the 'mix' of children and adults in play spaces, with adult use of equipment near children potentially placing children at risk, and co-location of child's play potentially leading to falls (Mitchell et al., 2007).

The high degree and acceptance of age segregation within our communities and institutions aggravate social issues, including generation-based stereotypes such as ageism (Vanderberk, 2007; Washington et al., 2019). Ageism involves explicit and implicit assumptions that group older adults into a homogenous cohort, defining them in an oversimplified and often unfavourable way (Minichiello et al., 2000) and facilitating intergenerational social distance and conflicts (Hauderowicz & Serena, 2020; Thang, 2013; Vanderbeck & Worth, 2014).

Age segregation can contribute to poorer mental health outcomes for older adults due to the effects of ageism as well as social disconnectedness and isolation. Ageism can lead to negative mental health among older adults, including depression, anxiety and even suicidal ideation (Chang et al., 2020; Marques et al., 2020). Age segregation can also contribute to the age homogeneity of social networks, which increases the risk of social disconnectedness and isolation (Hagestad & Uhlenberg, 2006; Steward & McDevitt, 2019). Both social disconnectedness and perceived social isolation in older adults are strongly linked to poor mental health outcomes in older adults (Santini et al., 2020), alongside functional and cognitive decline and dementia (Hilbrand et al., 2017; Xiang et al., 2021).

Benefits of intergenerational play

Intergenerational engagement can serve to alleviate these negative impacts and, at the same time, provide a raft of benefits for older adults. Intergenerational engagement has been shown to reduce age segregation, and the experience of ageism and social isolation (Parkinson & Turner, 2019). Interaction with younger people can improve mental, physical, cognitive and other health and wellbeing outcomes for older adults and improve self-worth; provide crucial channels for sharing knowledge, ideas and values; decrease social isolation and improve quality of life (MacCallum et al., 2006; Flora & Faulkner, 2007; Sànchez, 2007; Newman & Hatten-Yeo, 2008; Springate et al., 2008; Park, 2014; Zhang & Kaufman, 2016; Martins et al., 2019; Minghetti et al., 2021; Peters et al., 2021). One consistent outcome of intergenerational engagement for older people is a notable reduction in emotional and social anxiety, thus contributing to better mental health (Krzeczkowska et al., 2021). Intergenerational engagement also extends the lifespan, with a 2017 study showing that older adults are 37% more likely to survive the next 20 years if they babysit their grandchildren (Hilbrand et al., 2017).

Intergenerational *play* as a form of intergenerational engagement both enables and extends on these benefits. First, play provides a free, intuitively understood and multifaceted mechanism for engaging with others (Huizinga, 1955). Second, engagement in play provides the benefits attributed to engaging in play at all stages of life, including improvements in physical fitness, cognitive development, emotional wellbeing, positive feelings and relief from stress, psychological health[1] and social development and connection (Yarnal, 2006; Yarnal & Qian, 2011; Agate et al., 2018; Dankiew et al., 2020). Intergenerational play is also a vehicle for social interaction and learning between younger and older generations (Zhang & Kaufman, 2016), exposing younger and older generations to different perspectives (Davis et al., 2002). Overall, there are increasing bodies of evidence of the many mental and physical health and other benefits of intergenerational engagement for all generations involved (Giraudeau & Bailly, 2019).

Enabling intergenerational play in the physical and social environment

Play spaces are dedicated sites in the public realm for fostering play. While playgrounds were originally designed as mechanisms of positive social and physical engineering for children living in cities, the role of play spaces is increasingly important across the lifespan to meet health and wellbeing outcomes needed as cities grow (Shephard-Simms, 2012; Frost, 2015; Hope et al., 2017). Intergenerational play spaces can create spaces and opportunities for younger and older people to collaboratively participate in play activities and to gain the health and wellbeing benefits of engagement in this play (Fitzgerald, 2021).

However, there is an absence of literature on the design of intergenerational play spaces. The exception is Fitzgerald's (2021) thesis, which provides design guidelines for intergenerational playgrounds, including guidelines for site planning, programme, safety, engagement and choice. Our first stage design project both responds to and builds on Fitzgerald's guidelines with the involvement of a diverse range of subject matter experts, stakeholders and older adult experts through a co-design and service design process.

Method

To address the key challenge of designing an intergenerational play space when there is a paucity of literature on intergenerational – and particularly 'relational' – play space design, a lack of intergenerational play space exemplars, and multiple and complex barriers to older adult engagement in play spaces, the research and stakeholder team chose to facilitate a co-design workshop with older adults. Co-design provides designers with insights from users as 'experts of their experiences', making design success more likely if the unique knowledge, needs, challenges and aspirations of older adults as users of this space are captured and understood (Mahr et al., 2014).

The team developed the workshop structure and content using Woodcock et al.'s (2020) four guiding 'considerations' for designing older adults, informed by literature relating to these considerations:

Individual: acknowledging the heterogeneity of older adults and their contexts (Reyes, 2016) by involving them without stigmatising or making assumptions, and by ensuring that the process reinforces autonomy and agency (Gibson, 2018).
Empathic: recognising that older adults may be unused to co-design practice, and thus embedding co-design approaches that are accessible and engaging to enhance efficacy; creating an environment of equal and equitable collaboration (Sakaguchi-Tang et al., 2021) and mutual learning (Fischer et al., 2021); and ensuring that older adults are physically and emotionally comfortable during the session.
Practical: using inclusive materials and methods of communication designed for a range of abilities.
Methodological: using visual methods such as visual aids to create common ground between participants and enabling narrative modes that align with older adult preferences and strengths, such as reflections on life experience and knowledge (Sakaguchi-Tang et al., 2021).

Participants

The co-design workshop was delivered during the COVID-19 pandemic, and thus it was necessary to run the workshop online. In light of Woodcock et al.'s practical considerations and the difficulties of generating organic communication online, the research team capped participant numbers at ten. As few older adults currently live in Ginninderry, participants were recruited using snowball methods via the research and Ginninderry teams. Nine participants over the age of 65 signed up for the workshop but only seven attended on the day – with two unable to attend for family and health reasons.

Procedure

Seven participants met online for a two-hour workshop with members of the research team and Ginninderry. The workshop was divided into two sections with a midway break for participant comfort. As this workshop was held online, the team used Sanders' (2002) 'say' rather than 'do' or 'make' approach to co-design, actively listening and documenting input from the participants. A presentation using images, icons with large and minimal text, provided a visual aid to support engagement. A graphic illustrator was employed to capture the workshop in succinct and appealing visual form as an artefact and gift for participants. Section one of the workshop embedded Woodcock et al.'s (2020) individual, empathic and methodological considerations by:

- Asking each participant to introduce themselves, provide details of their relationship with Canberra, and their favourite play experience.
- Creating an equal and equitable collaborative environment through sharing key findings from the literature review to empower participants to contribute and help them understand the role and value of their input.
- Connecting participants with 'play' through comparison of their own childhood play experiences with their perceptions of play in childhood now.

Section two generated data about intergenerational play. Participants were asked (i) what they enjoy playing with children and young people, (ii) why they enjoy playing with children and young people, (iii) what are the challenges of playing with children and young people are? Finally, participants were asked to identify the amenities, equipment, activities and natural elements they needed and wanted in an intergenerational playground. Data was captured through workshop transcripts and graphic illustration.

Data analysis

The data from the workshop was analysed using Agate et al.'s (2018) intergenerational framework. An empathy map was generated from the workshop data, as empathy maps are tools to better understand participant perspectives from their point of view (Ferreira et al., 2015). Finally, design researchers in the team produced three 'personas'. Personas are a user modelling technique involving the creation of hypothetical user archetypes detailing their characteristics and needs (Ferreira et al., 2015).

Findings

The findings in the co-design workshop reinforced many key findings in the literature and are outlined below using Agate et al.'s (2018) categories: motivations, functions, constraints, negotiation/affordances and mechanisms.

- **Motivations:** participants were motivated to engage in intergenerational play by helping family, by being another important adult in a child's life, and of broader social use, and by the many benefits intergenerational play brings to themselves and others – including their own children, grandchildren and community.

  I think being another adult who's involved in their life is incredibly valuable. (Workshop participant)

... it's also good for my health. And my well being. ... And it's the participation. That's, that's really important. (Workshop participant)

- **Functions:** participants recognised the many benefits of intergenerational play. This included physical, cognitive and creative or imaginative benefits, as well as multiple psychosocial benefits – including a sense of purpose, achievement, social connection from participation and 'complete joy' – that contribute to better mental and physical health outcomes, as the literature review shows.

You're having to continuously use your brain, you're having outsmart them because they're tricky. (Workshop participant)
Playing with the kids also makes you feel young. It gives you that sense of accomplishment that you haven't lost those skills. (Workshop participant)

- **Constraints:** a key psychological constraint for participants is the perceived stigma of older adults visiting and engaging in play in spaces that are 'for children'.

When my grandson was born ... I couldn't wait for him to be big enough so that I could legitimately go on the merry go round in [Canberra city]. Because we don't think we should do it as adults, but if we've got a child in tow it's OK. (Workshop participant)

Participants also identified physical constraints relating to access into play spaces, to engaging in child-directed play activities for periods of time, and with the physical and behavioural challenges associated with being responsible for children's safety.

Two and three-year-olds, they react so quickly that it's hard to supervise them sometimes. My reaction time isn't as quick so it's hard to keep up with the kids. (Workshop participant-)

Other key constraints related to access and amenity include travel to the play space; access into and within the play space; and access to essential amenities such as toilets, water, seating and shade.

- **Negotiation/affordances:** the primary method for negotiating the perceived stigma of visiting and playing in play spaces was by accompanying known and willing children (e.g. grandchild). Simply enjoying watching children play was not enough to reduce the experience of stigma. Physical constraints were negotiated through passive participation such as watching and 'acknowledging skills'; following children on their play journey; facilitating activities in which both generations can participate; and recognising and adapting when activities are too challenging.

I'm always walking around because my grandson, he wants to go over to the flying fox and then he wants to go over here. (Workshop participant)

Affordances included maintaining physical health and a youthful outlook, and being open to the challenges that playing with children brings.

- **Mechanisms:** participants identified multiple mechanisms for enabling engagement in intergenerational play, including teaching lessons and focused time. In terms of intergenerational design, mechanisms for enabling intergenerational play included accessible amenities, and 'relational' equipment customised to meet older adult needs alongside children's needs.

And maybe that's where they could interact [in sandpits] going from high to low and low to high. You know, if the kids had some sort of digger that they can load into the high and Grandpa can dig it out and they can do it again. (Workshop participant)

Discussion

The findings in this workshop and literature review support Kaplan et al.'s (2020) holistic framework for informing intergenerational play design with a multi-dimensional – physical, temporal, psychological, sociocultural, political, institutional and ethical – understanding of spaces and how they impact and shape the zones of contact between generations.

Older adults are made of heterogeneous individuals, coming from different contexts and enjoying a diverse range of activities. Older adults in this study enjoy playing with children and recognise the many benefits and value of interacting in play for both generations. However, there are also physical, cognitive, psychosocial and socio-cultural challenges and barriers to older adults both visiting and engaging in play spaces.

These barriers are captured in the two 'personas' developed from the data. The first, 'George', has grandchildren but is not very mobile, experiences physical challenges with engaging in play and tires easily. As a result, George observes his grandchildren rather than connecting and cooperating through play. The second, Helen, does not have children or grandchildren; is physically mobile and enjoys watching children play but does not know how to engage with other people's children; and experiences loneliness.

The analysis of the data led to two outputs: the development of guidelines for enabling 'relational' activity in intergenerational play spaces based on the co-design workshop and interdisciplinary literature review, and the development through service design of a pilot intergenerational programme that addressed external barriers to participation and engagement in play in the play space.

Part I: Design guidelines for an intergenerational play space

Below is a summary of the 'Intergenerational Essentials' and 'Relational Activity' Guidelines developed to inform the design of intergenerational play space (Table 17.1).

Relational activity

Physical 'relational' activity guidelines:

- Physical activity is a key health and wellbeing benefit of play for children and older adults.
- Older adults and younger children have similar neuromuscular performance (Granacher et al., 2010) and physical activity needs such as strength and balance. Target these performances and needs using parallel or cooperative equipment, for example, parallel balance beams. Ensure physical play elements respond to culturally diverse user needs at Ginninderry (e.g. badminton).
- Create opportunities to engage in different levels of physical challenge, as 'light' exercise for some might be moderate to strenuous exercise for others.
- Include traditional equipment such as swings, see-saws, slides, sandpits and monkey bars because both generations understand how to use this equipment, but customise them to facilitate engagement by older adults. Examples include cooperative, customised swings where players face each other, or two-tiered sandpits including a seat, sandbox and sand toys for the older adult in the above sandpit.

Table 17.1 Summary of the 'Intergenerational Essentials' and 'Relational Activity' Guidelines

Intergenerational Essentials	
Co-locate with essential amenities	Both older adults and children require access to toilets, water, seating and shade to be comfortable and to spend time in play spaces.
Co-design with users	Co-design custom play elements and activities with older adults, children, designers, play experts and occupational therapists ensure design efficacy and success.
Offer diverse play elements and choices	The heterogeneity of users and diversity of user interests and abilities require a range of play experiences and play types the different types to offer multiple entry points to engagement.
Minimise possible hazards	Use materiality such as a soft surface to minimise the risk of falls. Boost older adult confidence by thoughtful allocating of play activity types to minimise possible dangerous intersections of play.
Provide wayfinding and signage	Facilitate intergenerational play by ensuring that people feel comfortable navigating their way around (Kaplan et al., 2007), through clear wayfinding signage at eye and ground level. Also include visual signs for key play elements to show users how to undertake relational play.

- Enable intergenerational play through walking together, such as adventure walking trails with co-located obstacle courses, environmental experiences or storytelling prompts.
- Layer physical activity with graduated challenges so that both younger children and older adults are incentivised to return to the park and improve their skills (Frost et al., 2004).
- Where older adults cannot or do not want to engage in physical activity, promote intergenerational interaction that enables children to engage older adults as 'help agents' (Hayes, 2003). Ensure there is safe and adequate space, and possible seating options, for older adults to comfortably engage through watching, narrativising and acknowledging children's play.

Cognitive 'relational' activity guidelines:

- Older adults enjoy imparting and sharing knowledge and skills (Reyes, 2016). Embed play experiences that enable the generations to cooperatively share skills and knowledge – whether this is about nature, or through cognitive activity. Examples include building a sandcastle together or talking about the environment.
- Older adults and children share a love of games (Zhang & Kaufman, 2016). Games provide an accessible mechanism for enabling meaningful engagement between the generations. Older adults can teach children the rules and tactics for games, providing another avenue for knowledge and skill sharing. Facilitate game spaces (on soft surfaces on the ground; at tables with comfortable seating; against a wall) and provide loose parts that enable relational activity. Ensure that game spaces are open-ended to facilitate culturally diverse play.
- Sensory engagement is a highly inclusive form of play and one with wellbeing benefits both for older adults, including those with dementia (Haigh & Mytton, 2016), and for children including neurodiverse children (Kianfar & Brischetto, 2021). Facilitate relational play by including natural and built sensory elements on a play journey, with dwell-in-place (e.g. seating) or signage prompts to engage with these elements in relational ways.
- Cultural heritage, storytelling and creative play: both older adults and children have a strong connection with storytelling. Stories are a critical mode of communication for older adults to connect to identity, legacy and memory (Balyasnikova & Gillard, 2018). Embed a storytelling circle or storytelling prompts at key play sites in the park. Build a 'street' library managed by play space visitors that includes children's stories from around the

world. Include changeable mats on tables that enable socio-dramatic play such as medical, teaching, chef/cooking, fairy, pirate.

Part II: Design guidelines for an intergenerational programme

Part II of the guidelines employs service design to address external barriers that prevent older adults from visiting an intergenerational play space and engaging in intergenerational play. Service design is:

> the process of planning and organising people, infrastructure, communication and material components of a service, with the goal of improving the service's quality, the interactions between a provider and its customers, and the customers' experiences.
>
> (Steen et al., 2011)

These guidelines are for a whole-of-service intergenerational play programme to be piloted at the Ginninderry intergenerational play space and surrounding parkland in Macnamara Park.

Service design tools, including customer journey maps and service blueprints, were used by the core research team to develop this pilot programme that utilises the intergenerational play space and surrounding parkland currently being built in Ginninderry, ACT, Australia.

These Part II guidelines include six categories developed from a service design perspective – awareness, sign-up, event time, transportation, activities and amenities – to address the following questions:

1. How will older adults, including isolated adults, learn of the programme?
2. How will older adults, including isolated adults, get to and from the programme?
3. What activities can be provided that enable intergenerational interactions?
4. How do you make participants feel safe when participating in the activities?

Awareness

A public event will only attract engagement if the community is aware that the event is taking place. Raising awareness becomes more difficult when one target demographic may not use digital communication tools or platforms. Utilising existing communication tools that the different target demographics are familiar with and that are trusted sources of information, such as community and retirement village notice boards, community and seniors centres, Ginninderry and other social media pages, child-care centres, newsletters and community-based apps can help reach more members of the community.

The communication channels identified for an event in Ginninderry were:

The GX app: this app was developed by the Joint Venture (JV) and is already being used to promote events around Ginninderry.

The Link: the Link is the Ginninderry community and information centre.

Capital Region Community Service (CRCS): the CRCS services North Canberra and provides services that assist isolated older adults with transportation to and from events. Partnering with an existing and trusted community organisation provides a level of assurance to the community that the play day will be a safe and welcoming environment. It also allows the project to utilise existing social capital to reach more community members.

Social Media: the Ginninderry Community Facebook page and the Strathnairn Playgroup are useful for reaching parents in the local community.

Signup

The event should be free to prevent financial exclusion and to encourage the widest diversity of possible attendees. An online platform such as Eventbrite allows for the creation and management of events and tracking interest to ensure numbers are manageable. For older adults unfamiliar with online event services, signup sheets can be placed in physical sites like community centres where staff can assist with the signup process.

Time of event

In line with Kaplan et al.'s (2020) temporal intergenerational contact zone, event timing must take into account the needs of all target demographics. For the event in Ginninderry, school holidays were chosen as the optimal time to host the event. During this time, children are free during the day and grandparents are tasked with childcare while parents work. The best time for the event was identified as between 10:00 am and 2:30 pm, allowing time to get to and from the event after morning pick up and aligning with available transportation (see below).

Transportation

Facilitating transportation to and from the event is critical to its success. Older people who cannot drive and do not feel safe catching public transport need access to safe transportation. The event should be accessible by public and private transportation with sufficient parking and safe access to the event from public transportation stops. For the event in Ginninderry, the Capital Region Community Service was identified as the best form of transportation for older, possibly isolated, adults. This service provides access to community cars and buses that provide transportation to social and recreational activities.

Activities

The activities need to align with the intergenerational design guidelines and actively promote the building of relationships between the generations. Intergenerational specialists such as the ACT Intergenerational Play Group should be employed to develop and guide the activities. The Ginninderry event consists of:

1. Introduction.
2. Icebreaker activity.
3. The main activity.
4. Lunch.
5. Free play on an intergenerational playground.
6. Feedback and wrap-up session.

Amenities

Key amenities are essential for an event involving an older and younger demographic – including toilets, water, seating, food and shade. These amenities enable older adults to feel safe spending time in public spaces, and for longer periods. The Ginninderry intergenerational play space will provide access to all of the above amenities. Co-design workshop participants also recommended inviting a coffee and food van to intergenerational play spaces. This helps people who do not want to, or can't, provide their own food and makes the event more accessible.

Mapping the service

Utilising service design methodology, the team mapped out the journey of an isolated older adult. The service blueprint and touchpoint diagram highlight the different touchpoints the user has with the service, the stakeholders involved in providing the service, the different stakeholders' roles and the required support processes that ensure the user's needs are met.

In the touchpoint diagram (Figure 17.1), the service is broken down into five different stages that the user will go through while they use the service. The stages are awareness, sign-up, transportation, the event and exiting the event. During awareness, sign-up, transportation and exit there are multiple ways a user might interact with the service. Each path that can be taken must be considered by the design team to ensure that whatever choice the user makes, they can seamlessly move through the service. Below is an example of how an older adult might move through the service, informed by the personas developed from the co-design workshop.

Mapping the service through service blueprinting ensures that no background or foreground processes are overlooked and that each stakeholder understands their role in the service. The graphical representation below (Figure 17.2) shows how an older adult who cannot drive and does not feel comfortable using public transportation might interact with the service. The service blueprint has five elements: from customer actions to support processes. Customer actions are actions the customer performs while interacting with the service, touchpoints are where the interactions occur and frontstage staff are employees who are interacting with the customer. The line of interaction shows the direct interactions between the customer and the organisation. The line of visibility shows which service activities are visible to the customer and which are invisible. Finally, backstage staff and support processes are employees who support the service but are not in direct contact with the customer.

Limitations and recommendations

This research project focused on intergenerational play from the perspective of older adults because their relationship with play is less well understood. Most participants in the co-design workshop were actively engaged in play in play spaces, which meant we were unable to explore the barriers, challenges and enablers of relational play with older adults who are not engaged in play in play spaces. Further, as children are the other key target demographic of the intergenerational play spaces, their input into developing relational activities is critical. We recommend that Stage 2 of this project involves a co-design workshop with older adults who do not play in play spaces; and a workshop of grandparents and grandchildren involving 'make' and 'do' design activities (Sanders, 2002). Finally, we recommend that custom play equipment and elements for older adults are co-designed with these users, in conjunction with designers, occupational therapists and aged healthcare experts and play experts.

Conclusion

Designing spaces for generations to play alongside each other is insufficient to break down age-related barriers. Intergenerational play elements and programmes need to focus on encouraging *relational* activity that challenges age segregation and ageism and facilitates social integration

Stages

Touchpoints

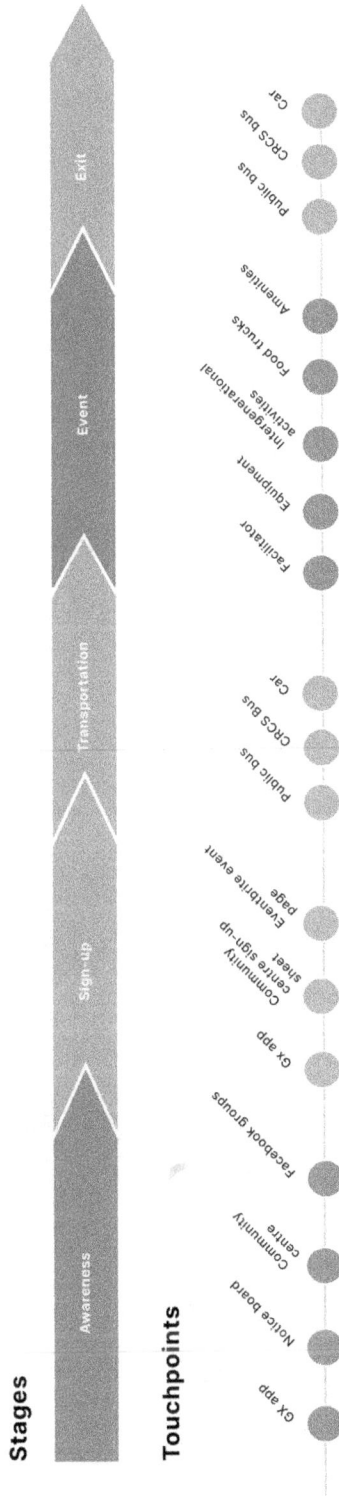

Figure 17.1 Touchpoint diagram for an isolated older adult accessing the service

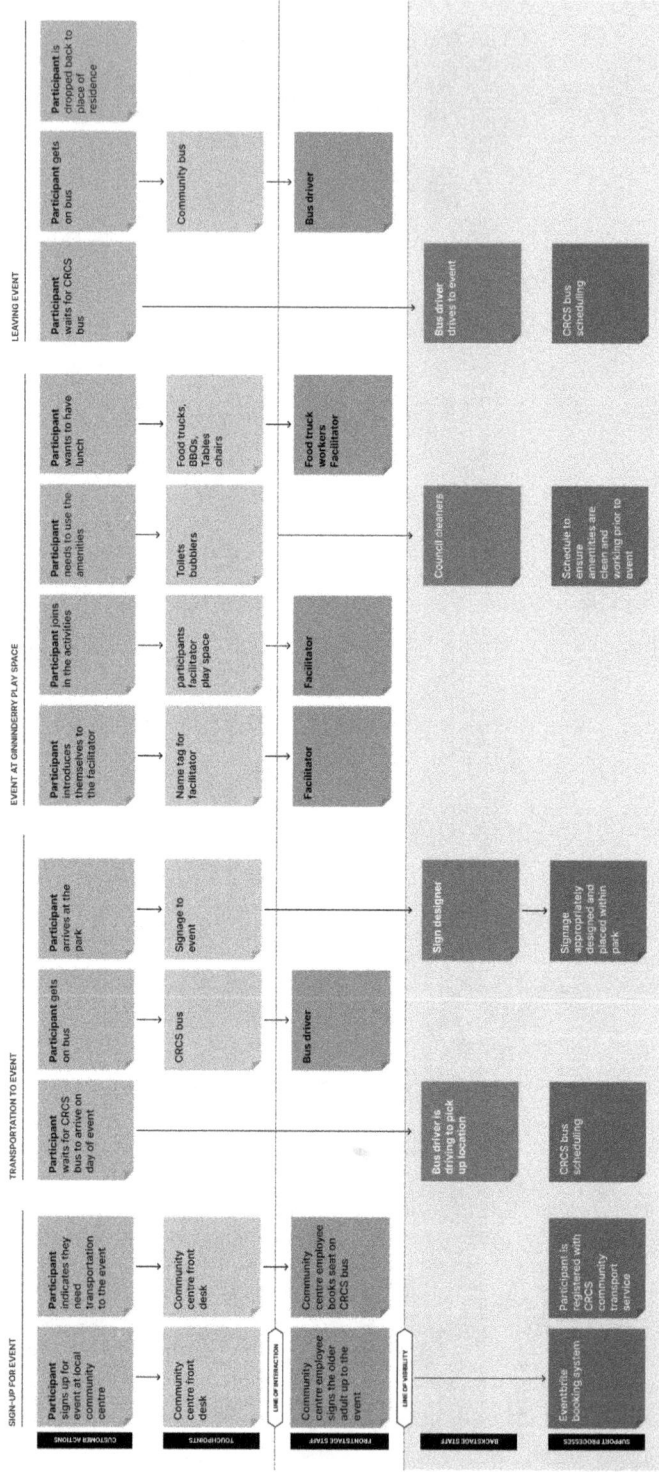

Figure 17.2 Service blueprint for isolated older adults accessing the service

and cross-generational understanding. Providing a play space and whole-of-service programme directed at creating and fostering these relationships is an innovative way to bridge the gap between generations and, at the same time, improve the mental health of older adults, including isolated members of the community. Using service design and co-design methods allowed for a more holistic and user-centred approach to creating the play space and programme, which is important to enhance efficacy. This chapter showed that it is possible to add layers to public play spaces to make them more inclusive, engaging and beneficial for older adults as 'players' with children. Mapping the service showed that an intergenerational activity is only one part of the service and organisations also need to consider transportation, availability of amenities and how to reach intended demographics. Activating spaces with structured activities can help the community learn how to use and interact with the space and with other community members.

Acknowledgement: The authors would like to acknowledge Ginninderry – and particularly Tulitha King – for supporting this project. We would also like to acknowledge Nathan D'Cunha and Daniela Castro de Jong for their contribution to this project.

Note

1 Emotional wellbeing refers to a person's awareness and understanding of their emotions and their ability to control their emotions when confronted with different scenarios. Psychological health encompasses emotional, behavioural and social health aspects of someone's life.

References

ACT Health. (2016). Health and Wellbeing of Older Persons in the Australian Capital Territory. Canberra: ACT Government.

Agate, J. R., Agate, S. T., Liechty, T., & Cochran, L. J. (2018). 'Roots and wings': An exploration of intergenerational play. *Journal of Intergenerational Relationships*, *16*(4), 395–421. https://doi.org/10.1080/15350770.2018.1489331

Australian Bureau of Statistics. (2021). *Strathnairn. 2021 census All persons QUickStats*. https://www.abs.gov.au/census/find-census-data/quickstats/2021/801011143

Balyasnikova, N., & Gillard, S. (2018). "I love to write my story": Storytelling and its role in seniors' language. *Canadian Journal for the Study of Adult Education*, *30*(2). https://cjsae.library.dal.ca/index.php/cjsae/article/view/5428/4535

Borzenkova, G. (2021). *Designing play equipment to develop the social competence of children with cerebral palsy*. University of Wolverhampton.

Burr, B., Atkins, L., Bertram, A. G., Sears, K., & McGinnis, A. N. (2019). "If you stop playing you get old": Investigating reflections of play in older adults. *Educational Gerontology*, *45*(5), 353–364. https://doi.org/10.1080/03601277.2019.1627058

Cajamarca, G., Herskovic, V., Lucero, A., & Aldunate, A. (2022). A co-design approach to explore health data representation for older adults in Chile and Ecuador. *Proceedings of the 2022 ACM designing interactive systems conference* (pp. 1802–1817). https://dl.acm.org/doi/pdf/10.1145/3532106.3533558

Chang, E. S., Kannoth, S., Levy, S., Wang, S. Y., Lee, J. E., & Levy, B. R. (2020). Global reach of ageism on older persons' health: A systematic review. *PLoS One*, *15*(1), Article e0220857. https://doi.org/10.1371/journal.pone.0220857, PubMed: 31940338, PubMed Central: PMC6961830

Community Services. (2019). Age-Friendly Canberra: a Vision for our City. Canberra: ACT Government.

Cosco, S. L. (2017). *A study of play across the lifespan* (Masters Dissertation), Centre for Health Promotion Studies. University of Alberta. https://doi.org/10.7939/R3Q81547R

Cushing, D., Washington, T., Mackenzie, J., Buys, E., Trost, S., Mortensen, W., Volbert, T., Nieberler-Walker, K., Hughes, S., Sutherland, A., & Boyd, B. (2022). *Inter-generational parks: Design guide for physical activity and social engagement across generations*. Queensland University of Technology. https://eprints.qut.edu.au/235562/1/Intergenerational_parks_design_guide_2022_reduced.pdf

Dankiew, K. A., Tsiros, M. D., Baldock, K. L., & Kumar, S. (2020). The impacts of unstructured nature play in early childhood development: A systematic review. *PLoS One, 15*(2), Article e0229006. https://doi.org/10.1371/journal.pone.0229006, PubMed: 32053683, PubMed Central: PMC7018039

Davis, H., Vetere, F., Gibbs, M., & Francis, P. (2011). Come play with me: Designing technologies for intergenerational play. *Universal Access in the Information Society, 11*(1), 17–29. https://doi.org/10.1007/s10209-011-0230-3

Davis, L., Larkin, E., & Graves, S. B. (2002). Intergenerational learning through play. *International Journal of Early Childhood, 34*(2), 42–49. https://doi.org/10.1007/BF03176766

Eberle, S. G. (2014, Winter). The elements of play: Toward a philosophy and a definition of play. *American Journal of Play, 6*(2), 214–233. https://psycnet.apa.org/record/2014-22060-003

Ferreira, B., Silva, W., Oliveira, E., & Conte, T. (2015). Designing personas with empathy map. *SEKE 2015.* https://doi.org/10.18293/SEKE2015-152

Fischer, B., Östlund, B., Dalmer, N. K., Rosales, A., Peine, A., Loos, E., Neven, L., & Marshall, B. (2021). Co-design as learning: The differences of learning when involving older people in digitalization in four countries. *Societies, 11*(66). https://doi.org/10.3390/soc11020066

Fitzgerald, M. (2021). *Together: Design guidelines for intergenerational playgrounds.* Kansas State University.

Flora, P. K., & Faulkner, G. E. (2007). Physical activity: An innovative context for intergenerational programming. *Journal of Intergenerational Relationships, 4*(4), 63–74. https://doi.org/10.1300/J194v04n04_05

Frost, J. L. (2015). Designing and creating playgrounds: Journal of engineering Johnson. In S. G. Eberle, T. S. Henricks, & D. Kuschner (Eds.). *The handbook of the study of play* (Vol. 2., pp. 425–434). Rowman & Littlefield.

Frost, J. L., Brown, P. S., Sutterby, J. A., & Thornton, C. D. (2004). The developmental benefits of playgrounds. *Childhood Education, 81*(1), 42–44. https://doi.org/10.1080/00094056.2004.10879012

Gibson, S. C. (2018). "Let's go to the park." an investigation of older adults in Australia and their motivations for park visitation. *Landscape and Urban Planning, 180*, 234–246. https://doi.org/10.1016/j.landurbplan.2018.08.019

Ginninderry. (2021). *Ginninderry project vision.* https://ginninderry.com/wp-content/uploads/2021/09/55003_Project_Vision_Factsheet.pdf

Giraudeau, C., & Bailly, N. (2019). Intergenerational programs: What can school-age children and older people expect from them? A systematic review. *European Journal of Ageing, 16*(3), 363–376. https://doi.org/10.1007/s10433-018-00497-4

Goldmintz, Y., & Schaefer, C. E. (2007). Why play matters to adults. *Psychology and Education, 44*, 12–25.

Granacher, U., Muehlbauer, T., Gollhofer, A., Kressig, R. W., & Zahner, L. (2011). An intergenerational approach in the promotion of balance and strength for fall prevention–a mini-review. *Gerontology, 57*(4), 304–315. https://doi.org/10.1159/000320250

Gray, P. (2017). What exactly is play, and why is it such a powerful vehicle for learning? *Topics in Language Disorders, 37*(3), 217–228. https://doi.org/10.1097/TLD.0000000000000130

Hagestad, G. O., & Uhlenberg, P. (2005). The social separation of old and young: A root of ageism. *Journal of Social Issues, 61*(2), 343–360.

Hagestad, G. O., & Uhlenberg, P. (2006). Should we be concerned about age segregation?: Some theoretical and empirical explorations. *Research on Aging, 28*(6), 638–653. https://doi.org/10.1177/0164027506291872

Haigh, J., & Mytton, C. (2016). Sensory interventions to support the wellbeing of people with dementia: A critical review. *British Journal of Occupational Therapy, 79*(2), 120–126. https://doi.org/10.1177/0308022615598996

Hauderowicz, D., & Serena, K. L. (2020). Everyday encounters in publics spaces: Spatial potentials for intergenerational relationships. In M. Kernan & G. Cortellesi (Eds.), *Intergenerational learning in practice: Together old and young* (1st ed.). Routledge.

Hayes, C. L. (2003). An observational study in developing an intergenerational shared site program: Challenges and insights. *Journal of Intergenerational Relationships, 1*(1), 113–132. https://doi.org/10.1300/J194v01n01_10

Henricks, T. (2006). *Play reconsidered: Sociological perspectives on human expression*. University of Illinois.

Hilbrand, S., Coall, D. A., Gerstorf, D., & Hertwig, R. (2017). Caregiving within and beyond the family is associated with lower mortality for the caregiver: A prospective study. *Evolution and Human Behavior, 38*(3), 397–403. https://doi.org/10.1016/j.evolhumbehav.2016.11.010

Hope, C., Bishop, K., Turner, B., Mews, G., Montana-Hoyos, C., & Fuller, G. (2017). *Canberra play space study, play, creativity and culture project*. University of Canberra.

Hughes, B. (2002). *A playworker's taxonomy of play types* (2nd ed.). PlayLink.

Huizinga, J. (1955). *Homo ludens: A study of the play element in culture*. Beacon.

Kaplan, M., Haider, J., Cohen, U., & Turner, D. (2007). Environmental design perspectives on intergenerational programs and practices: An emergent conceptual framework. *Journal of Intergenerational Relationships, 5*(2), 81–110. https://doi.org/10.1300/J194v05n02_06

Kaplan, M., Thang, L. L., Sánchez, M., & Hoffman, J. (2020). *Intergenerational contact zones: Place-based strategies for promoting social inclusion and belonging*. Taylor & Francis Group. http://ebookcentral.proquest.com/lib/anu/detail.action?docID=6111166

Kianfar, K., & Brischetto, A. (2021). All play together: Design concepts of a sensory play equipment aimed to an inclusive play experience. In C. S. Shin, G. Di Bucchianico, S. Fukuda, Y. G. Ghim, G. Montagna, & C. Carvalho (Eds.), *Advances in industrial design*. AHFE 2021. Lecture Notes in Networks and Systems (Vol. 260). Springer. https://doi.org/10.1007/978-3-030-80829-7_54

Krzeczkowska, A., Spalding, D. M., McGeown, W. J., Gow, A. J., Carlson, M. C., & Nicholls, L. A. B. (2021). A systematic review of the impacts of intergenerational engagement on older adults' cognitive, social, and health outcomes. *Ageing Research Reviews, 71*, 101400. https://doi.org/10.1016/j.arr.2021.101400

Levinger, P., Sales, M., Polman, R., Haines, T., Dow, B., Biddle, S. J. H., Duque, G., & Hill, K. D. (2018). Outdoor physical activity for older people-the senior exercise park: Current research, challenges and future directions. *Health Promotion Journal of Australia: Official Journal of Australian Association of Health Promotion Professionals, 29*(3), 353–359. https://doi.org/10.1002/hpja.60

Link, J. (2017). *Intergenerational playgrounds unite the young and old*. Goric Marketing Group USA, Inc. https://goric.com/intergenerational-playgrounds-unite-the-young-and-old/

MacCallum, J. A., Palmer, D., Wright, P., Cumming-Potvin, W., Northcote, J., Brooker, M., & Tero, C. (2006). *Community building through intergenerational exchange programs: Report to the National Youth Affairs Research Scheme (NYARS)*. Australian Government Dept. of Families, Community Services and Indigenous Affairs on behalf of NYARS. http://www.facs.gov.au/internet/facsinternet.nsf/vIA/youthpubs/$file/community_building.pdf

Marques, S., Mariano, J., Mendonça, J., De Tavernier, W., Hess, M., Naegele, L., Peixeiro, F., & Martins, D. (2020). Determinants of ageism against older adults: A systematic review. *International Journal of Environmental Research and Public Health, 17*(7), 2560. https://doi.org/10.3390/ijerph17072560

Martins, T., Midão, L., Martínez Veiga, S., Dequech, L., Busse, G., Bertram, M., McDonald, A., Gilliland, G., Orte, C., Vives, M., & Costa, E. (2019). Intergenerational programs review: Study design and characteristics of intervention, outcomes, and effectiveness: Research. *Journal of Intergenerational Relationships, 17*(1), 93–109. https://doi.org/10.1080/15350770.2018.1500333

Minghetti, A., Donath, L., Zahner, L., Hanssen, H., & Faude, O. (2021). Beneficial effects of an intergenerational exercise intervention on health-related physical and psychosocial outcomes in Swiss preschool children and residential seniors: A clinical trial. *PeerJ, 9*, e11292. https://doi.org/10.7717/peerj.11292

Minichiello, V., Browne, J., & Kendig, H. (2000). Perceptions and consequences of ageism: Views of older people. *Ageing and Society, 20*(3), 253–278. https://doi.org/10.1017/S0144686X99007710

Mitchell, V., Elton, E., Clift, L., & Moore, H. (2007). *Do older adults want playgrounds?* https://repository.lboro.ac.uk/articles/online_resource/Do_older_adults_want_playgrounds_/9338732

Newman, S., & Hatton-Yeo, A. (2008). Intergenerational learning and the contributions of older people. *Ageing Horizons, 8*(10), 31–39. https://www.ageing.ox.ac.uk/download/50

Park, A. L. (2014). Do intergenerational activities do any good for older adults well-being? A brief review. *Journal of Gerontology and Geriatric Research, 3*(5), 181. https://doi.org/10.4172/2167-7182.1000181

Parkinson, D., & Turner, J. (2019). Alleviating social isolation through intergenerational programming: DOROT's summer teen internship program. *Journal of Intergenerational Relationships*, *17*(3), 388–395. https://doi.org/10.1080/15350770.2019.1617606

Peters, R., Ee, N., Ward, S. A., Kenning, G., Radford, K., Goldwater, M., Dodge, H. H., Lewis, E., Xu, Y., Kudrna, G., Hamilton, M., Peters, J., Anstey, K. J., Lautenschlager, N. T., Fitzgerald, A., & Rockwood, K. (2021). Intergenerational Programmes bringing together community dwelling non-familial older adults and children: A systematic review. *Archives of Gerontology and Geriatrics*, *94*, 104356. https://doi.org/10.1016/j.archger.2021.104356

Reyes, S. (2016). *Intergenerational interactions: Designing for the young & old*. University of Florida.

Rogoff, B., Morelli, G. A., & Chavajay, P. (2010). Children's integration in communities and segregation from people of differing ages. *Perspectives on Psychological Science*, *5*(4), 431–440. https://doi.org/10.1177/1745691610375558

Sakaguchi-Tang, D. K., Cunningham, J. L., Roldan, W., Yip, J., & Kientz, J. A. (2021). Co-design with older adults: Examining and reflecting on collaboration with aging communities. *Proceedings of the ACM on Human-Computer Interaction*, *5*(CSCW2), 1–28. https://doi.org/10.1145/3479506

Sànchez, M., Butts, D. M., Hatton-Yeo, A., Henkin, N. A., Jarrot, S. E., Kaplan, M. S., Martínez, A., Newman, S., Pinazo, S., Sáez, J., & Weintraub, A. P. C. (2007). *Intergenerational programmes: Towards a society for all ages* (No. 23; Social Studies Collection). La Caixa Foundation.

Sanders, E. B. N. (2002). From user-centred to participatory design approaches. In J. Frascara (Ed.), *Design and the social sciences: Making connections* (pp. 1–8). Taylor & Francis

Santini, Z. I., Jose, P. E., York Cornwell, E., Koyanagi, A., Nielsen, L., Hinrichsen, C., Meilstrup, C., Madsen, K. R., & Koushede, V. (2020). Social disconnectedness, perceived isolation, and symptoms of depression and anxiety among older Americans (NSHAP): A longitudinal mediation analysis. *The Lancet. Public Health*, *5*(1), e62–e70. https://doi.org/10.1016/S2468-2667(19)30230-0

Shackell, A., Butler, N., Doyle, P., & Ball, D. (2008). *Design for play: A guide to creating successful play spaces*. Department for Children, School and Families.

Sheppard-Simms, E. (2012, August 2012). The evolution of play spaces. *Landscape Architecture Australia* (135). https://landscapeaustralia.com/articles/the-evolution-of-playspaces-1/

Sicart, M. (2014). *Play matters*. MIT Press.

Springate, I., Atkinson, M., & Martin, K. (2008). *Intergenerational practice: A review of the literature* (LGA Research Report F/SR262). National Foundation for Educational Research. https://www.nfer.ac.uk/publications/LIG01/LIG01.pdf

Steen, M., Manschot, M., & De Koning, N. (2011). Benefits of co-design in service design projects. *International Journal of Design*, *5*(2). http://www.ijdesign.org/index.php/IJDesign/article/view/890/346

Steward, A., & McDevitt, K. (2019). A phenomenological perspective of intergenerational engagement, social isolation and age segregation. *Innovation in Aging*, *3*(Suppl. 1), S153. https://doi.org/10.1093/geroni/igz038.550

Thang, L. L., & Kaplan, M. S. (2013). Intergenerational pathways for building relational spaces and places. In G. D. Rowles & M. Bernard (Eds.), *Environmental Gerontology: Making meaningful places in old age* (pp. 225–251). Springer.

Transport Canberra and City Services (2018). Better Suburbs Play spaces forum, Canberra: ACT Government.

United Nations. (2006). *Convention on the rights of persons with disabilities*. https://www.un.org/development/desa/disabilities/convention-on-the-rights-of-persons-with-disabilities.html

United Nations. (n.d.). *Ageing*. https://www.un.org/en/global-issues/ageing

Van Vleet, M., & Feeney, B. C. (2015). Play behavior and playfulness in adulthood: Play and playfulness. *Social and Personality Psychology Compass*, *9*(11), 630–643. https://doi.org/10.1111/spc3.12205

Vanderbeck, R. M. (2007). Intergenerational geographies: Age relations, segregation and re-engagements. *Geography Compass*, *1*(2), 200–221. https://doi.org/10.1111/j.1749-8198.2007.000012.x

Vanderbeck, R. M., & Worth, N. (2014). *Intergenerational space*. Taylor & Francis Group. http://ebookcentral.proquest.com/lib/anu/detail.action?docID=3569497

Villar, F. (2007). Intergenerational or multigenerational? A question of nuance. *Journal of Intergenerational Relationships*, *5*(1), 115–117. https://doi.org/10.1300/J194v05n01_11

Washington, T. L., Flanders Cushing, D., Mackenzie, J., Buys, L., & Trost, S. (2019). Fostering social sustainability through intergenerational engagement in Australian neighborhood parks. *Sustainability*, *11*(16), 4435. https://doi.org/10.3390/su11164435

Whitebread, D., Basilio, M., Kuvalja, M., & Verma, M. (2012). *The importance of play*. University of Cambridge, Toy Industries of Europe.

Woodcock, A., Moody, L., McDonagh, D., Jain, A., & Jain, L. C. (Eds.) (2020). *Design of assistive technology for ageing populations*. Springer International.

World Health Organisation. (2011). *Age friendly world*. https://extranet.who.int/agefriendlyworld/network/canberra/

World Health Organisation. (2022). *Ageing and health*. https://www.who.int/news-room/fact-sheets/detail/ageing-and-health#:~:text=At%20this%20time%20the%20share,2050%20to%20reach%20426%20million

Xiang, X., Lai, P. H. L., Bao, L., Sun, Y., Chen, J., Dunkle, R. E., & Maust, D. (2021). Dual trajectories of social isolation and dementia in older adults: A population-based longitudinal study. *Journal of Aging and Health*, *33*(1–2), 63–74. https://doi.org/10.1177/0898264320953693

Yarnal, C. M. (2006). The Red Hat Society: Exploring the role of play, liminality, and communitas in older women's lives. *Journal of Women and Ageing*, *18*(3), 51–73. https://doi.org/10.1300/J074v18n03_05

Yarnal, C. M., & Qian, X. (2011). Older-adult playfulness: An innovative construct and measurement for healthy aging research. *American Journal of Play*, *4*(1), 52–79. https://www.museumofplay.org/app/uploads/2022/01/4-1-article-yarnal-older-adult-playfullness.pdf

Zhang, F., & Kaufman, D. (2016). A review of intergenerational play for facilitating interactions and learning. *Gerontechnology*, *14*(3), 127–138. https://journal.gerontechnology.org/currentIssueContent.aspx?aid=2216

Part 3
Policy and design

Introduction

Designing policy and regulations for better design

Tom Dening, Kristina Niedderer, Geke Ludden and
Vjera Holthoff-Detto

Policy

First of all, what do we mean by policy? Readers may have somewhat different expectations. This is unsurprising as the word policy has several definitions. For example, just trawling a few definitions on the internet, we see that policy may be regarded as a set of ideas or a plan; a principle of action or conduct; a system of guidelines; a course of action; or a law, regulation, procedure or administrative action. Some definitions emphasise the high-level nature of policies, whereas others allow for policy to be made at an individual level. Some suggest that the term policy applies especially in politics, economics and business, and certainly many definitions mention governments and government bodies. Some definitions are expanded by mention of the importance of developing policy among alternative approaches and taking into consideration current circumstances. Another point raised is that policy may apply to either current or future circumstances. Furthermore, policies are often not made in an area that is totally novel. They augment or supplant existing policies, so the theoretical basis of policy change is probably as important as considering the basis of developing new policies (Cerna, 2013).

The purpose of a policy seems to be to guide decision-making, set a course of action, and to achieve desired outcomes. In theory, this suggests that outcomes of policies could be measured to see if they have worked. In practice, especially perhaps with political policies, this rarely happens as the government may not wish to make the results too public. Or, given how policies are usually launched in a changing social context, there may simply be too many variables to measure meaningful outcomes (like social benefit). However, process outcomes can be measured, even if the value of some of these may be questionable. For other types of policy, such as health policy, numerous measures are available (Allen et al., 2020), so perhaps the issue in that context is selecting the most relevant outcomes. In the following, we look more closely at policy and its relationship with design. In this process we distinguish the role of design within policy development on the one hand, and on the other the role of policy for driving developments in design.

Policy design

Policy development is often referred to as policy design. This is perhaps slightly unhelpful, as it conflates development with design, and they are not quite the same thing. Policies, after all, stem from politicians, who are not generally regarded as designers. Their interests lie more in political impact and getting re-elected, so any creative elements of policy development lie somewhere downstream.

DOI: 10.4324/9781003318262-23

However, undoubtedly some aspects of developing policies may use design principles, for example in order to get the message across in a compelling manner. It is also the case that 'policy design' is a major topic within the field of political science. In this context, the term policy design applies to the act of defining policy aims and the policy tools to deliver them (Cairney, 2021). Policies emerge in a variety of ways, for example in how they may originate from political dogma or in response to objective empirical data. Howlett (2014) set out a useful list of questions regarding policy design, which loosely adapted include the following: What is being designed? Who are the designers? Why do they design what they do? (in other words, what is the mix of political imperative versus technical ideas?) How is the design conducted? How do designs evolve? Probably in recent years, such questions would be augmented by asking what is the input of members of the public into policy design, since methods such as focus groups play an important part in political activity and political science (Stanley, 2016).

However, policy development is generally focused on political activity, generating statements of intent for political parties and being an important aspect of delivering government once the party has gained power. This is relevant to this book, but our scope is broader as we are interested the interaction of policy and design. So not just how policies are designed, but how design can assist the delivery of policies, and how people from the distinct worlds of policymaking and design can work together to achieve desired outcomes. And, within this particular book, how that can occur with particular relevance to mental wellbeing and involving service user groups from the worlds of mental health, dementia and neurodiversity.

The interaction of policy and design

Design may interact with policy at any of the stages of the policy lifecycle. There is no generally agreed model of the stages of policy development, and indeed using a model with stages implies a more rational and linear process than is often the case. Nonetheless, it may be useful to consider policy development as a set of stages from conceptualisation to evaluation (Hoefer, 2021). In short, policy starts with identification of need, identifying who needs to be involved, and gathering relevant information. This is followed by drafting and consultation prior to deciding how it will be published and presented. The policy then needs to be implemented and, ideally, to be evaluated, though this last stage is sadly often missing in the world of political policy.

At each of these stages, design has an important part to play. It probably has always been important but, in the past, the design elements of policy development, presentation and implementation have been covert and implicit, and it is only more recently that policymakers have paid more attention to the design aspects of their work. Inevitably, the work of identifying a topic for policy development, forming a team and producing drafts is a design process, but there is potential for formal inputs from design theory and practice. The more devolved and inclusive policy design becomes, the more there is scope for citizen inclusion and involvement. This is valuable as input from the public is likely to make the policy more relevant to people's lives, enhance a sense of ownership (rather than being done to) and improve the chances of successful implementation. It is therefore unsurprising that a model like Arnstein's (1969) ladder of citizenship is cited more than once in this section of the book.

In practical terms, where might designers be actively involved in policy design? And what might policymakers usefully learn about design? This section provides some real-life examples of how design has been worked into policy. Designers are involved in the conception and creation of plans for the appearance and function of products, structures and systems, which in this context includes policy. Key areas of engagement include establishing the process by which the policy is to be generated; for example, how public voices are to be engaged in co-design and co-production. But the detail of how things are to be done is also a design task, including the formatting of any documents for a lay readership or producing materials for people with limited literacy.

Once a policy has been drafted, it needs to be published and promoted, otherwise nobody will be aware of its existence. Again, this is increasingly an area to involve designers, since we have moved a long way from simply printing many hard copies of reports. Design can be involved in films, animations, use of social media, bespoke approaches to target specific communities, e.g. youth or people from minority ethnic backgrounds. Ideally, a policy under development should consider how it will be implemented and how it will be evaluated, so these are also design tasks.

A theme of this book, and of the chapters in this final section, is the fundamental importance of co-design and co-production. This has to be genuine, not tokenistic, and needs to run throughout any project like a golden thread. The MinD–*Designing for People with Dementia* project, which involved the editors and several authors of this book, produced guidelines on designing with and for people with dementia (Dening et al., 2020). These would be broadly applicable to other contexts, such as those of neurodiversity and mental health problems, which are covered in this book. A summary of the guidance was produced for different stakeholder groups, including policymakers (Niedderer et al., 2020).

Examples of policy design in practice

The extent to which different governments have embraced multidisciplinary design into policy-making appears quite variable, certainly in terms of available resources on the internet. A small selection of examples is described here, with the expectation that this is a rapidly changing area, and further evidence of the influence of design upon policy will emerge in the near future.

The European Union (EU) hosts the EU Policy Lab (European Commission, 2024), which is described as a collaborative and experimental space for innovative policy-making. It is linked to the EU Joint Research Centre, which provides independent, evidence-based science and knowledge, which the *Policy Lab* works to bring into the sphere of policy-making. In its own words, the EU *Policy Lab* is both a mindset and a way of working together that combines stories and data, anticipation and analysis, imagination and action. Currently, there are three main strands of work: Foresight, Design for Policy and Behavioural Insights. The Competence Centre on Foresight provides strategic and future-oriented input, developing an anticipatory culture within the European Commission, developing and using different methods and tools to bring foresight into decision-making processes. The Design for Policy team acts as the catalyst for innovation in policy-making. This work includes research, analysing information and testing new ideas to challenge assumptions and tackle complex problems in a collaborative manner. It also involves identifying and involving relevant stakeholders and promoting work across teams and disciplines. Behavioural Insights refers to work that supports EU policy-making by identifying behavioural elements in policies and testing behavioural levers that may increase policy effectiveness.

The UK government is clearly committed to the importance of design in policy-making, as evidenced by the Public Policy Design (Gov.UK, 2023a) and *Policy Lab* blogs (Gov.UK, 2023b). The Public Policy Design blog is intended for a wide audience of whoever may be interested in how policy-making is being modernised and incorporating design ideas. It uses the examples provided in its blogposts how multidisciplinary policy design teams contribute innovative ways of involving people. The blog is supported by a multidisciplinary policy design group across the UK government. So far, this community has worked with over 40 central and local government organisations, including all the major government departments. *Policy Lab*, established in 2014, is committed to bringing innovative approaches to policy-making. This creates collaboration across many different disciplines, including science, social sciences, arts and humanities. Some methods used are now regarded as entrenched in mainstream policymaking, e.g. design and film ethnography, while others are still to find their place. Chapter 19 is written by authors from *Policy Lab* and provides more detail on their work.

A third example of design firmly at the heart of policy-making is provided by the Australian Government Policy Hub (2023). This uses a model called Delivering Great Policy that has been developed using co-design with people within and outside the civil service. The model has four core elements: clear on intent, well-informed, practical to implement and influential. These elements sit on top of four so-called foundations for readiness: culture, mindsets, skills and tools and processes. Desired mindsets include qualities such as being humble, proactive, curious, timely, collaborative and practical. The web presentation of the model bears evidence of attention to design details, including infographics and a video.

Policy influence in design through standards and regulation

While design thinking may help support policy development, in return, policy can direct design development. Policy may be handed down to the practising designer in form of regulations and design standards. For example, there are regulations and standards for cars or ladders, for building houses and medical equipment, for care home and hospital design. These come in different formats and for different purposes. Often, they have user safety at heart, such as the NEN regulations in the Netherlands (NEN, 2023), and the UK's General Product Safety Regulations (Legislation.gov.uk, 2023) which are supported by standards issued by the Department for Business, Energy & Industrial Strategy (2022).

It is important to understand the differences between the two. 'In simple terms, a regulation is a set of rules outlined by the government that must be followed as a minimum standard. A regulation is enforceable by law, so as workers, following regulations is mandatory' (Scannable, 2023). By comparison, product standards can be established by government bodies or by private sector bodies. 'Standards are agreed specifications for products, processes, services, and performance. They are generally voluntary but can be mandatory when cited in Acts, regulations or other legislative instruments' (Standards New Zealand, 2023). The purpose of standards is, amongst others, to keep people safe by preventing accidents and injuries; they can help to avoid inconsistencies in processes and minimise duplication; and they can save time and money. Standards can offer an effective, consensus-based alternative to legislation and 'set a benchmark for best practice' (Standards New Zealand, 2023). For example, the UK government (Gov.UK, 2023c) offers a list of 'standards that businesses can use to show their products, services or processes comply with essential requirements of legislation.' Where no sector standards exist, interim standards may be created, e.g. by relevant sector bodies, to offer guidance. Specifications may be used as audit tools (Standards New Zealand, 2023).

However, there are few regulations or standards for design outside safety and liability. There have been legislations for design in some areas for a long time: for example, for play equipment for children and increasingly strict regulations for medical devices (Medical Device Regulations) that includes regulations on documenting the design process. More recently, attention for effects on user experience and psychosocial effects of products has risen, especially relating to user experience and its psychosocial effects. Examples include taking into consideration the effects of the brightness and quality of lighting on certain user groups, perhaps people with an autism spectrum disorder or epilepsy, or creating comfortable spaces in airports for children with autism that give them a 'refuge' from the sensory overload of such places (as discussed in two of the chapters in this part of the book). Similarly, research and recommendations exist for safe, social spaces for people with dementia in hospitals to reduce the need for restraint (e.g. Büter & Marquart, 2019). With a few selected examples, this part of our book aims to put a spotlight on the need to consider better what ways can lead from policy to its successful translation into tangible designs. There still remain shortcomings and the need for further development of such standards to ensure that our manifold social and physical environments support people in their wellbeing.

Chapters in this section

The seven chapters in the third and final section of the book examine various aspects of the interaction of design and policy. The authors approach these issues from several different angles, sometimes as policymakers or policy influencers, sometimes as academics reviewing the field of policy-making and sometimes as designers providing worked examples of how design expertise and co-design/co-production have been applied to successful projects.

In Chapter 18, Andy Bell and Sarah Hughes, now both chief executives of UK mental health third sector organisations, describe how mental health policies are made in England. They involve many stakeholders and mental health policies often also cut across other areas of legislation, such as education and justice. Bell and Hughes conclude that mental health policy is inherently political, intensely competitive and hotly contested. These qualities are unlikely to be limited to England, but probably apply in many other countries too.

Chapter 19 is an account by Camilla Buchanan and colleagues of their work for *Policy Lab* in the UK. This sets out their commitment to participatory design and co-design approaches, as well as how they use techniques such as film ethnography. This account is illustrated by a case study of a project with the Disability Unit.

Chapter 20, written by Jennifer Lim, focuses on dementia, but especially issues of culture, and how to use a cultural adaptation framework in service development. The CAST-ID framework has five aspects: Components, Adaptation Strategies, Training, Involvement and Documentation, all of which need to be addressed for dementia interventions to appropriate and effective in diverse cultural groups. Lim's review of the literature suggests that there is still a long way to go.

A third chapter on dementia is Chapter 21, by Thomas Engelsma and colleagues. The challenge here is the patchy uptake of mobile health (mHealth) applications for people living with dementia. The work described in this chapter uses a model (MOLDEM-US) to characterise the barriers to effective mHealth use and provide a set of principles (cognition, perception, frame of mind and speech and language) that can be used by future software designers and researchers to promote inclusive mHealth design principles and guidance for people with dementia.

The final two chapters provide two excellent, contrasting examples of projects that have employed good design principles along with inclusive co-design, involving end-users as much as possible. In Chapter 22, Elena Bellini and Alessia Macchi present three case studies of work in different hospital departments: emergency care, maternity and psychological services. The emphasis here is on flexibility and customisation. Although the design often starts from considering the needs of people with neurodiversity or mental health problems, the authors point out that appropriate sensory designs offer advantages to everyone involved with health or care environments. Jill Corbyn and colleagues, in Chapter 23, discuss how hospital lighting may have profound effects on people with neurodiversity, notably how the widespread adoption of LED lighting may cause sensory overload and distress to this group. The chapter describes a series of collaborative co-design projects to develop guidance about sensory-friendly LED lighting that meets the needs of people with autism and other forms of neurodiversity.

This section of the book may thus be regarded as a circular walk, starting with how policy is made and how policy-making is influenced, moving through several examples, finally returning to policy being made on the basis of evidence derived from collaborative design projects.

References

Arnstein, S. (1969). A ladder of citizen participation. *Journal of the American Planning Association*, *35*(4), 216–224. https://doi.org/10.1080/01944366908977225

Allen, P., Pilar, M., Walsh-Bailey, C., et al. (2020). Quantitative measures of health policy implementation determinants and outcomes: A systematic review. *Implementation Science*, *15*, 47. https://doi.org/10.1186/s13012-020-01007-w

Australian Government Policy Hub. (2023). *Introduction to delivering great policy*. Policy Hub.

Büter, K., & Marquardt, G. (2019). *Demenzsensible Krankenhausbauten*. DOM Publishers. ISBN 978-3-86922-716-0

Cairney, P. (2021). The politics of policy design. *EURO Journal on Decision Processes*, *9*, 100002. https://doi.org/10.1016/j.ejdp.2021.100002.

Cerna, L. (2013) *The nature of policy change and implementation: A review of different theoretical approaches*. OECD. Retrieved September 18, 2023, from Cerna 2013 The Nature of Policy Change and Implementation.pdf

Dening, T., Gosling, J., Craven, M., & Niedderer, K. (2020). *Guidelines for designing with and for people with dementia mind: Designing for people with dementia*. Retrieved September 18, 2023, from https://designingfordementia.eu/

Department for Business, Energy & Industrial Strategy. (2022). *Notice of publication 0072/22: References to standards in support of the general product safety regulations 2005 (S.I. 2005/1803)*. Retrieved September 18, 2023, from https://assets.publishing.service.gov.uk/government/uploads/system/uploads/attachment_data/file/1113073/ds-0072-22-gpsr-notice.pdf

European Commission. (2024). *EU policy lab*. Retrieved January 29, 2024, from https://policy-lab.ec.europa.eu/index_en

Gov.UK. (2023a). *Public policy design blog at: Public policy design*. Retrieved September 18, 2023, from blog.gov.uk

Gov.UK. (2023b). *Policy lab blog*. blog.gov.uk

Gov.UK. (2023c). *Guidance: Designated standards*. Retrieved September 18, 2023, from https://www.gov.uk/guidance/designated-standards

Hoefer, R. (2021). The surprising usefulness of the policy stages framework. *Journal of Policy Practice and Research*, *2*(3), 141–145. https://doi.org/10.1007/s42972-021-00041-2

Howlett, M. (2014). From the 'old' to the 'new' policy design: Design thinking beyond markets and collaborative governance. *Policy Sciences*, *47*(3), 187–207. https://doi.org/10.1007/s11077-014-9199-0.

Legislation.gov.uk. (2023). *The general product safety regulations 2005. At: The general product safety regulations 2005*. Retrieved September 18, 2023, from legislation.gov.uk

NEN Royal. (2023). *Netherlands standardization institute*. Standard for Progress. Retrieved September 18, 2023, from https://www.nen.nl/en

Niedderer, K., Dening, T., & Powell, K. (2020). *Recognising design as a means for enhancing quality of life, self-empowerment and social engagement for people with dementia: Recommendations for funders & policymakers, designers, design researchers & design educators, design regulators & voluntary organisations. Mind: Designing for people with dementia*. Retrieved September 18, 2023, from https://designingfordementia.eu/

Scannable (2023). *Standards and regulations. What are the differences?* Retrieved September 18, 2023, from https://www.scannable.io/blog-posts/standards-and-regulations-what-are-the-differences

Standards New Zealand. (2023). *Explaining standards*. Retrieved September 18, 2023, from https://www.standards.govt.nz/about/explaining-standards/

Stanley, L. (2016). Using focus groups in political science and international relations. *Politics*, *36*(3), 236–249. https://doi.org/10.1177/0263395715624120.

18 Designing and influencing mental health policy

Bringing evidence and experience to decision-making

Andy Bell and Sarah Hughes

Introduction

This chapter focuses on how mental health policies are made, drawing from our experience of working in England over the last two decades. It explores the processes by which policy decisions are made, who makes and influences them, and how policies relating to mental health intersect with many others. It explores both national policy-making and how decisions are made at levels below national government.

Mental health policy inevitably covers a broad canvas. Most often, it is understood in relation to the provision of mental health (treatment) services and the legal frameworks that govern how and when people can be deprived of their liberty for assessment or treatment. These are crucial topics. But mental health policy also relates to decisions about promoting and protecting mental health and preventing mental illness as well as policies that affect people living with mental illness. In reality, they all overlap within the social policy space.

Who makes mental health policy?

Policy-making in England centres on the national 'Westminster' government. Unlike in Scotland, Wales or Northern Ireland, there is very little devolution in England (with some partial exceptions). The vast majority of major spending decisions are made in Whitehall by the Treasury and the major spending departments of the national government, including the Department of Health and Social Care.

The existence in the UK of a National Health Service (NHS) means that the vast majority of health care is available free at the point of use, funded by national taxation. This also means that the major decisions about how NHS funds are spent are made nationally. Since 2013, this has been overseen by a national executive agency, NHS England. As a result, the last two major mental health policies in England (the Five Year Forward View for Mental Health and the NHS Long Term Plan) have been produced by the NHS rather than by the government.

While national policies determine the overall structures and priorities of the NHS, decision-making about how resources are deployed locally has been delegated to a series of different bodies over the last 20 years. At the time of writing, responsibility for allocating NHS funding locally is being transferred to new bodies known as Integrated Care Systems. These cover geographical areas with populations averaging one million each (but with a wide range) and are governed by an Integrated Care Board, there will be 42 in England. Recent lobbying by mental health charities led to a change in the legislation creating these new boards as statutory bodies, requiring that they all include at least one member with expertise in mental health.

DOI: 10.4324/9781003318262-24

Unlike previous arrangements over the last three decades, Integrated Care Systems break down the divide within the NHS between 'purchasers' and 'providers': where separate organisations are responsible for commissioning services on behalf of local people and for providing the majority of those services. The new Integrated Care Boards will include representatives of NHS provider organisations (known as 'trusts') as well as local authorities and some other partners, which means that decisions about resource allocation will be made collectively rather than by commissioning bodies alone.

Local authorities in England have no direct power over the provision of health care services but they do have responsibility for public health (which includes substance misuse services, health Visiting and school nursing), social services for both children and adults, housing and many other services that are relevant to mental health. They also have powers of scrutiny over local NHS organisations and are required to set overall health and wellbeing strategies for their local areas that the NHS is expected to heed when making its plans for healthcare provision. In some, mostly metropolitan, areas, local authorities have also coalesced into combined authorities, such as in the West Midlands, or separate regional structures have been created between the national and local level – such as in Greater London and Greater Manchester. With the exception of Greater Manchester, these do not hold powers relating to health and care services, but they have influence over many of the determinants of mental health, for example through their powers relating to economic development, housing and transport.

Who influences mental health policy?

While mental health policy is 'made' by a relatively small group of people and organisations that hold political and administrative power, the process of influencing policy includes a much wider range of actors that all seek to be heard and factors that determine what gets prioritised.

Political policymakers in particular (nationally and locally) are influenced by either actual or perceived public opinion on any given topic. As most political officers in England represent local constituencies or wards, the feedback they receive from the voting public in those places has an important impact on their priorities and choices. A growing perception that mental health 'matters' to constituents is one important aspect of why it gained in its political profile in the decade up to 2020 – a position which is now at risk as other health policy priorities have gained ground since the start of the COVID-19 pandemic.

The ways in which public opinion is articulated can include direct contact with individual constituents (for example, through local 'surgeries', letters and casework requests) as well as hearing from community organisations – including campaign groups – and mediated contact, for example, through local media. Social media contact with constituents, campaigners and 'influencers' is also increasingly informing policymakers' perceptions of public pressure and interest.

Mental health policymakers are also exposed to advice and lobbying from a range of advocacy and interest groups. These include professional associations representing groups of people who work in mental health and other adjacent services; charities and think-tanks specialising in mental health; commercial interests, such as the pharmaceutical industry or for-profit mental health service providers; and campaign groups led by people who have used mental health services. Influence is also wielded by academics and researchers, people in the public eye with personal experience of mental health difficulties, and media organisations and commentators. This makes it a highly contested and congested field. And it means that policymakers need to be aware of who they are hearing from, how they are funded and whose interests they may represent.

The relationships between policymakers and institutional influencers are complex. They are often bidirectional – decision-makers may reach out to trusted 'experts' for advice and counsel when they need it, while those seeking to influence policy will reach out to policymakers to assert their views and ideas. The question of who wields influence at any time will depend on the political 'weather', the resources, skills and knowledge of those seeking influence, how to negotiate power structures and cultures and the esteem in which their organisations or the groups they represent are held.

The ways in which policy is influenced are also subject to regulations governing organisations. Charities, for example, are required to work within legislation that governs the scope of their influencing activity, with oversight from the national regulator, the Charities Commission. At a local level, charities seeking to influence decisions about how services are commissioned may also encounter difficulties advocating for their community when they are also seeking funding for their services from the same agencies they are trying to influence.[1]

In mental health policy-making in England, professional voices have tended to be given precedence over those of people who have experienced mental health difficulties or used mental health services. Among the professions, as with most health policy areas, medical voices (psychiatry in particular) have been held in higher esteem than other professional groups. This is not consistently the case: medical bodies have at times held views contrary to the government of the time and had less influence as a result. However, power structures within the health system more broadly do tend generally to be reflected in the extent of routine influence on mental health policy-making over time.

A less well recognised factor in both the making and influencing of mental health policy is that of philanthropy and charitable trusts. Philanthropic funding – from more traditional family charities to modern, professional organisations such as Comic Relief and the National Lottery Community Fund – can have a major impact on policy-making by investing in new types of service provision or campaigns that seek to generate social change. This can include setting up and supporting organisations (including the Sainsbury Centre for Mental Health – a precursor of the current Centre for Mental Health), funding service provision that later gets adopted into policy, or funding campaign groups and coalitions, such as the highly successful Maternal Mental Health Alliance. Decisions made by philanthropic organisations and individuals can therefore have a significant long-term impact on policy, albeit in almost all cases at one remove.

What influences mental health policy?

The factors that determine 'what' influences policymakers are also wide and complex. The 'evidence' that informs policy can come from academic or clinical research, from reports produced by interested parties, from narratives articulated by individuals or groups, or from surveys. None of these types of evidence is entirely (and sometimes not at all) objective – though they will often claim to be. They are the product of actors' choices about what to observe and articulate. And these are based on power structures that determine what evidence is created, who by, and how it is communicated.

Within the field of research, for example, power relationships determine what topics are regarded as important enough to receive funding and what kind of activity will be supported. Mental health research funding in the UK is dominated by a small number of organisations which disburse a mixture of public and charitable funds to organisations – predominantly universities – that carry out research. The decisions they make determine not just what topics get researched but who will be involved in that work (either as researchers or participants) and how decisions will be made about how the research is conducted.[2]

And once research is carried out, the ways in which it is communicated are also pivotal to the level and type of influence it will wield. For example, publication in academic journals may increase the chances of a study wielding influence in clinical decision-making (through bodies such as the National Institute for Health and Care Excellence) but not necessarily exert influence on political processes (at least not without mediation through press coverage or direct advocacy). Implementation science attempts to overcome many of these obstacles by incorporating the research, communication and translation for policy and practice.

While there is a diverse range of organisations that produce mental health research in England – from major international charities such as the Wellcome Trust to community groups and networks based in localities or around communities of interest – the ways in which it is translated into policy influence favour those with the means to communicate their findings effectively. Media coverage of research can increase its influence considerably, and competition for media attention is intense and favours organisations with access to professional media relations infrastructure.

It is not just evidence from research that influences mental health policy, however. Evidence from experience and the efforts of advocates also make a major impact. Experiential evidence can exert a significant impact on mental health policy by shedding light on systemic issues through a tragic event. The death of Olaseni Lewis in police custody following the use of physical restraint was the inspiration for 2018 legislation to regulate the use of force against people in custody. Alongside other tragic deaths of Black men in custody, it also highlighted the disproportionate use of coercion against people from racialised communities in the mental health and criminal justice systems. While this inequity has been in plain sight in routine data and research for many years, policy action has tended to be prompted by high profile individual cases that have made it harder to ignore the issue.

Experiential evidence has also prompted policy activity in relation to the risk factors for deaths by suicide. Most recently, campaigns by bereaved families have highlighted the risks of unregulated social media spaces to young people at risk of suicide. These have prompted national policymakers to attempt to tighten online safety legislation to protect children from harmful content.

Some campaigns of this kind have been led entirely by individuals and families, either singly or in groups, often facilitated by networks created through social media interactions. Others have been supported by charities or other lobby groups that have worked alongside those affected and have drawn on their experiences to make the case for systemic change.

The many actors and factors that influence mental health policy are illustrated by the diverse and competing imperatives that bear on the Mental Health Act. The current Act for England and Wales dates mostly from 1983 (itself an updated version of legislation from 1959) with amendments, most notably those made in 2007. It was reviewed by an independent panel in 2018, most of whose recommendations are due to be implemented in legislation expected (at the time of writing) to be introduced into Parliament in 2022.

The Mental Health Act has been influenced over the years by concerns about public safety, most notably in the late 1990s and early 2000s following a number of high-profile homicides involving people with a mental illness. It is also influenced by concerns about the human rights of people who (uniquely) are detained in hospital for assessment or treatment. Latterly, concerns about the growing and disproportionate use of the Act among Black communities were a major imperative behind the 2018 independent review.[3]

With such competing and contradictory imperatives, multiple different interest groups have sought to influence the shape and tone of the Mental Health Act. These include professional groups, charities, homicide victims' families and a range of campaign groups, including those speaking from personal experience of being subject to the Act. An analysis of Parliamentary debates in the run up to the 2007 Act noted that the influences cited by MPs and Peers were predominantly those of medical or clinical professionals, which had the effect of narrowing the scope of debate and normalising the use of coercion.[4] More recently, experts by experience have been more prominent – for example, having been in key roles in the independent review.

How far this will extend when new legislation is debated in Parliament will denote how far the balance of power has shifted since 2007 and whose views and voices are given prominence when decisions are made. Then, not a single sitting MP had ever acknowledged that they had ever experienced a mental health difficulty. Since 2012, a number of MPs have spoken about their experiences of mental ill health and how they have incorporated their lived experience into their understanding of the issues they are debating. This has at the very least, changed the tenor of Parliamentary debates about mental health – from being a topic that affects other people to being something of personal relevance and universal significance.

Intersections with other/adjacent/overlapping policies

Mental health policy intersects with a wide range of adjacent, overlapping and cross-cutting topics. All public policies have intersections, and few exist in isolation. But mental health policy has a pronounced level of connectivity across multiple policy areas.

Most evidently, mental health policy is located within the wider world of health and social policy. Decisions made about public health, health services and social care inevitably affect mental health. It is rare that such decisions are made with mental health in mind. For example, the recent UK Government decision to require large restaurant chains to display calories on their menus did not appear to have considered the risks this poses to people with eating disorders (or if it was considered, it was dismissed as a major concern). Decisions about health and care service funding or reform are seldom made with mental health as a major consideration.

Mental health policy also intersects significantly with justice policies, on numerous levels. There are specific policies that combine health and justice, most notably the Mental Health Act, including within it the statutory frameworks for the police to detain people in an emergency, for the courts to make hospital orders in relation to serious offences, and for people in prison to be transferred to hospital for treatment. The Mental Health Act also intersects with national and international Human Rights frameworks (not always comfortably), with Mental Capacity legislation, and it depends on key legal safeguards such as the role of the Tribunal service in reviewing the use of detention. The Mental Health Act is also shaped in practice by case law, meaning that court decisions and interpretations of the Act can have a major impact over time on how the letters of the law are enacted and how it intersects with human rights and other imperatives.

Policies relating to social security, education, employment, housing, equality and the economy as a whole also intersect with mental health in significant ways. Decisions made in these areas can all affect the public's mental health. For example, policies that reduce entitlements to social security benefits have been shown to lead to increases in mental ill health, while policies that improve employment protections can improve mental health at a population level.[5] And new policy intersections emerge over time – as seen in the recent rise of online safety as a mental health policy concern.

Some policy decisions have direct and specific impacts on people living with a mental illness. Policies about disability benefits, for example, affect people with mental health conditions – in the ways people's needs and entitlements are assessed. Many mental health charities and campaign groups have actively engaged in this area to seek changes to policies that are seen to disadvantage and discriminate against people with mental health problems. They include the process by which people's disabilities are assessed and the application of benefit 'sanctions' against people who are out of work.

While these adjacent and intersecting policy areas have a very significant impact on mental health, it is rare for policies to be designed with people's mental health in mind. In the absence of a policy-making framework that ensures the mental health impacts of policies are actively considered, decisions made in government departments that have little mental health expertise can cause significant harm.

Devolved nations

The vast majority of mental health policies and those adjacent to them are devolved to the separate governments and assemblies in Scotland, Wales and Northern Ireland. A partial exception is Wales, where justice policies and the Mental Health Act continue to be determined in Westminster. This creates a potential dissonance – where health policies are made in Cardiff but they intersect with justice policies that are made in England. The Welsh Assembly Government has sought to address this through actions such as the Mental Health Measure, which adds to the Mental Health Act an additional entitlement to an assessment of needs for anyone requiring mental health support in the community.

Recent and future trends

Mental health policy has always been a keenly contested territory, subject to complex and competing imperatives, ideologies and understandings. It is inherently political. It competes for attention with many other overlapping policy areas and is subject to the vagaries of decisions made across government with little regard to their impacts on mental health.

While that will never change, there are some noticeable trends in mental health policy and how it gets made that could have a significant impact over time. These include:

Recognition of intersectionality: as with many other policy areas, there is a growing understanding that mental health policy needs to address systemic and structural issues in society in order to make an impact on people's wellbeing. In local government in particular, there is a recognition that improving mental health is linked to addressing racism, violence against women and girls and poverty.

Voice of lived experience: people living with mental health difficulties have campaigned for decades to be heard by those who make and influence mental health policy. This is beginning to happen, though not systematically. National bodies including NHS England, the major mental health charities and professional associations have set up mechanisms for incorporating lived experience perspectives into their decision-making. How far this represents the start of a genuine and sustained shift in power remains to be seen. Power structures are largely unchanged, and progress can be quickly undone if it is not embedded.

Policy research: while the vast majority of mental health research funding is dedicated to clinical research, a small but growing minority is being used for research relating to policy, service development and implementation. This includes the government-funded Mental Health Policy Research Unit, led by a consortium of universities, whose work has included investigations relevant to the reform of the Mental Health Act and the use of digital technology in mental health services.

Social media: mental health policy debates increasingly take place on social media platforms, most notably X (formerly Twitter). The majority of actors within the mental health policy sphere have some presence on social media. These include large numbers of policymakers, the organisations that seek to influence them, and people with lived experience of mental ill health or being a caregiver. Networks of individuals are increasingly raising concerns that organisations have neglected or not noticed – sometimes prompting charities to pay attention to a topic they have not engaged in previously.

Rise and fall? There is no doubt that mental health rose in profile as a policy priority in the decade up to 2020. That decade featured a much higher volume than before of government policy documents and initiatives relating to mental health, of media coverage about mental health and of activity in local areas to address mental health concerns. But this upward trajectory is not guaranteed to continue, and there are signs that it is waning. And while mental health may be higher profile now, there are concerns that service provision is falling behind rising demand. This risks creating an air of fatalism – that even when mental health gets a fairer share of the policy spotlight, and more money is invested into services, that it still doesn't resolve itself.

System changes: the creation of Integrated Care Systems is the latest of a series of system changes in and around the NHS. The place of mental health within each of the 42 systems will inevitably vary, and the ways in which local policies are made and investments are prioritised will lead to very different outcomes across the country. It is highly unlikely that the new system will lead to any power shift in the way policies are made and who makes them; this will still very largely be dominated by clinical and managerial professionals in employed or non-executive roles in the NHS and to a lesser extent local government.

Prevention and promotion: the vast majority of policy-making about mental health in England has focused on service provision. The two most significant national policies relating to mental health in the last decade (the Five Year Forward View for Mental Health and the NHS Long Term Plan) were created by and for the NHS, with scant attention paid to the wider world. Mental health policies have largely ignored the determinants of mental health or opportunities to influence them.[6] And policies relating to the determinants have mostly ignored mental health as a major area of concern. This may be changing. The UK Government is consulting, at the time of writing, on a ten-year cross-government mental health plan, including exploring ways of promoting mental wellbeing and preventing mental illness. Local and combined authorities in England are also paying more attention to the determinants of mental health and seeking ways of promoting wellbeing.

Conclusions

Mental health policy is complex and dynamic. Decisions that affect our mental health are made across government, in a whole range of public services (including but going far beyond health and care) and in local government. Mental health services do not exist in isolation; they are part of a much wider system of health and social services with connections to schools, the justice system, employers and communities. This means that mental health policy is affected by many other policies and decisions, often made with little thought to the effects they might have on people's mental health or the mental health system.

The ways mental health policies are designed, made and implemented are equally complex. The power structures that determine who is able to 'make' policy and whose voices are heard in that process remain largely unchanged over many decades. While people with personal experience of mental ill health have fought with increasing success to be heard and heeded, power and influence remains largely with traditional actors and organisations: professional bodies, major philanthropic and research funders, academic institutions, government agencies and elected politicians. Others may from time to time be co-opted into decision-making roles, but centres of power do not shift significantly.

The organisation we work in, Centre for Mental Health, is an active participant in this system. The Centre seeks to influence policy and has worked with successive governments and executive agencies to support decision-making about mental health. Its research is created with a view to informing policy decisions, using evidence (from personal narratives to economic analyses) to influence choices about how resources are used and priorities are set. It works with other organisations, including academic and professional bodies, user-led and community groups, and other charities and trusts, to have its voice and views heard. Inevitably, it is not always successful. No single part of the system ever can (or should) be. But it seeks to use the influence it has to put inequalities centre stage, to highlight lived experience as well as more traditional types of evidence, and to inform policies across the full range that have an impact on our mental health.

Mental health policies and the ways they are influenced will continue to evolve as the world we're living in changes, along with our understandings of what will enable people to have better mental health. While power structures are highly resistant to change, mental health policy is the product of the dynamics between the people and institutions that make policy and those that seek to influence it from outside. It is, therefore, inherently political, intensely competitive and hotly contested.

Note on authorship

Dr Sarah Hughes is now chief executive of Mind but co-wrote this chapter while chief executive of Centre for Mental Health, and the insights provided are drawn from the authors' work at the Centre.

Notes

1 https://www.centreformentalhealth.org.uk/publications/arm-arm
2 https://www.centreformentalhealth.org.uk/publications/fit-for-purpose
3 https://www.gov.uk/government/groups/independent-review-of-the-mental-health-act
4 https://pubmed.ncbi.nlm.nih.gov/32930654/
5 https://www.nationalelfservice.net/populations-and-settings/poverty/social-security-evidence-benefits-mental-health/
6 https://www.centreformentalhealth.org.uk/publications/mental-health-for-all

19 How can policymakers design for mental health and wellbeing?

Camilla Buchanan, Vanessa Lefton and Kate Langham

Introduction

The chapter explores the 'how' and 'what' of design work in a policy space. It considers how design methods contribute a different kind of 'material' to policy decision-making and what impacts this has on policy initiatives, with reference to a project from the UK *Policy Lab*. Firstly, context about where the work described takes place is given. Secondly, ideas about co-design and wellbeing from the academic literature are explored. Thirdly, a specific case of policymakers engaging with design methods is discussed with reference to a *Policy Lab* project working with the UK Cabinet Office. Finally, some considerations for policymakers are suggested and conclusions made.

Design has long been understood as a human-centred discipline. However, the places where designers and design are appearing, and the types of problems and needs being addressed through design have expanded enormously in recent years. The new contexts for design include government agencies, healthcare systems, business and organisational strategy, as well as complex systems that encompass several different fields (Banerjee, 2014: Irwin, 2015: Lurås, 2016).

In the past two decades, the public sector and other organisations or networks delivering social systems and services – including foundations and charities – have been places of huge growth for design (Bason, 2010: Mulgan, 2014: Sangiorgi & Prendiville, 2017). Latterly, design has also percolated into the worlds of policy-making and strategy development where, although it is now more present, it is still underdeveloped in theory and practice (Clarke & Craft, 2019).

This chapter looks at how policymakers are working with designers to gain insights about citizens. Often, although by no means always, the kind of insights that designers/design researchers generate when working on public/social policy relate to issues of mental health and wellbeing. And, more specifically, how these two factors are affected by policy decisions. Gaining knowledge about granular human experiences as they relate to policy outcomes has been a major motivator for policymakers to work with designers, and a desire to understand 'lived experience' can often be the first step for a policy team to engage with design approaches.

A note on context

The ideas in this chapter are drawn from an applied context where policymakers are engaging with design, through the work of the UK *Policy Lab*. The *Lab* was established in 2014 as a multidisciplinary team which has now grown to around 30 people and works across the UK government – bringing skills including ethnography, systems thinking, art, futures and design to policy-making. The team aims to apply these varied skills to policy challenges and, although design is only one of a number of disciplines represented in the team, it provides an underpinning framework and way of working for the *Lab*. The team operates on a 'cost recovery basis', meaning it is funded directly

DOI: 10.4324/9781003318262-25

through commissions from departments as well as local government and, on occasion, outside organisations. To date, *Policy Lab* has worked on around 180 projects as well as a range of other thought leadership and training initiatives across the UK civil service and beyond.

The mission of the *Policy Lab* team is 'to radically improve policymaking through design, innovation and people-centred approaches', and a major pillar of *Policy Lab*'s work is about anchoring policy-making in a deep understanding of people and their everyday lives. Throughout its history, *Policy Lab* has used its methods and approaches to consider how different groups experience government policy and to gain detailed 'lived experience' insights that inform policy development. We use a range of different disciplines and approaches to achieve this understanding, including, ethnography, co-design and other participatory and observational techniques. We have also intentionally developed the *Lab* team to include anthropology, design and ethnographic skills. *Policy Lab* researchers and designers often spend time engaging directly with the people affected by government policies. This might include engaging people in co-design workshops or projects and using film footage and other 'artefacts' such as photographs and maps to collect observational data about research participants.

Participatory, co-design and ethnographic strategies can help policymakers to understand in more detail the drivers behind quantitative evidence and to meaningfully connect to people affected by policy decisions. However, these methods are still relatively niche in policy-making, both in the UK and internationally. Through this chapter, we aim to share more of our understanding of design methods from their practical use with policy teams in *Policy Lab*'s work.

Theories of participation, co-design and ethnography

Design is, in many ways, a fundamentally participatory discipline. Stakeholders provide inspiration in the form of evidence from their own lives when they participate in design processes. They also dictate whether a design output is fit for purpose by choosing to use, amend or reject design products – although there may be less flexibility for people to do this with government services where there is usually only one choice of 'provider'. Participation by non-designers in the design process is a prominent theme in contemporary design literature. In applied contexts, designers working in governments and other design teams 'borrow' heavily from anthropology disciplines to bring a participatory lens to their design work. To understand these trends, it is useful to outline concepts of participation, co-design and ethnography and their significance in present-day design activity, particularly as it relates to policy development. The following section looks at ideas from the academic literature.

Participation

Over the course of several decades, as the design field has matured, emphasis on participation has grown, and the involvement of non-designers in the design process is now a common feature of contemporary design. As Hyysalo and Hyysalo (2018) argue, 'User involvement in design is no longer a fringe activity. Industry, the public sector, peer-to-peer initiatives, and academia alike have begun to see citizens as important actors in various development and innovation activities' (p. 42).

There is significant diversity in concepts and definitions of participation and co-design. Burford et al. (2013) suggest that although participatory approaches in design have significant potential to transfer to other fields, current barriers include a 'diversity of approaches' and 'lack of common vocabulary' (p. 41). Similarly, Steen (2013) notes that despite its prominence as a working practice, the concept of co-design receives 'little scholarly attention' and projects are often loosely named co-design resulting in 'conceptual dilution' (p. 16). In the context of

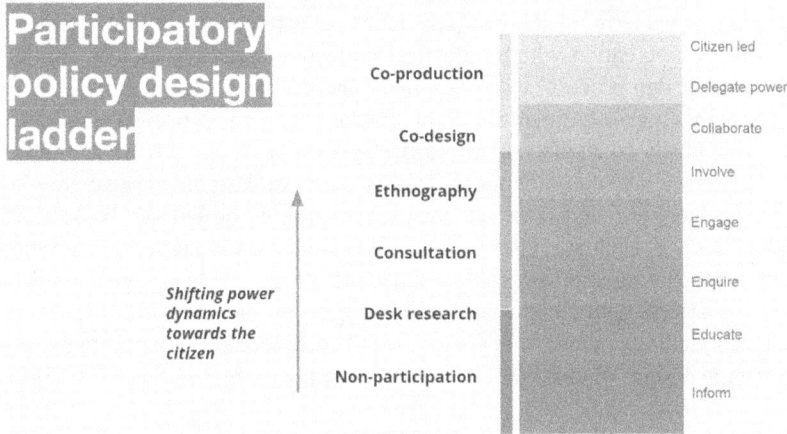

Figure 19.1 Participatory policy design ladder, illustrating a spectrum of non-participation to citizen-led action, adapted from Arnstein (1969), by *Policy* Lab

policy-making, ideas about how participatory and co-design strategies can inform the policy process are even less developed.

Sherry Arnstein's (1969) work helps to clarify ideas of participation. Arnstein's 'Ladder of Citizen Participation' (Figure 19.1) illustrates potential levels of citizen participation; it establishes a dynamic between power and participation. For Arnstein, citizen participation is citizen power. In the diagram below, *Policy Lab* has mapped how design in a policy-making context can enable citizen engagement.

Elizabeth Rocha (1997) builds on this through her 'Ladder of Empowerment', which describes how individuals and collectives can undermine or contribute to the building of power. At the lowest rung of her ladder lies the 'Atomistic Individual Empowerment' actor. She argues that:

> At the heart of empowerment lie the needs of socially and economically marginalised populations and communities. As recent and ongoing economic restructuring and welfare state retrenchments continue, planners will increasingly be required to address the needs of such communities.
>
> (p. 31–44)

Participation is an inherently social process that focuses on engagement, creativity and decision-making to improve end-users' satisfaction in the long term (Steen, 2013).

Co-design

Designers often create end products or services. In co-design, the overall process becomes an output. It is an umbrella term to describe participatory methods applied in a design-led context. Co-design means tailoring specific participatory methods to a project and audience, empowering stakeholders to become the experts. It is not a linear process and changes throughout the course of a project (McKercher, 2020). This aspect of co-design often makes developing a co-design project proposal challenging, as the outcome should be led and defined by the overall design process.

Sanders and Stappers (2008) provide a helpful definition of co-design activity. They argue that co-creation is a broad term referring to 'any act of collective creativity', whereas co-design is a specific form of co-creation which indicates 'collective creativity as it is applied across the whole span of a design process' with 'designers and people not trained in design working together' (p. 6). They observe an increase in the uptake of these approaches and argue that, to date, co-design has mostly taken place in the early stages of the design process, but the involvement of non-designers in decision-making at the later stages of designing is also growing (p. 5).

Drawing on the literature, and from our own experience, co-design can be seen as a joint inquiry to explore, discuss, evaluate and develop design solutions. It is a process that brings people together to improve their own or other people's situations. When people engage in co-design they also participate in a process with social qualities. Participants are empowered to express and share ideas, engage in storytelling to draw from their own and other people's thoughts and experiences, to explore and define design solutions that influence future policy design. Steen (2019) states:

> Co-design can be understood as a process of collaborative design thinking: a process of joint inquiry and imagination in which diverse people jointly explore and define a problem and jointly explore and evaluate solutions. It is a process in which participants are able to express and share ideas, experiences, to discuss and negotiate their roles and interests, and to jointly bring about positive change.
>
> (p. 28)

The experience of co-designing generates a sense of belonging and wellbeing by prioritising relationships. It brings people together, inviting future users to participate, discuss and illustrate their design ideas. There is no 'one-size-fits-all' to co-design. It is about tailoring the right processes and tools to the project. Methods and materials should be aligned to the audience and their ability to strengthen communication and invite engagement to shape policy. Through a co-design activity, new knowledge is created that results in co-learning. This ensures users' voices are heard and that their opinions are taken into consideration. Such projects are a form of individual and community engagement and empowerment, with the outcome sometimes being less of a priority than the overall experience.

To optimise the benefits created through the co-design process, designers have adopted new methods and tools that invite stakeholders to play a central part in the design of a solution. Using accessible, engaging tools enables non-designers to visually illustrate their ideas and engage in a design process. Providing the opportunity to 'make' something, whether it's policy change or something more tangible, is seen as having a positive impact on wellbeing. Activities such as designing and creating are often referred to as sources of enjoyment which can lead to engagement and a sense of achievement (De Couvreur et al., 2013, p. 58). Co-design enables participant empowerment by involving people as experts and employing their competencies throughout the project process. Research shows that stakeholder involvement in an iterative process impacts on wellbeing. Participants often feel empowered with outcomes such as feeling a sense of community affiliation (Sanoff, 2006, p. 61). This specifically relates to people being listened to, feeling valued and being able to contribute something of worth that impacts on their future.

The wellbeing created by the 'active' integration of stakeholders in an iterative co-design process is not a by-product but a key component of the design process (Sangiorgi, 2010). Design research has outlined the potential of participatory design processes to serve as a means for social transformation by passing power to stakeholders for them to influence the creation of user-centred services and products. By considering and managing not only the impacts of what is being designed but also the social impacts of the design process, designers can work to enhance the overall influence of co-design on participants' wellbeing.

The features of participatory and co-design approaches, including genuine inclusion and collaboration, are a major reason for *Policy Lab* to draw on design approaches in its work with citizens. In turn, the alternative skills that innovation teams like the *Lab* bring to policy development initiatives, particularly those involving citizen engagement, are a major motivator for policymakers to work with designers.

Ethnography

Ethnography gathers in-depth insights from spending time with people. Other qualitative research methods like focus groups and surveys are valuable for providing a bird's eye view of an issue; they reveal experiences that repeat across groups of people (in other words, large-scale patterns). Ethnography enables the researcher to 'zoom' into those patterns (Siodmok, 2022). Fieldwork takes place over a period of time and involves building trust between the researcher and participant. Rapport is built by researchers being empathetic, warm, understanding and non-judgemental. They are led by the participant, rather than following predefined questions. As a result, insights can reveal issues researchers might not know to ask about.

External context, including living arrangements, interpersonal interactions and the wider locality, can all be captured in ethnographic research via small, production-quality video cameras. This enables data to be captured in an unobtrusive way. Film research, used by *Policy* Lab, provides a detailed record of fieldwork and enables the *Lab* to revisit the research repeatedly to conduct comprehensive, iterative analysis. Film can also be used as a device to explore wider aspects of a person's life than a researcher would access through a typical research interview (Pink & Morgan, 2013).

Participation, co-design and ethnography applied to policy-making

The promise of increased knowledge and engagement from specific social groups has been a central objective for policymakers to engage with designers and approaches from ethnography. From our experience, participation in the policy process, through design approaches, focuses on providing tools that empower people to jointly reflect on their ideas and experiences, to communicate and help solve real design problems. In a policy context, co-design enables groups to empathise with one another, form new relationships and constructively explore ideas; it is an approach to designing with, not for, people, involving sharing power, managing and maintaining communication with local stakeholders (McKercher, 2020). Ethnography, and other approaches from anthropology, offer policymakers rich insights about the 'what' that sits behind the 'how' of qualitative data and at *Policy Lab* are being used as part of the design process.

However, analyses about how these methods are used in strategic contexts like policy-making are relatively limited. Ideas of ethics, power dynamics and protocols around increased participation are in their infancy. Although the *Policy Lab* team has been working with co-design, and participatory and ethnographic approaches for a number of years, these are still relatively niche practices in relation to policy-making as a whole. This chapter aims to share some of our practical experience in response to the current knowledge gaps.

How *Policy Lab* uses design for wellbeing

A core principle in *Policy Lab's* ways of working is to involve people outside traditional policy-making in evidence-gathering, idea-generation and decision-making. Policymakers use *Policy Lab*'s tools and techniques as a way to understand the lives of people affected by government policy and to engage them.

Policy Lab *participatory and co-design approaches*

By using engaging experiences to test ideas and see what works, *Policy Lab* works with research participants to co-design future ideas. This has been a core practice of the *Policy Lab* team since it was established in 2014. Visual design tools often enable policy ideas to be presented in more accessible ways, as well as supporting conversations and facilitating ideas in more engaging formats (Cottam, H. & Leadbeater, C. 2004). Design tools also allow information to be broken down into forms that can overcome language barriers and communicate patterns of information concurrently; providing hands-on tools empowers people to reflect jointly on their ideas and experiences, to communicate and cooperate and help solve real policy problems using a language that everyone can understand. Psychologists who use art in their practice understand that what emerges from using our hands is often quite different from that of the written word (Rojas, J. & Kamp, J. 2022). More tangible experiences provide a level playing field for participation, exploration and experimentation, often improving people's openness and readiness to engage. For the participant, it is a process of reflection and growth, using simple tools they tell their story to an engaged listener (Cottam, H. 2018). This is particularly relevant to policy-making where the types of information policymakers use can be technical and inaccessible, as are many of the buildings and spaces where policy-making typically takes place.

Selecting research participants to include in public engagement work is about understanding the policy scope and challenges in order to prioritise groups and relationships that need to be built. An important aspect of co-design is managing and maintaining communication with participants to support the challenges that inherently arise in this process. Challenges and misunderstandings between participants need to be sensitively managed and most require the rethinking or editing of a plan. Listening to participant frustrations and requirements is key to co-design to build trust and maintain reciprocal relationships. It is imperative that participants are kept on board throughout the project process to support negotiations and help maintain interest and enthusiasm in a project. Often, being actively involved and engaged throughout the process enables participants to understand why decisions have been made.

Policy Lab ethnography and film ethnography

Policy Lab uses ethnographic methods and film ethnography to enable policymakers to understand the lived experience of citizens. We have been using these approaches since 2014 and have deployed them on around 30 of the projects within our overall portfolio. In *Policy Lab*, ethnographic research means spending time with participants in their own environment, in order to gain a deep understanding of their world. Our ethnography is based on observation interspersed with unstructured, empathetic interviewing. By observing participants, we capture what people actually do as well as what they say they do. Immersing ourselves in the participant's world allows us to understand them in context. External factors such as culture, environment and social networks are often crucial determinants of behaviour. Lots of behaviour is implicit, unconscious or rationalised *post hoc*. This means that observing participants in the moment gives the richest understanding of real life.

> Observation is the best form of education in my book … We can just be us, we can share our views and we can just give you a tiny little glimpse into our world. Because we don't expect you to know it, because you're not living it.
>
> (*Policy Lab* participant, 2020)

Policy Lab uses ethnographic material and ethnographic films as a tool in policy-making to represent research findings. Films create a way of transferring peoples' voices into the room with policymakers, rather than in a mediated form through written reports or by government researchers. Ethnographic films bring evidence to life, providing a channel to communicate participants' emotions, attitudes and beliefs within the context of their own lives.

> *Policy Lab*'s ethnography of asylum seekers told a compelling story about journeys, customer needs and the every-day challenges they face. It provided a rich source of insight which has undoubted value in helping us design and produce customer-centric solutions.
>
> (*UKVI Immigration and Protection, Senior Transformation Manager*)

Ethnography can bring lived experience to the design of new strategies so that the government can focus on what is important to members of the public. It can be used to reveal aspects and impacts of a policy that might otherwise have been missed. Ethnography can also be used to test prototypes of new policies, to observe how changes to policy would happen in practice. Finally, because ethnography can capture how people experience government as a whole, it can also highlight to policymakers where cross-government collaboration is needed.

Project snapshot, Windrush Lessons Learned Review (2019-20)

Wendy Williams, His Majesty's Inspectorate of Constabulary and Fire & Rescue Services and review Chair, commissioned *Policy Lab* to create thematic films about the experience of five individuals from the Windrush generation and an ethnographic report. These were included as case studies in the Lessons Learned Review's report and a summary film communicating the experiences of those affected was published alongside the report. This work centred the experiences of the individuals affected and meant that their stories could be told in their own terms.[1]

Not only does ethnography help to improve the range of material available to policymakers, but it can also engage participants positively. Testimony from individuals involved in *Policy Lab*'s research projects illustrates the beneficial effect of feeling listened to. This has been particularly impactful on projects working with individuals who may feel marginalised.

> I am very grateful to have been given the opportunity to be a part of this important research project and hope my small contribution has provided some valuable insight.
>
> (*Covid* Diaries Project, 2021)

> It was a pleasure to do the interviews and I was made to feel that my views mattered. It is important that chronically ill and disabled people are given the opportunity to have their say and for policymakers to take on board the effects that their decisions have on people's daily lives.
>
> (*Ethnographic research with disabled people, 2020/21*)

Project snapshot, Independent Review of Children's Social Care (2021–22)

Policy Lab created an innovative yet robust methodology for putting families and young people at the heart of understanding the children's social care system. Work focused on exploring the lived experience of parents or legal guardians of children with a 'child in need plan' or a 'child protection plan', capturing their experiences through short films, backed by analytical reports.

Participants were asked to undertake remote interviews to build rapport and understand their experiences of the system. They were then asked to journal their experiences as video diaries. This created space for people to narrate their stories in their own terms. As COVID-19 guidelines were relaxed, remote engagement was combined with face-to-face interactions, including research visits to London and Cumbria. Participants shared personal stories, at times painful to recount, including experiences of abuse, loss and mental health difficulties. The recruitment practices, research methods and final outputs were conducted in a way that prioritised participant privacy and wellbeing.[2]

A core aspect of the ethnographic research undertaken by *Policy* Lab is empathy and rapport building with participants. This can help the researcher to uncover deeper insights and understanding about a person's life. It also serves to create a more equal power dynamic between researcher and participant.

Overall, *Policy Lab* uses this and other practices as a core part of its offer to policymakers, in order to bring different types of evidence and experience to bear on policy development, as well as to test policy ideas in dynamic and engaging formats.

Case study: Disability Unit

The following section explores a specific case of policymakers engaging with design methods with reference to a *Policy Lab* project working with the UK Cabinet Office.

In March 2019, a newly formed Disability Unit within the UK government was tasked with starting a programme of 'lived experience research' to ensure disabled people's lived experience shaped future policy development. While incomplete, the pre-existing evidence base clearly showed that disabled people experience worse outcomes in all areas of life compared to non-disabled people.

Policy Lab – with its combination of design and research skills – partnered with the Disability Unit to understand the daily experiences of disabled people. The Disability Unit's stated aim for the work was to 'identify problems that could be resolved through policy change' (Cabinet Office, Disability Unit, 2021). The work illustrated the policy team's desire to inform policy intent using design methodologies which capture lived experiences.

The first stage of the project created a picture of daily experiences of life in the UK with a disability. From June to October 2019, *Policy Lab* recruited and worked with 12 disabled people in England, developing film research material to understand their lives. Researchers used a range of methods, including in-depth interviews, ethnographically led film work, journey mapping and diary writing. Policy Lab spent around 70 hours engaged in deep listening, observation and participation. Areas of focus emerged from participant-led interviews and journey maps that were conducted at the start of the project. The film research focused on identity, health,

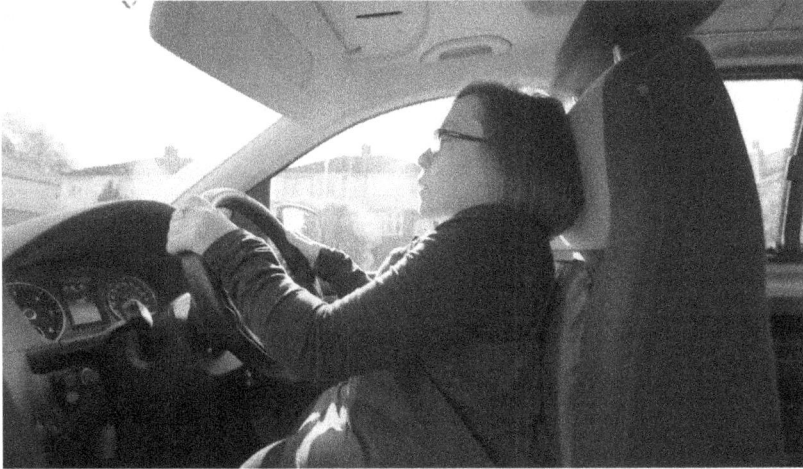

Figure 19.2 Still from film ethnography commissioned by the Disability Unit, showing our participant Donna in her car (2019)

relationships and society, as well as experiences of the built environment. Following fieldwork, researchers undertook a process of grounded thematic analysis to codify the data, turning individual stories into a body of evidence for the Disability Unit (Figure 19.2).

During the first summer of COVID-19, *Policy Lab* and the Disability Unit returned to participants to understand their changed realities resulting from COVID-19, using insights from the first project as a baseline. The second research project took place over six weeks between July and September 2020. Researchers used new remote methods, comprising longer interviews, weekly tasks and check-ins conducted over WhatsApp as well as a final speculative design exercise to develop imagined futures with the participants. These creative future visions were converted into animations by *Policy* Lab. Although the work was largely remote, material aspects of design were still in place – represented by video clips, audio recordings, photographs and sketches. At a time of social disconnection, during the COVID-19 pandemic, the range of research approaches was designed to create a sense of direct engagement for participants (Figure 19.3).

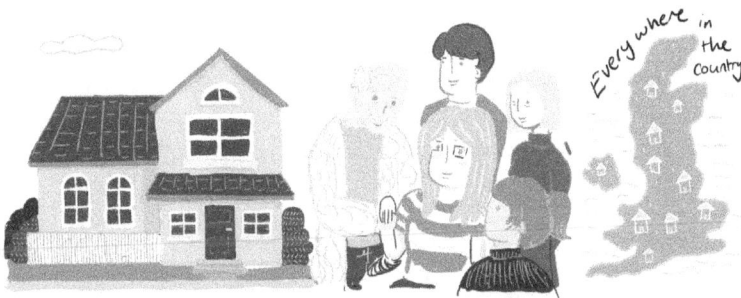

Figure 19.3 Future speculative sketch created by a designer working with a research participant, 2020

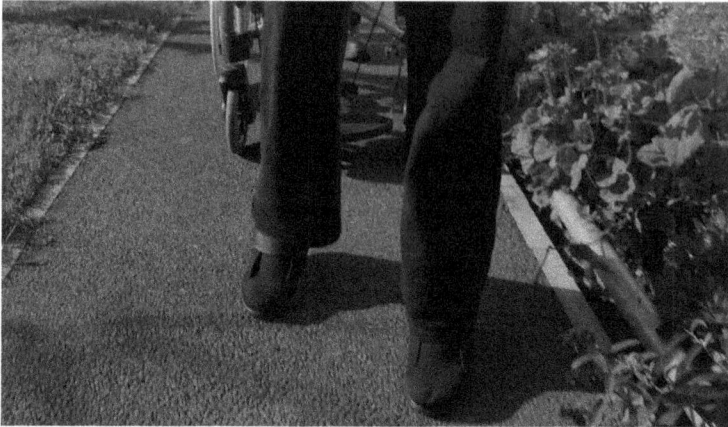

Figure 19.4 Still from film ethnography commissioned by the Disability Unit, with a research participant (2019)

The themes uncovered were, in part, a set of polarities around feelings such as 'dependence/independence', 'intimacy/functionality' and 'safety/risk'. The research also resulted in granular and practical knowledge about aspects of everyday life, including feelings of increased vulnerability when receiving social care or healthcare and uncertainty around the changing COVID-19 rules. There were occasional moments of positivity, and some participants even sought ways to enhance their independent living during the lockdowns (Cabinet Office, Disability Unit, 2021).

Through the research, further knowledge about disabled people's daily experiences was developed, focussing on impacts associated with COVID-19. More broadly, the project developed near real-time insights into how the pandemic was being experienced at the individual and human level. It foregrounded the personal situations of a group of individuals, at a time when at least some of the existing data about how people live had been quickly invalidated by the disruptions associated with COVID-19. Overall, the data consistently indicated that disabled people face enormous challenges and barriers to living a socially valued life of inclusion compared with non-disabled people. Participants said that they believed in opportunities for change, given the radical reformulation of every aspect of life brought about by COIVD-19, and subsequent empathy and understanding about the experiences of disabled people.

The Disability Unit applied this emerging research to inform immediate and longer-term policy development, as well as shape its strategy for evidence on disability. Insights were also used to understand the experiences behind data, and quotes from the research were used by the Office for National Statistics to illustrate their statistical data releases about the lives of disabled people during this time (Office for National Statistics, 2020). The research was also published in full by the Disability Unit (Cabinet Office, 2021) (Figure 19.4).

Conclusions

Design work in strategic contexts can enable policy teams to profoundly improve their knowledge of people's lived experience. In *Policy Lab* projects, we frequently see that working with ethnographers and designers results in far deeper understanding for policymakers about experiences relating to mental health and wellbeing amongst their stakeholders. Gaining insights about lived experience is also a common entry point for policymakers to engage with and commission designers and can result in design work being used more widely and in other ways by an organisation or policy team.

Participatory, co-design and ethnographic approaches are frequently used at the early stages of *Policy Lab* projects, for example, as a means to provide inspiration on how to progress an idea. The people involved can be highly varied, including leaders, policymakers, frontline service staff as well as service users and less-visible stakeholders such as family members or friends. Engagement and participation can have a fundamental impact on the design process, knowledge generated for policymakers and the role of the designer – which in policy contexts increasingly involves facilitating the participation and engagement of citizens in policy development.

However, in strategic environments – where multiple and competing needs exist – the relationship between policy and design is nuanced. In these situations, designers – or people leading the design process – are empowered to make decisions about which groups are engaged in design activity and how they are represented. The decision-making agency that designers have raises questions about the ethics and values of participatory and co-design work in policy-making contexts, which need further exploration. Although teams like *Policy Lab* are often commissioned to redress and reframe power dynamics by representing marginalised groups in institutions and systems where their experiences are often hidden from view, the power that designers hold has not typically been made explicit by the champions of design work in policy-making – it requires further interrogation to establish the rigour and transparency of the field. The reverse can of course also be true, that designers can uncover insights and develop ideas in policy contexts that would improve citizen experiences but with limited ability to act on these.

This chapter has explored a range of approaches deployed by designers and researchers relating to policy development. It discussed how these approaches are being used by *Policy Lab* and its commissioners – policy teams inside the UK government, and beyond – to develop new understandings of policy challenges, to foreground the micro experiences of individuals in policy decisions and as a way of working that is inclusive and clear through its materiality. The chapter has also referred in depth to a specific case study of *Policy Lab*'s work with the Disability Unit at the UK Cabinet Office.

Overall, the chapter has highlighted how *Policy Lab* has adapted design and ethnography for a policy-making context. It has aimed to show the enormous benefits of these approaches to both policymakers and participants, including new evidence generated for policy decision-making and positive feelings of being 'listened to' by participants. *Policy Lab* projects, such as the work for the Cabinet Office, explore new challenges and opportunities for the use of participation, co-design and ethnographic approaches to improve policy for citizens. Designers and policymakers continue to play with the potential of these methods, as well as new and emerging tools and approaches. But they also need to be persistent and aware in order to address ethical considerations and make use of the full spectrum of possibilities offered by design in a policy-making context.

Notes

1 The ethnographic film for the Policy Lab project commissioned by the Windrush Lessons Learned Review is here: https://www.youtube.com/watch?v=xEJksQpWkaE
2 *Policy Lab* blog. An independent review of Children's Social Care: appreciating the wider Family Context: https://openpolicy.blog.gov.uk/2022/06/09/an-independent-review-of-childrens-social-care-appreciating-the-wider-family-context/

References

Arnstein, S. (1969). A ladder of citizen participation. *Journal of the American Planning Association, 35*(4), 216–224.

Banerjee, B. (2014). Innovating large scale transformations. In C. Bason (Ed.), *Design for policy*. Gower.

Bason, C. (2010). *Leading Public Sector Innovation: Co-creating for a better society*. Policy Press.

Bason, C. (Ed.). (2014). *Design for policy*. Gower.

Burford, G., Harder, M. K., & Hoover, E. (2013). What is participation? Design leads the way to a cross-disciplinary framework. *Design Issues, 29*(4), 41–57.

Cabinet Office & Disability Unit. (2021). *Exploring the everyday lives of disabled people*. Online Reporter. Retrieved June 2023, from https://www.gov.uk/government/publications/exploring-the-everyday-lives-of-disabled-people

Clarke, A., & Craft, J. (2019). The twin faces of public sector design. *Governance, 32*(1), 5–21.

Cottam, H. (2018). *Radical help. How can we make relationships between us and revolutionise the welfare state?* Virago Press.

Cottam, H., & Leadbeater, C. (2004). *RED health: Co-creating services. Review of education* (Working Paper No. 1). Design Council.

De Couvreur, L., Dejonghe, W., Detand, J., & Goossens, R. (2013). The role of subjective well-being in co-designing open-design assistive devices. *International Journal of Design, 7*(3), 57–68.

Dewey, J. (1917). *The need for a recovery of philosophy, in creative intelligence: Essays in the pragmatic attitude*. Henry Holt and Co.

Hyysalo, V., & Hyysalo, S. (2018). Mundane and strategic work in collaborative design. *Design Issues, 34*(3), 42–58.

Irwin, T. (2015). Transition design: A proposal for a new area of design practice study, and research. *Design and Culture, 7*(2), 229–246.

Lurås, S. (2016). Systems intertwined: A systemic view on the design situation. *Design Issues, 32*(3), 30–41.

McKercher, K. (2020). *Beyond sticky notes*. Amazon.

Mulgan, G. (2014). *Design in Public and Social Innovation: What works and what could work better*. Nesta. Retrieved June 2023, from https://media.nesta.org.uk/documents/design_in_public_and_social_innovation.pdf

Office for National Statistics. (2020). *Coronavirus and the social impacts on disabled people in great Britain: July 2020*. Retrieved June 2023, from https://www.ons.gov.uk/peoplepopulationand community/healthandsocialcare/disability/articles/coronavirusandthesocialimpactsondisabledpeoplei ngreatbritain/july2020

Pink, S., & Morgan, J. (2013). Short-term ethnography: Intense routes to knowing. *Symbolic Interaction, 36*(3), 351–361.

Rocha, E. (1997). A ladder of empowerment. *Journal of Planning Education and Research, 17*(1), 31–44.

Rojas, J., & Kamp, J. (2022). *Dream play build*. PRESS.

Sanders, E., & Stappers, J. P. (2008). Co-creation and the new landscapes of design. *Codesign, 4*(1), 5–18.

Sangiorgi, D. (2010). *Transformative services and transformation design*. Nordic Service Design Conference, Linkoping, Sweden.

Sangiorgi, D., & Prendiville, A. (Eds.). (2017). *Designing for service*. Bloomsbury.

Sanoff, H. (2006). Multiple views of participatory design. *Middle East Technical University Journal of the Faculty of Architecture, 23*(2), 131–143.

Siodmok, A. (2022). Lab long read: Human-centred policy? Blending 'big data' and 'thick data' in national policy - policy lab. *Openpolicy.blog*. Retrieved June 2023, from gov.uk. https://openpolicy .blog.gov.uk/2020/01/17/lab-long-read-human-centred-policy-blending-big-data-and-thick-data-in -national-policy/

Steen, M. (2013). Co-design as a process of joint inquiry and imagination. *Design Issues, 29*(2), 16–28. The MIT Press.

20 Developing culturally appropriate dementia interventions for people from culturally diverse backgrounds

Jennifer N. W. Lim

Setting the scene

There are 900,000 people aged 65 years and over living with dementia in the UK (Alzheimer's Society, 2023). Calculated based on the 2011 census data, 25,000 people of culturally diverse backgrounds[1] have dementia and this is an underestimated figure (All-Party Parliamentary Group on Dementia, 2013). Dementia has a huge economic cost, with two thirds (£17.4 billion) of the total cost of £36.7 billion shouldered by the people with dementia and their families, and £10.3 billion and £4.3 billion by the social care and NHS respectively (Alzheimer's Society, 2023).

Increasing age is the biggest risk factor for dementia, with a prevalence of 7.1%, or 1 in every 14 people aged 65 years and over. By 2051, it is predicted that over 2 million people of the UK population (Alzheimer's Society, 2023), and 269,800 people from culturally diverse backgrounds will have dementia[2]. However, approximately 5% of cases of dementia in the UK (about 42,000 though this number may be an underestimate) present before the age of 65 and are referred to as having young onset dementia. The impacts of this condition on the lives of the individuals and their families are significantly different and more disruptive (Dementia UK, 2022), and financially profound (Kandiah et al., 2016). Young onset dementia seems to be more common in the culturally diverse population with a 6% occurrence (Knapp et al., 2007; Bothongo et al., 2020); this is likely due to the higher risk of comorbidity conditions such as vascular disease and diabetes as well as social deprivation and poverty experienced in this population (Bothongo et al., 2022; Bajekal, 2004; Evandrou, 2000; Evandrou et al., 2016).

The number of people of culturally diverse background living with dementia is underestimated. There are persistent problems of delayed help-seeking in this population because of poor awareness, understanding and conceptualisation of the condition, language barriers, social stigma, negative experiences of accessing and navigating the health and social care services; leading to under-diagnosis (Mukadam et al., 2013; Baghirathan et al., 2020; Roche et al., 2021; Co et al., 2021). Underdiagnosis of dementia is further exacerbated by a lack of culturally appropriate interventions and screening tools, and a lack of culturally trained health care professionals (Mukadam et al., 2011; Moriarty et al., 2011; Kenning et al., 2017). This has resulted in differing diagnostic outcomes – and referral pathways to support services – for people from culturally diverse backgrounds compared to their white counterparts (Wilson et al., 2020; Dodd et al., 2020).

The number of people of culturally diverse backgrounds living with dementia will likely be larger than predicted in 2051. Apart from the continued migration of people escaping harsh regimes and war, and for economic purposes, the recent UK government's policy of granting residence to the population of its former colony, Hong Kong, has seen a dramatic increase of Chinese people in the country – with over 100,000 people moving to the UK by 2023 (UK Home Office, 2023a). To date, around 170,000 Ukrainians have arrived in the UK under the

DOI: 10.4324/9781003318262-26

government family scheme and sponsorship visas (UK Home Office, 2023b). Britain's multi-cultural society is becoming ever more diverse, and an inclusive healthcare system is needed to meet everyone's needs.

Since 2010, numerous policy documents have suggested ways in which local services need to develop and be more responsive to the needs of culturally diverse communities in their locality (Moriarty et al., 2011). In 2016, the Prime Minister's Challenge on Dementia 2020 called on key players – NHS, Public Health England, Care Quality Commission, Health Education, Alzheimer's Research UK, Alzheimer's Society – to reduce dementia inequalities as a priority area. The implementation guidance (National Collaborating Centre for Mental Health, 2018) pledged consistent support and care for each person and their family and carer after diagnosis and to improve staff training. More fundings are being allocated to understand dementia in the 'underserved groups' and for the evaluation of interventions and services in these populations (e.g. Alzheimer's Society, 2022). We now have a better understanding of dementia experienced by the Black and South Asian ethnic groups (Blakemore et al., 2018; Dodd et al., 2020; Roche et al., 2021), but we know little about other ethnic groups. For example, there is currently only one study reporting the experience of a small Chinese community (Baghirathan et al., 2020) and one brain health intervention being delivered in the Chinese communities in five cities (Alzheimer's Research UK, 2022). The diversity within ethnic groups also means that the dementia experience and needs of subcultural groups are different. A Sikh female carer speaking Punjabi is likely to have a different background and needs from another South Asian male Muslim carer speaking a different language. Two Chinese persons with dementia who speak Cantonese may have different health needs due to different historical experience and countries of migration. It is not just ethnicity; there is also the issue of intersectionality that divides people: class, socio-economic status, gender, religion, sexuality and many other factors together play a role. The design and development of dementia interventions to address disparities in these communities will have to be sensitive to all these factors.

The diversity of the UK population highlights the importance of careful attention to the distinctive cultural characteristics and needs of the communities in developing and implementing interventions to improve dementia outcomes, particularly given the health disparities that they are facing. Furthermore, even in the best-developed interventions, there are often differences in community environments and target populations or communities that really do necessitate certain kinds of modifications of an intervention. There is also considerable evidence that culture and context influence almost every aspect of an intervention (Marsiglia & Booth, 2015). Hence, cultural tailoring or adaptation of interventions intended for communities from diverse backgrounds is therefore critical and urgent to improve early diagnosis and quality of life of people with dementia and families.

Terminologies: cultural sensitivity, cultural tailoring, cultural adaptation and cultural appropriateness

Cultural sensitivity is defined as the extent to which ethnic/cultural characteristics, experiences, norms, values, behavioural patterns and beliefs of a target population as well as relevant historical, environmental and social forces are incorporated in the design, delivery and evaluation of targeted health promotion materials and programmes (Resnicow et al., 1999).

Cultural tailoring is 'the adaptation of the study design, materials and other components of the intervention to reflect cultural needs and preferences at the population level' (Torres-Ruiz et al., 2018). The features of a tailored intervention include: (a) its collection of messages or strategies that are intended for a particular person rather than a group of people, and (b) these messages or strategies are based on individual level factors that are related to the health or behavioural outcome of interest (Kreueter & Skinner, 2000; Kreueter et al., 2004). According to these authors, true culturally tailored approaches identify cultural dimensions relevant to health (e.g. religiosity, racial pride), measure individual differences on those dimensions and deliver individualised health promotion messages matching an individual's endorsement of cultural dimensions.

Cultural adaptation has been defined as 'the systematic modification of an evidence-based treatment or intervention protocol to consider language, culture, and context in such a way that it is compatible with the client's cultural patterns, meanings, and values' (Bernal et al., 2009). Backer (2001) defined adaptation of programme as deliberate or accidental modification of the programme that includes, a) deletions or additions (enhancements) of programme components; b) modifications in the nature of the components that are included; c) changes in the manner or intensity of administration of programme components called for in the programme manual, curriculum or core components analysis; or d) cultural and other modifications required by local circumstances.

Culturally appropriate interventions have the following characteristics: a) incorporating the cultural values of the group, (b) with strategies that reflect the subjective culture (attitudes, expectancies, norms) of the group and (c) with components that reflect the behavioural preferences and expectations of the group's members (Marín, 1993).

The above terms describe deliberate actions to develop and/or adapt strategies that fit and are congruent with the psychological, social, cultural, behavioural and environment of the target individual, population group or community. These terms are used interchangeably in the literature and are taken to have a similar meaning in this chapter.

Five principles guiding development and implementation of cultural strategies

When considering adaptation or tailoring an intervention, three main questions are often asked. What are the components of an intervention that can be adapted to make it culturally appropriate without affecting the intervention's fidelity? What aspects of the target community/group need to be considered for tailoring/adaptation for an intervention to be culturally appropriate? What features are needed to develop and implement the culturally appropriate intervention? Presented below are five key elements or principles that determine the development and implementation of a culturally appropriate intervention successfully (Figure 20.1). For a sustainable and future replication of the intervention, all these principles should be met fully.

Determining the components to adapt: core components and peripheral components of intervention

'What components to adapt in an intervention?' is a question about the fidelity of the intervention. Intervention fidelity refers to the degree to which a specific intervention is implemented as intended (An et al., 2020). It is also referred to as the degree of fit between the developer-defined components of a programme and its actual implementation in an organisational or community setting (Backer, 2001). Adherence, intensity, strength of treatment, integrity, dosage, intensity, quality of intervention delivery, participant responsiveness, compliance and programme differentiation are also terms referring to fidelity (Backer, 2001; An et al., 2020).

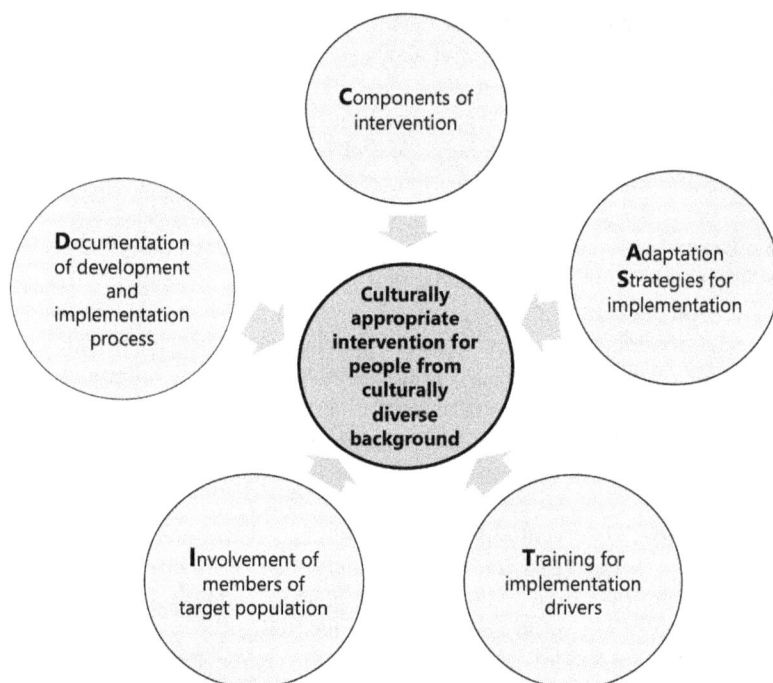

Figure 20.1 The five principles of cultural adaptation (CAST-ID)

An intervention consists of core and peripheral components. Core components are theory-driven and derived from empirical principles. They are the essential functions or principles, and associated elements and intervention activities that are judged necessary to produce desired outcomes. They are directly related to a programme's theory of change, which proposes the mechanisms by which an intervention or programme works. They are intended to positively impact the proximal outcomes that address the identified needs and that increase the likelihood that longer-term outcomes will be achieved. (Blasé & Fixsen, 2013). Core components are often equated with measures of fidelity, defining the effectiveness of an intervention or programme. Therefore, core components should not be modified or adapted (Castro et al., 2004) since interventions are more effective when implemented with fidelity (Durlak & DuPre, 2008). Backer (2001) provided there is guidance to determine the core components of an intervention, by examining its theoretical framework for its theory of change and by conducting an analysis of core components. Having knowledge of the core components will ensure that they are implemented accordingly.

Peripheral components are elements, processes or activities that are required to support the implementation of the core components. Peripheral components are implementation strategies which are methods and tools used to change policies, administrative procedures and the environment; they are the *how* of implementation, the means through which core components are put into practice (NASEM, 2019). According to Fixsen and colleagues (2001), there are (1) intervention processes and outcomes, and (2) implementation processes and outcomes in every intervention. Implementation outcomes refer to fidelity (Are they doing the programme as intended?) while effectiveness outcomes refer to the outcomes of a fully implemented intervention (Yes, they are, and it is/is not resulting in good outcomes). The effectiveness of an intervention therefore depends on how well the peripheral components are supporting or delivering the core components.

Chu and Leino (2017) described peripheral components as culturally adapted materials and activities that engagement and delivery of the core components of an intervention. For an intervention targeted at people from diverse backgrounds, cultural adaptation of the peripheral components has been reported to maintain the fidelity of the core components and deliver positive outcomes of dementia interventions (Chu et al., 2012; Aguilera et al., 2010). Adapting peripheral elements of an intervention so that they meet the needs of diverse communities while retaining the core components is key to successful implementation. Strong evidence indicates that engaging communities closely in the development and implementation of interventions is critical to their success and sustainability (Gallagher-Thompson et al., 2000; Vila-Castelar et al., 2022).

Developing and tailoring implementation strategies: what aspects of the target community/ group need to be adapted for an intervention to be culturally appropriate?

Several frameworks have been proposed to guide cultural adaptation. The earliest model, the ecological validity model (EV), describes eight dimensions (Bernal et al., 1995), later summarised into three dimensions by Castro and colleagues (2001). Resnicow and colleagues (1999) provided a similar model with two dimensions to guide the development of adaptation strategies: surface structure and deep structure adaptation. They argued that cultural adaptation must move beyond surface structure (changing the ethnicity or the appearance of role models), to deep structure by addressing the core values, beliefs, norms and other more significant aspects of the cultural group's world views and lifestyles. These earlier frameworks, however, were not explicit about community or target group's involvement and the use of existing evidence; these additional factors are included in the five-dimension framework introduced by Kreueter and colleagues (2003). Table 20.1 provides details of the frameworks.

Identifying the training needs of implementation drivers

People or staff who competently use or implement core intervention components in their interaction with the target group can positively influence the outcomes of the intervention (Fixsen et al., 2001). They need the required skillsets and knowledge to perform their role to implement the intervention successfully (Wandersman et al., 2008). This includes knowledge of the core components of the intervention, the mechanisms of change, the needs of the population and social and cultural influences, and research skills for data collection. For culturally appropriate interventions, implementors need to be culturally competent and culturally safe.

Cultural competence is a range of cognitive, affective and behavioural skills that lead to effective and appropriate communication with people of other cultures (Deardorff, 2009). Cultural competence is also the ability to resolve differences and identify solutions that reduce interference from various cultural factors (Leininger & McFarland, 2002). *Cultural safety* requires individuals and organisations to examine themselves and the potential impact of their own culture on clinical interactions and healthcare service delivery. This requires individual healthcare professionals and healthcare organisations to acknowledge and address their own biases, attitudes, assumptions, stereotypes, prejudices, structures and characteristics that may affect the quality of care provided. Cultural safety requires healthcare professionals and their associated healthcare organisations to influence healthcare to reduce bias and achieve equity within the workforce and working environment (Curtis et al., 2019).

Table 20.1 Cultural adaptation frameworks

Cultural adaptation framework	Dimensions	Details
Bernal et al., 1995	Ecological Validity model – 8 dimensions	1.Language 2.Persons 3.Metaphors 4.Content 5.Concepts 6.Goals 7.Methods 8.Context
Resnicow et al., 1999	2 dimensions	1. Surface structure refers to the extent to which interventions meet the target population where they are, how well they fit within their culture and experience. Adaptation to match intervention materials and messages to observable, 'superficial' (though nonetheless important) characteristics of a target population, such as involving people, places, language, music, food, product brands, locations and clothing familiar to and preferred by the target audience. It also includes identifying what channels (media) and settings (churches, schools) are most appropriate for the delivery of messages and programmes. For cultural competence or interpersonal sensitivity, using ethnically matched staff to recruit participants as well as to deliver and evaluate programs. 2. Deep structure refers to how socio-demographic and racial/ethnic populations differ in general (i.e. core cultural values) as well as how ethnic, cultural, social, environmental and historical factors may influence specific health behaviour. In a broad sense, this entails understanding how members of the target population perceive the cause, course and treatment of an illness (i.e. explanatory models). More specifically, this includes investigating perceptions relating to how religion, family, society, economics and government (policy) might influence target behaviour.
Castro et al., 2001	Ecological model (refined) – 3 dimensions	1.Cognitive information processing characteristic – language and age/developmental level 2. Affective motivational characteristics – gender, ethnic background, religious background, socio-economic status 3. Environmental characteristics – ecological aspects of the local community
Krueter et al., 2003	5 dimensions	1. Peripheral strategies – modifying the observable properties of intervention materials by using certain colours, images, fonts, pictures of group members or declarative titles that overtly convey relevance to the group 2. Linguistics strategies – altering the language used in intervention materials to make them comprehensible 3.Constituent-involving strategies – utilising the cultural knowledge and experience of members of the subcultural group 4.Sociocultural strategies – recognising, reinforcing and building upon a subcultural groups cultural values, beliefs and behaviours 5.Evidential strategies – using 'evidence' such as epidemiological data for a specific subcultural group or experiences from individuals with similar backgrounds to increase the perceived relevance of information

Organisations and staff involved in implementation need training to be competent and culturally safe in order to improve engagement, acceptability and receptivity of intervention – as well as to build trust and rapport with the target group/community.

Involving members of the target group/community/population

Culture is seldom uniformly experienced by all members of a given community (Weinstein, 1988); directly involving members of the community to design and develop tailored strategies is therefore critical to the efficiency and effectiveness of intervention (Resnicow et al., 1999; Krueter et al., 2003; NASEM, 2019; Peters et al., 2013). One of the five dimensions of Krueter's cultural adaptation model, constituent-involving strategies, advocates for the direct experience of members of the target group in developing or adapting intervention. Drawing on the experience and support from constituents to develop and implement intervention provides valuable insights into the cultural characteristics that are not easily observed – such as language, cultural dress or preferred colour schemes (Kreueter et al., 2003).

Furthermore, the procedures for cultural adaptation are argued to be an integration between both 'top-down' and 'bottom-up' approaches through a series of adaptation stages (Barrera et al., 2013). A top-down, universal approach views an original intervention's content as applicable to all groups – with no need for alterations – whereas a bottom-up approach is a culture-specific approach that emphasises culturally grounded content consisting of the unique values, beliefs, traditions and practices of a particular group (Falicov, 2009). Members of the target community should be involved as early as possible to maximise the benefits of their participation in design, planning and so on. The community-based participatory research (CBPR) is an example of such an integrated approach which emphasises reciprocal knowledge exchange and mutual benefit among partners from the start of the intervention (Minkler & Wallerstein, 2011); this approach has proved to be successful and sustainable in culturally adapted behavioural change interventions (Wilson & Miller, 2003; Kirby, 2002).

Documenting and reporting implementation strategies

As an implementation strategy, it is necessary to document culturally adapted strategies so that effective strategies can be replicated and scaled up. Implementation strategies need to be labelled and precisely described in sufficient detail to enable measurement and 'reproducibility' of their components (Michie et al., 2009; Davies et al., 2010). A framework is available for specifying and reporting implementation strategies – this asks for details of the strategy (such as name, definition); specifics in terms of the actors/developers; the type of action; the action target; when it was used; the dosage of implementation; the outcome affected; the theoretical and pragmatic justification for the choice of strategy – which allows for empirical testing (Proctor et al., 2013).

From here, the acronym CAST-ID (Components of intervention, Adaptation Strategies for implementation; Training for implementation drivers Involvement of members of target population; and Documentation of development and implementation process), will be used to refer to the five principles for cultural adaptation of intervention (as shown in Figure 20.1).

Culturally appropriate interventions in dementia: the state of the art

Many culturally appropriate interventions have been implemented to address the dementia disparities faced by people from culturally diverse backgrounds. Five systematic reviews focusing on prevention, caregiving and therapeutic interventions for people with dementia

Table 20.2 Characteristics of included systematic reviews

Authors of systematic reviews	Years searched, included studies	Country of studies	No. of studies with ethnic groups
Napoles et al. (2010)	1980–2009 18 studies included	18 US	10 African American 11 Latinx 1 Chinese American
Ma and Saw (2020)	2010–2019 9 out of 29 studies conducted in Western countries	4 US 3 Australia 1 Canada 1 Singapore & Australia	All Chinese
Huggins et al. (2021)	2015–2021 25 studies	21 US 3 UK 1 Australia	10 Black African American and Black Hispanic 11 Hispanic 3 South Asian (UK) 5 Chinese
James et al. (2021)	2010–2021 9 of 23 studies conducted between 2010 and 2019 in Western countries	9 US	Latinx, Chinese and African Americans (US)
Brijnath et al. (2021)	2010–2020 66 studies	57 US 5 Australia 2 UK 1 Netherlands	22 African American 21 Hispanic American 8 multi-ethnic population (including 4 Mexican and 4 Caribbean Americans) 2 Chinese American and Japanese American 1 Puerto Rico and Spanish American 3 Multi-ethnic Australian 1 Black African, Caribbean and Black British 1 South Asian (Indian and Pakistani British) 1 Turkish, Surinamese and Mixed-ethnic Dutch

have been conducted to date, to review primary studies implemented in Western countries (Table 20.2). The extent to which these interventions have been implemented – and to what effect – is unknown.

Implementation research seeks to understand what, why and how interventions work in 'real world' settings and to test approaches to improve them (Peters et al., 2013). Therefore, in this part, an umbrella review is performed to assess what cultural adaptations have been made, how they have been delivered, and what the results of the implementation in the dementia interventions are. The CAST-ID framework for cultural adaptation will be used to guide the synthesis of evidence.

Electronic search for systematic reviews

The databases – MEDLINE, CINAHL, PsycINFO and Psychology and Behavioural Sciences Collection, PUBMED and SCOPUS – were searched using terms such as 'dementia or Alzheimer's or cognitive impairment or memory loss', 'culturally' adapted or tailored or appropriate', 'intervention or strategies or best practices or treatment or therapy or progress or management', 'minority ethnic' and 'systematic review'. A total of 113 citations were yielded and of these, four systematic reviews that specifically addressed the provision of culturally appropriate interventions for dementia in diverse cultures were selected. Additional searches on Google Scholar were also performed and one systematic review published in 2021 was further located. These five systematic reviews, published between 2010 and 2021, examined the topics of promotion of dementia knowledge, caregiving, recruitment and therapeutic interventions (Napoles et al., 2010; Ma & Saw, 2020; Huggins et al., 2021; James et al., 2021; Brijnath et al., 2021).

Results

A total of 95 culturally tailored studies on dementia, covered in the systematic reviews, have been implemented between 1980 and 2020 (Table 20.2). The majority of the studies were conducted in the United States. Only five studies were based in the UK, targeting the Black African and Caribbean, and South Asian ethnic groups. No culturally appropriate intervention has been delivered to Chinese or other ethnic groups in the UK during the period of the reviews.

Outcomes of intervention

Although positive outcomes were reported in the reviews, the details reported are variable across the studies (Table 20.3). This is possibly due to poor documentation of the cultural adaptation or tailoring strategies in the primary studies and of the measurement of effectiveness of the adaptation strategies on outcomes.

Cultural adaptation principles

The systematic reviews did not provide any information on health theoretical models used in the primary studies; comparisons of effectiveness between studies and analyses of generalisation

Table 20.3 Outcomes of culturally appropriate dementia studies

Authors of systematic reviews	*Outcomes of studies reported in the review*
Napoles et al. (2010)	Mainly positive outcomes, but studies did not assess the effect of ethnicity effect with cultural tailoring. There were too few studies to allow for conclusive interpretations of the association between cultural tailoring of interventions and their effectiveness for specific ethnic groups.
Ma and Saw (2020)	Produced largely desirable/positive outcomes. Absence of significant treatment effect was noted, and only seven studies assessed follow-up treatment effects.
Huggins et al. (2021)	Improvement in outcomes in many studies (intervention content and outcome measures varied greatly across studies, few use standardised validated instruments.)
	High interest in participation despite stigma; targeted recruitment strategies but intervention was short in duration and failed to follow up with participants over time.
James et al. (2021)	Six out of the nine studies have a positive outcome; three with unclear feasibility (not all participants completed intervention)
Brijnath et al. (2021)	No outcome reported as the review aimed at recruitment and participation of minority ethnic people in dementia research. Only 38 out of 66 studies reported recruitment details, and only one study reported on retention.

thus are of less meaning. The theoretical model of an intervention defines the core components and behavioural change mechanisms; this information is useful to assess if the culturally tailored strategies (implementation) impact on the effectiveness of the intervention.

None of the reviews uses a cultural adaptation framework (Table 20.4) to extract the data; instead, cultural adaptation strategies were simply listed or described. The frameworks provide a tool to identify adaptation strategies at different dimensions and to evaluate if these strategies are meeting the cultural characteristics and needs of the target population. The types of culturally adapted strategies reported in the reviews can be identified as language-, culture-, community- and cultural competency-based. The majority of the strategies were adapted at the surface level. Only two reviews reported deep structure adaptation strategies which are essential to effect changes in the core components of the intervention (Napoles et al., 2010; Ma & Saw, 2020). It appears that a blended approach or a combination of culturally adapted strategies was implemented, but how much of each type of strategy or what combinations of strategies were used in the interventions is unknown since these details are not reported in the reviews. It is also unknown to what extent which adaptation was made to the intervention, what modifications were made, and whether there were additional or deletions of existing peripheral components/implementation materials.

Cultural sensitivity training was one of the strategies reported, but no details were provided on the extent to which these strategies were being adopted (or how they have impacted on the delivery and outcome of the intervention). None of the reviews uses a cultural competency or safety framework or discuss this aspect of delivery, considering its importance when interacting with culturally diverse communities.

On involvement of community members in the design and development of the intervention, studies that adopted a community-based participatory research approach reportedly produced positive and sustainable outcomes, but the extent of community members' involvement was not presented in the systematic reviews. Outreach and engagement strategies were used in some studies, but there was little detail reported in the reviews. This area of intervention appears to receive little attention in the studies; Brijnath and colleagues (2021) found that only 38 studies of the 66 included studies provided some details on the strategies they used to engage and recruit participants. Retention of participation is also a subject that is rarely covered in the systematic reviews; only one study reported strategies to retain participation in their study (Brijnath et al., 2021). For studies involving people with dementia, retention is a major issue due to their condition; strategies to address this issue and meet the needs of this unique group of participants are needed.

Apart from naming the strategies, most of the fundamental details required to empirically test implementation strategies – as recommended by Proctor and colleagues (2013) – are not reported in the five reviews.

Gaps and recommendations

The systematic reviews on cultural adaptation in dementia interventions focused mainly on listing the tailored strategies reported in the primary studies. They provided little information to assess if the CAST-ID principles of cultural adaptation have been followed to produce and deliver strategies that are congruent or fitting the needs of the members of the target community/group. Additionally, the aim of examining tailored strategies is to better understand the processes of implementation and the factors affecting the implementation of the intervention; this information is needed to empirically test the strategies, examine the impact of implementation and

Table 20.4 Types and level of cultural adaptation strategies

Authors	Categories	Types of tailored strategies	Level of tailoring: surface and core structure
Napoles et al. (2010)	Language-based	• Translated material • Simplified messages • Oral presentation • Written materials in simple language to fit target population's literacy needs and acceptability • Bilingual staff	Surface structure
	Culture-based	• Respecting custom by protecting elders • Focusing on familism value and custom • Recognising spiritual aspects of caregiving through prayers • Educational approach was non-stigmatising • Problem-solving approach stressing the use of faith to help work through stressful caregiving • In-home programme	Deep structure
	Community-based	• Training on self-empowerment through knowledge and advocacy for care and information-seeking	Deep structure
		• Addressing logistical barriers • Flexible sessions • Sessions begin with social conversation • Festive, celebration atmosphere	Surface structure
	Cultural-competency–based	• Bicultural staff • Staff training on cultural sensitivity • Training on interactive and personal approach to be consistent with *personalism*	Surface structure
Ma and Saw (2020)	Language-based	• Translated materials • Interactive videos with PowerPoint slides • Interpreter • Bilingual staff	Surface structure
	Culture-based	• Building rapport with one-month preparatory phase; survey on family structure, dynamics, strength and weaknesses, survey to assess needs for caregiving intervention-based on caregivers' prioritised areas • Portraying caregiver on vignettes as a mother, father or spouse with dementia, actors, grandchildren and adult children	Deep structure
	Community-based	• Use of community elderly social centres or community facilities or home • Information on local services and hospice care • Formed advisory committee • Recruiting NGOs • Recruiting from community care management centre	Surface structure
	Cultural-competency–based	• Use paraprofessional with psychology degree • Active partnership between nurse and caregiver to identify areas for intervention to build trust and alliance	Surface structure

(*Continued*)

Table 20.4 (Continued)

Authors	Categories	Types of tailored strategies	Level of tailoring: surface and core structure
Huggins et al. (2021)	Language-based	• Sessions delivered in the participant's preferred language • Translated materials	Surface structure
	Culture-based	• Cultural text messages that incorporate colloquialisms, idioms and content	Surface structure
	Community-based	• CBPR approach • Community committee advisory group • Focus group discussions	Surface structure
	Cultural-competency–based	• Cultural sensitivity training and community health	Surface structure
James et al. (2021)	Language-based	• Translated materials • Delivery in the local language • Increased use of visual aids • Oral presentation due to low literacy • Bilingual staff	Surface structure
	Culture-based	• Local metaphor • Reframing information to fit cultural values and practices • Meeting participants/clients' needs and cultural values (home, *familismo*) • Use of local actors in a video vignette, soap-opera-style approach to present intervention messages • Reframing intervention as providing better care than self-care • Role play • Use of the terminology 'memory problems' vs 'Alzheimer's' to avoid the stigma of mental health	Surface structure
	Community-based	• Offered at preferred location • In-house therapy • Classroom feeling to avoid the stigma of therapy	Surface structure
	Cultural-competency–based	• Bicultural staff • Rephrased 'assertive communication' with a more respectful phrase	Surface structure
Brijnath et al. (2021)	Language-based	• Translated material • Interpreter • Bilingual worker • Simplified materials	Surface structure
	Culture-based	• Participation based on preferences and needs (choosing time and frequency of engagement) • Culturally appropriate content	Surface structure
	Community-based	• Community presentation to facilitate recruitment • Community out-reach (health fairs, word-of-mouth) Monetary compensation • Recruit in churches, aged care facilities, local ethnic media and community organisations • Bilingual agencies • Through community surveys	Surface structure
	Cultural-competency–based	• Bicultural workers • Cultural sensitivity training for researchers • Recruiting researchers through specialist clinics with high ethnic-minority patient caseload	Surface structure

outcome of the intervention and conduct cost evaluation for improvement and scaling up. The CAST-ID principles discussed in this chapter – determining core and peripheral components in the intervention, developing culturally appropriate strategies for implementation, identifying skill sets and training for implementation drivers, involving members of the target community/ group and documenting and specifying details of strategies – can be used as guidance to successfully develop and implement effective and sustainable culturally appropriate interventions that can be replicated and tested.

The findings from the systematic reviews showed that there has been success in achieving surface-level tailoring (which aims to improve acceptability and receptivity of the intervention), but not in deep-level tailoring (which influences or impacts the efficacy of the intervention). Deep structure sensitivity requires an understanding of the cultural, social, historical, environmental and psychological forces that influence the target health behaviour in the proposed target population (Resnicow et al., 1999). Interventions with deep structure strategies have been shown to be more effective than those with surface level adaptations only (Jani et al., 2008; Huey et al., 2018). Furthermore, interventions that lack relevance to the needs and preferences of the target group – even if the intervention could be administered with complete fidelity – exhibit low levels of effectiveness. This principle suggests that a deep structure understanding of the target group/community is essential to develop a culturally relevant and efficient intervention. The dimensional cultural adaptation frameworks in Table 20.4 provide guidance to develop strategies at both surface structure and deep structure of cultural sensitivity; the systematic use of the framework for cultural tailoring can improve the outcome of an intervention targeting people from diverse cultures.

There is a persistent problem in recruiting and engaging people from culturally diverse backgrounds to participate in dementia research (Alzheimer's Research UK, 2021; Wright, 2020). Although minority ethnic communities make up about 14% of the UK population, only approximately 5% have ever participated in clinical research (Harrison & Smart, 2016). Similarly, only 5% of African Americans and 1% of Hispanic people have participated in research, even though they respectively make up 12% and 16% of the US population (The Society for Women's Health Research, 2011). Low participation of people from culturally diverse groups in research leads to limited generalisability and validity of the findings, affecting the equity in the distribution of resources for research and services (Oakley et al., 2003). Some of the reported barriers to participation in medical research are worries about the effectiveness of clinical trials, concerns related to financial and confidentiality issues and lack of knowledge of research trials (Mills et al., 2006; Shah et al., 2016, Harrison & Smart, 2016). A recent scoping review on factors influencing research participation of people from minority ethnic groups revealed barriers at both the surface- and deep-structure levels, namely barriers related to culture, language and ethnic beliefs, cultural congruence between investigators and participants and fear and mistrust of research (Anwuluorah et al., 2022). Employing bilingual staff is one common surface level adaptation strategy being used in dementia intervention studies, and some studies used outreach and engagement activities such as community fairs, liaison activities, recruiting from community centres, churches and elderly media to increase their presence and trust. Deep level adaptation strategies are needed to address issues of fear and mistrust of research in the community. Involving researchers from the same cultural background and experience as the participants in the study could improve congruence between investigators and participants.

People living with dementia need a familiar environment and trust to feel comfortable participating in the intervention (Lim et al., 2019). Strategies to gain their trust, such as involving familiar faces (e.g. their care workers or healthcare professionals) in the implementation and delivering of the intervention in a familiar venue, will increase participation and engagement as well as retention. In a previous study, Lim and colleagues (2019) completed their multicenter study with 99% participation from people with dementia by involving care workers and health-care professionals in the delivery of the intervention.

Cultural tailoring involves a planned, organised, iterative and collaborative process that often includes the participation of members of the targeted population for whom the adaptation is being developed (Bareera et al., 2013). Involving community members in the project from the start has many advantages. Apart from gaining and building trust and providing familiarity, it can empower the community to take ownership of the intervention and ensure sustainability. Community-based participatory research has been shown to produce these effects in dementia studies (Huggins et al., 2021).

The cultural competence of the investigator and of the cultural adaptation team is also important for conducting a deep structure analysis of the needs and preferences of a targeted cultural group, apart from implementing the strategies (Castro, 1998; Skaff et al., 2002). Documenting the strategies as well as the implementation process of the intervention is essential for measurement, evaluation and scaling up.

Conclusion

In this chapter, the CAST-ID – **C**omponents, **A**daptation **S**trategies, **T**raining, **I**nvolvement and **D**ocumentation – framework, which consists of five principles to develop and adapt interventions targeting people from culturally diverse backgrounds, is presented. For any intervention to have a good chance of success, and to be effective, sustainable and replicable, all the conditions of the CAST-ID principles must be met. The synthesis of the evidence from the five systematic reviews showed that much is still needed to be done to make the interventions in dementia culturally appropriate and effective for their target population.

Acknowledgements

The author is grateful to Professor Richard Cheston for his valuable comments and to Dr. Marc Chrysanthou for proofreading this work.

Notes

1 The collective terms, i.e. Black and Minority Ethnic groups (BME) and Black, Asian, Minority Ethnic groups (BAME) imply a single population and do not capture the heterogeneity and diversity of the characteristics of the ethnic groups and subcultures in the UK. These terms are replaced with phrases such as 'culturally diverse groups/population/communities' and 'people with culturally diverse background' in this chapter (NHS Race & Health Observatory, 2022).
2 Calculated based on 3.8 million people aged 65 years and over in the BME population (Lievesley, 2010).

References

Aguilera, A., Garza, M. J., & Munoz, R. F. (2010). Group Cognitive behavioral therapy for depression in Spanish: Culture-sensitive manualised treatment in practice. *Journal of Clinical Psychology*, *66*(8), 857–867.

All-Party Parliamentary Group on Dementia. (2013). *Dementia does not discriminate: The experiences of black, Asian and minority ethnic communities*. At: *Dementia does not discriminate: The experiences of black, Asian and minority ethnic communities*. Retrieved February 5 2024, from alzheimers.org.uk

Alzheimer's Research UK. (2021). *Dementia attitudes monitor: Wave 2 2021.* Retrieved October 31, 2023, from ALZ_DAM_long-Report_21_LR_WEB_FINAL2.pdf. alzheimersresearchuk.org

Alzheimer's Research UK. (2022). *Project at University of Wolverhampton to protect brain health in Chinese communities.* Retrieved October 31, 2023, from https://www.alzheimersresearchuk.org/project-at-university-of-wolverhampton-to-promote-brain-health-in-chinese-communities/

Alzheimer's Society. (2022). *Black, Asian and minority ethnic communities and dementia research.* Retrieved October 31, 2023, from https://www.alzheimers.org.uk/for-researchers/black-asian-and-minority-ethnic-communities-and-dementia-research

Alzheimer's Society. (2023). *Facts for the media about dementia. facts for the media about dementia.* Alzheimer's Society. Retrieved October 31, 2023, from alzheimers.org.uk

An, M., Dusing, S. C., Harbourne, R. T., Sheridan, S. M., & START-Play Consortium. (2020). What really works in intervention? Using fidelity measures to support optimal outcomes. *American Physical Therapy Association, 100*(5), 757–765.

Anwuluorah, Q. U., Lim, J. N. W., Chrysanthou, M., & Bauermeister, S. (2022, June 20). Factors affecting participation in medical/health research in black and minority ethnic groups: A scoping review. Annual Research Conference (ARC), Faculty of Education, Health and Wellbeing. Researchers' Week 2022 Programme.

Backer, T. (2001). Finding the Balance: Program fidelity and adaptation in substance abuse prevention (a state-of-art review). US Department of Health and Human Services: F&A 2002. csun.edu

Baghirathan, S., Cheston, R., Hui, R., Chacon, A., Shears, P., & Currie, K. (2020). A grounded theory analysis of the experiences of carers for people living with dementia from three BAME communities: Balancing the need for support against fears of being diminished. *Dementia (London), 19*(5), 1672–1691. https://doi.org/10.1177/1471301218804714

Bajekal, M., Blane, D., Grewal, I., et al. (2004). Ethnic differences in influences on quality of life at older ages: A quantitative analysis. *Ageing and Society, 24*(5), 709–728.

Barrera, M., Castro, F. G., Strycker, L. A., & Toobert, D. J. (2013). Cultural adaptations of behavioral health interventions: A progress report. *Journal of Consulting and Clinical Psychology, 81*(1), 196–205.

Bernal, G., Bonilla, J., & Bellido, C. (1995). Ecological validity and cultural sensitivity for outcome research: Issues for the cultural adaptation and development of psychosocial treatments with Hispanics. *Journal of Abnormal Child Psychology, 23*(1), 67–82.

Bernal, G., Jimenez-Chafey, M. I., & Domenech Rodríguez, M. M. (2009). Cultural adaptation of treatments: A resource for considering culture in evidence-based practice. *Professional Psychology: Research and Practice, 40*(4), 361–368.

Blakemore, A., Kenning, C., Mirza, N., Daker-White, G., Panagioti, M., & Waheed, W. (2018). Dementia in UK South Asians: A scoping review of the literature. *BMJ Open; 8*(4), e020290

Blasé, K., & Fixsen, D. (2013). *Core intervention components: Identifying and operationalizing what makes programs work. ASPE research brief.* US Department of Health and Human Services.

Bothongo, P. L. K., Jitlal, M.,Parry, E., Foote, E. F., Waters, S., et al. (2020). *Ethnic and socioeconomic determinants of dementia risk: A nested case-control study in the population of East London.* Alzeihmer's and Dementia. https://doi.org/10.1002/alz.037869

Bothongo, P. L. K., Jitlal, M., Parry, E., Foote, E. F., Waters, S., et al. (2022). Dementia risk in a diverse population: A single-region nested case-control study in the east end of London. *Lancet Regional Health, 15,* 100321.

Brijnath, B., Croy, S., Sabates, J., Thodis, A., Ellis, S., de Crespigny, F., Moxey, A., et al. (2021). Including ethnic minorities in dementia research: Recommendations from a scoping review. *Alzheimer's & Dementia: Translational Research & Clinical Intervention, 8*(1), e12222.

Castro, F. G. (1998). Cultural competence training in clinical psychology: Assessment, clinical intervention, and research. In A. S. Bellack & M. Hersen (Eds.), *Comprehensive clinical psychology: Sociocultural and individual differences* (Vol. 10, pp. 127–140). Pergamon.

Castro, F. G., Barrera, M., & Martinez, C. R. (2004). The cultural adaptation of prevention interventions: Resolving tension between fidelity and fit. *Prevention Science, 5*(1), 41–45.

Castro, F. G., Rawson, R., & Obert, J. (2001, December 6–7). *Cultural and treatment issues in the adaptation of the Matrix model for implementation in Mexico.* Paper Presented at the Centros de Integracion Juvenil Conference on Drug Abuse Treatment, Mexico City, Mexico.

Chu, J. P., Huynh, L., & Aean, P. (2012). Cultural adaptation of evidence-based practice utilizing an interative stakeholder process and theoretical framework: Problem solving therapy for Chinese older adults. *International Journal Geriatric Psychology, 49,* 255–263.

Chu, J. P., & Leino, A. (2017). Advancement in the maturing science of cultural adaptations of evidence-based interventions. *Journal of Consulting and Clinical Psychology, 85*(1), 45–57.

Co, M., Couch, E., Gao, Q., Mac-Ginty, S., Das-Munshi, J., & Prina, M. (2021). Access to health services in older minority ethnic groups with dementia: A systematic review. *Journal of American Geriatric Society, 69*(3), 822–834.

Curtis, E., Jones, R., Tipene-Leach, D., Walker, C., Loring, B., Paine, S. J., & Reid, P. (2019). Why cultural safety rather than cultural competency is required to achieve health equity: A literature review and recommended definition. *International Journal for Equity in Health, 18*(1), 174.

Davies, P., Walker, A. E., & Grimshaw, J. M. (2010). A systematic review of the use of theory in the design of guideline dissemination and implementation strategies and interpretation of the results of rigorous evaluations. *Implementation Science, 5,* 1–6.

Deardorff, D. K. (2009). *The sage handbook of intercultural competence.* Sage Publications.

Dementia UK. Young Onset Dementia. (2022). Retrieved October 31, 2023, from https://www.dementiauk.org/about-dementia/young-onset-dementia/

Department of Health and Social Care. (2016). *Challenge on dementia 2020: Implementation Plan. Challenge on dementia 2020: Implementation plan - GOV.UK.* Retrieved October 31, 2023, from www.gov.uk

Dodd, E., Pracownik, R., Popel, S., Collings, S., Emmens, T., & Cheston, R. (2020). Dementia services for people from Black, Asian and minority ethnic and white-British communities: Does a primary care based model contribute to equality in service provision? *Health and Social Care in the Community, 30*(2), 622–630.

Durlak, J. A., & DuPre, E. P. (2008). Implementation matters: A review of research on the influence of implementation on program outcomes and the factors affecting implementation. *American Journal of Community Psychology, 41*(3–4), 327–350.

Evandrou, M. (2000). Social inequalities in later life: The socio-economic position of older people from ethnic minority groups in Britain. *Population Trends, 101,* 11–18.

Evandrou, M., Falkingham, J., Feng, X., & Vlachantoni, A. (2016). Ethnic inequalities in limiting health and self-reported health in later life revisited. *Journal of Epidemiology and Community Health, 70*(7), 653–662.

Falicov, C. J. (2009). Commentary: On the wisdom and challenges of culturally attuned treatments for Latinos. *Family Process, 48*(2), 292–309.

Fixsen, D. L., Naoom, S. F., Blasé, K. A., Friedman, R. M., & Wallace, F. (2001). *Implementation Research: A Synthesis of the Literature. Implementation Research: A Synthesis of the Literature | NIRN.* Retrieved October 31, 2023, from unc.edu

Gallagher-Thompson, D., Arean, P., Coon, D., Menedez, A., Takagi, K., et al. (2000). Development and implementation of intervention strategies for culturally diverse caregiving populations. In R. Schultz (Ed.), *Handbook on dementia caregiving: Evidence-based intervention for family caregiver.* Springer Publishing Co, 151–185.

Harrison, E. K., & Smart, A. (2016). The under-representation of minority ethnic groups in UK medical research. *Ethnicity and Health, 22*(1), 65–82. https://doi.org/10.1080/13557858.2016.1182126

Huey, S. J., & Tilley, J. L. (2018). Effects of mental health interventions with Asian Americans: A review and meta-analysis. *Journal of Consulting and Clinical Psychology, 86*(11), 915–930. https://doi.org/10.1037/ccp0000346

Huggins, L. K. L., Min, S. H., Dennis, C.-A., Ostbye, T., Johnson, K. S., & Xu, H. (2021). Interventions to promote knowledge among racial/ethnic minority groups: A systematic review. *Journal of the American Geriatrics Society, 70,* 609–621.

James, T., Mukadam, N., Sommerlad, A., Cebellos, & Livingston, G. (2021). Culturally tailored therapeutic interventions for people affected by dementia: A systematic review and new conceptual model. *Lancet Healthy Longev.*, *2*(3), e171–e179.

Jani, J. S., Ortiz, L., & Aranda, M. P. (2008). Latino outcome studies in social work: A review of the literature. *Research on Social Work Practice*, *19*(2), 179–194.

Kandiah, N., Vivian, W., Xuling, L., Mei Mei, N., Lim, L., Ng, A., et al. (2016). Cost related to dementia in the young and the impact of etiological subtype on cost. *Journal of Alzheimer's Disease*, *49*(2), 277–285. https://doi.org/10.3233/JAD-150471

Kenning, C., Daker-White, G., Blakemore, A., Panagioti, M., & Wahee, W. (2017). Barriers and facilitators in accessing dementia care by ethnic minority groups: A meta-synthesis of qualitative studies. *BMC Psychiatry*, *17*(1), 316. https://doi.org/10.1186/s12888-017-1474-0

Kirby, D. (2002). Effective approaches to reducing adolescent unprotected sex, pregnancy, and childbearing. *Journal of Sex Research*, *39*(1), 51–57.

Knapp, M., Prince, M., Albanese, E., Banerjee, S., Dhanasiri, S., Fernandez, J.-L., Ferri, C., McCrone, P., Snell, T., & Stewart, R. (2007). The full report. alzheimers_16425.

Kreuter, M. W., Lukwago, S. N., Bucholtz, D. C., Clark, E. M., & Sanders-Thompson, V. (2004). Achieving cultural appropriateness in health promotion programs: Targeted and tailored approaches. *Health Education and Behavior*, *30*(2003), 133–146. https://doi.org/10.1016/j.ypmed

Kreuter, M. W., & Skinner, C. S. (2000). Tailoring: What's in a name? *Health Education Research*, *15*(1), 1–4. https://doi.org/10.1093/her/15.1.1

Leininger, M., & McFarland, M. R. (2002). *Transcultural nursing: Concepts, theories, research, and practice* (3rd ed.). McGraw Hill.

Lievesley, N. (2010). *The future ageing of the ethnic minority population of England and Wales. The future ageing of the ethnic minority population of England and wales. Pdf.* Retrieved October 31, 2023, from cpa.org.uk

Lim, J. N. W., Almeida, R., Holthoff-Detto, V., Ludden, G. D. S., Smith, T., Niedderer, K., & The MinD Consortium. (2019). What is needed to obtain informed consent and monitor capacity for a successful study involving people with mild dementia? Our experience in a multi-centre study. In K. Niedderer, G. D. S. Ludden, R. Cain, & C. Woelfel (Eds.), *Designing with and for people with dementia: Wellbeing, empowerment and happiness. Proceedings of the international mind conference.* MinD & TUD Press. Designing with and for People with Dementia. core.ac.uk

Ma, K. P. K., & Saw, A. (2020). An international systematic review of dementia caregiving interventions for Chinese families. *International Journal of Geriatric Psychiatry*, *35*(11), 1263–1284.

Marín, G. (1993). Defining culturally appropriate community interventions: Hispanics as a case study. *Journal of Community Psychology*, *21*(2). https://doi.org/10.1002/1520-6629(199304)21:2<149::AID-JCOP2290210207>3.0.CO;2-Y

Marsiglia, F. F., & Booth, J. M. (2015). Cultural adaptation of interventions in real practice settings. *Research on Social Work Practice*, *25*(4), 423–432.

Michie, S., Fixsen, D. L., Grimshaw, J. M., & Eccles, M. P. (2009). Specifying and reporting complex behaviour change interventions: The need for a scientific method. *Implementation Science*, *4*, 1–6.

Mills, E., Seely, D., Rachlis, B., Griffith, L., Wu, P., Wilson, K., Ellis, P., & Wright, J. (2006). Barriers to participation in clinical trials of cancer: A meta-analysis and systematic review of patient-reported factors. *Lancet Oncology*, *7*(2), 141–148.

Minkler, M., & Wallenstein, N. (2011). *Community-based participatory research for health: From process to outcomes.* Jossey-Bass.

Moriarty, J., Sharif, N., & Robinson, J. (2011). *Black and minority ethnic people with dementia and their access to support and services. Social care institute for excellence, research briefing, black and minority ethnic people with dementia and their access to support and services.* Retrieved October 31, 2023, from kcl.ac.uk

Mukadam, N., Cooper, C., & Livingston, G. (2011). A systematic review of ethnicity and pathways to care in dementia. *International Journal of Geriatric Psychiatry*, *26*(1), 12–20. https://doi.org/10.1002/gps.2484

Mukadam, N., Cooper, C., & Livingston, G. (2013). Improving access to dementia services for people from minority ethnic groups. *Current Opinion in Psychiatry*, *26*(4), 409–414. https://doi.org/10.1097/YCO.0b013e32835ee668

Napoles, A. M., Chadiha, L., Eversley, R., & Moreno-John, G. (2010). Developing culturally sensitive dementia caregiver interventions: Are we there yet? *American Journal of Alzheimer's Disease and Other Dementias*, *25*(5), 389–406.

NASEM (National Academy of Sciences, Engineering and Medicine). (2019). *Effective Implementation: Core components, adaptation and strategies*. National Academies Press.

National Collaborating Centre for Mental Health. (2018). *Dementia care pathway: Full implementation guidance. Nccmh-dementia-care-pathway-full-implementation-guidance.pdf*. Retrieved October 31, 2023, from rcpsych.ac.uk

NHS Race & Health Observatory. (2022). *The power of language: A consultation report on the use of collective terminology at the NHS race & health observatory*. Retrieved October 31, 2023, from https://www.nhsrho.org/publications/nhs-race-health-observatory-terminology-consultation-report/

Oakley, A., Wiggins, M., Turner, H., Rajan, l., & Barker, M. (2003). Including culturally diverse samples in Health Research: A case study of an urban trial of social support. *Ethnicity and Health*, *8*(1), 29–39.

Peters, D. H., Adam, T., Alonge, O., Agyepong, I. A., & Tran, N. (2013). Implementation research: What it is and how to do it. *BMJ*, *347*, f6753. https://doi.org/10.1136/bmj.f6753

Proctor, E. K., Powell, B. J., & McMillen, J. C. (2013). Implementation Strategies: Recommendations for specifying and reporting. *Implementation Science*, *8*, 139–150.

Resnicow, K., Baranowski, T., Ahluwalia, J. S., & Braithwaite, R. L. (1999). Cultural sensitivity in public health: Defined and demystified. *Ethnicity and Disease*, *9*(1), 10–21.

Roche, M., Higgs, P., Aworinde, J., & Cooper, C. (2021). A review of qualitative research of perception and experiences of dementia among adults from black, African, and Caribbean background: What and whom are we researching? *Gerontologist*, *61*(5), e195–e208. https://doi.org/10.1093/geront/gnaa004

Roche, M., Mukadam, N., Adelman, S., & Livingston, G. (2021). The IDEMCare Study – Improving dementia care in Black African and Caribbean groups: A feasibility cluster randomised controlled trial. *International Journal of Geriatric Psychiatry*, *33*(8), 1048–1056. https://doi.org/10.1002/gps.4891

Shah, H., Albanese, E., Duggan, C., Rudan, I., Langa, K., Carrillo, M., et al. (2016). Research priorities to reduce the global burden of dementia by 2025. *Lancet Neurology*, *15*(12), 1285–1294. https://doi.org/10.1016/S1474-4422(16)30235-6

Skaff, M. M., Chesla, C. A., Mycue, V. D., & Fisher, L. (2002). Lessons in cultural competence: Adapting research methodology for Latino participants. *Journal of Community Psychology*, *30*(3), 305–323.

Society for Women's Health Research United States Food and Drug Administration Office of Women's Health. Dialogues on Diversifying Clinical Trials: Successful Strategies for Engaging Women and Minorities in Clinical Trials. (2011). Retrieved October 31, 2023, from White Paper on the Dialogues on Diversifying Clinical Trials Conference. fda.gov

Torres-Ruiz, M., Robinson-Ector, K., Attinson, D., Trotter, J., Anise, A., & Clauser, S. (2018). A portfolio analysis of culturally tailored trials to address health and healthcare disparities. *International Journal of Environmental Research and Public Health*, *15*(9), 1859. https://doi.org/10.3390/ijerph15091859

UK Home Office. (2023a). *Statistics on Ukrainians in the UK. Statistics on Ukrainians in the UK - GOV. UK*. Retrieved October 31, 2023, from www.gov.uk

UK Home Office. (2023b). *How many people come to the UK each year (including visitors)? How many people come to the UK each year (including visitors)? - GOV.UK*. Retrieved October 31, 2023, from www.gov.uk

Vila-Castelar, C., Fox-Fuller, J. T., Guzman-Velez, E., Schoemaker, D., & Quiroz, Y. T. (2022). A cultural approach to dementia: Insights from US Latino and other minoritized groups. *Nature Reviews – Neurology*, *18*(5), 307–314. https://doi.org/10.1038/s41582-022-00630-z

Wandersman, A., Duffy, J., Flaspohler, P., Noonan, R., Lubell, K., Stillman, L., et al. (2008). Bridging the gap between prevention research and practice: The Interactive Systems Framework for dissemination and implementation. *American Journal of Community Psychology*, *41*(3–4), 171–181.

Weinstein, N. (1998). The precaution adoption process. *Health Psychology*, *7*, 4.

Wilson, A., Bankar, J., Regen, E., Phelps, K., Agarwal, S., Johnson, M., et al. (2020). Ethnic variations in referrals to the Leicester memory and dementia assessment service, 2010 to 2017. *BJPsych Open, 6*(5), e83. https://doi.org/10.1192/bjo.2020.69

Wilson, B. D. M., & Miller, R. L. (2003). Examining strategies for culturally grounded HIV prevention: A review. *AIDS Education and Prevention, 15*(2), 184–202. https://doi.org/10.1521/aeap.15.3.184.23838

Wright, L. (2020). Arts engagement, mortality and dementia: What can the data say? *Journal of Epidemiology and Community Health, 74*(9), 764. https://doi.org/10.1136/jech-2020-214227

21 Design principles and guidelines for inclusive mHealth design for people living with dementia

Thomas Engelsma, Monique W. M. Jaspers and Linda W. P. Peute

Introduction

Mobile health or mHealth applications aim to fulfil innovative functions in providing effective and efficient care. They have the potential to, for example, provide resources and strategies to support people living with dementia and their loved ones (Yousaf et al., 2019). These people can be supported with cognitive training and activities of daily living, screening, health and safety monitoring, leisure and socialisation, or navigation (Yousaf et al., 2019). However, mHealth tools do not always meet the capabilities, needs and preferences of the users, which might be due to poor usability.

Defined by the International Organization for Standardization, or ISO, usability is: 'the extent to which a system, product or service can be used by specified users to achieve specified goals with effectiveness, efficiency and satisfaction in a specified context of use' (International Organization for Standardization, 2013). Poor usability of mHealth can be caused by a lack of inclusive design and may result in low acceptability and uptake. When applying inclusive design, tools for universal audiences or specified users are designed to be accessible for all potential users with their wide ranges of (in)capabilities, caused by, for example, cognitive or visual impairments. Without an inclusive design approach, mHealth can be considered easy to use and intuitive for a universal audience but might not be sufficiently designed nor tested with more vulnerable populations such as those living with dementia. For those people, poorly designed mHealth can introduce the previously mentioned usability issues.

Inclusive mHealth design efforts must be built on evidence, to increase willingness to use, alongside enhancing the accessibility, usability and retention rates of mHealth technologies. A first step to support inclusive mHealth design is to provide context-specific principles and guidelines for both user-interface and user-experience design that are aligned with the capabilities, needs and wishes of the end-users. From the users' perspective, a well-designed user-interface is easy to understand and operate, allowing them to execute tasks successfully and efficiently while also feeling competent and content. Human interface design principles provide high-level considerations that are seen as foundations for good design and are used to create effective user interfaces of tools. Existing design principles are based on research in the field of cognitive psychology, human-computer interaction and best practices of design (Constantine & Lockwood, 1999; Cooper & Reimann, 2003; Gerhardt-Powals, 1996; Lidwell et al., 2010; Shneiderman et al., 2017; Nielsen, 1994). Design guidelines show how to apply design principles in practice (Wang & Huang, 2015).

The development of mHealth for people living with dementia is highly complex and brings challenges. These people experience unique combinations of (1) types of dementia, (2) stage of dementia and (3) comorbidities, leading to varying patterns of symptoms that can hamper mHealth use. To contribute to this challenge, we identified and captured these barriers to

DOI: 10.4324/9781003318262-27

mHealth use in a literature-based model utilising a human factors approach. 'Human factors' is defined as: 'the scientific discipline concerned with the understanding of interactions among human and other elements of a system, and the profession that applies theory, principles, data and methods to design in order to optimise human well-being and overall system performance' (International Organization for Standardization, 2011). Human-factors design thus aims to improve the interactive components of products to decrease the potential for human error.

Scientific literature on studies applying human-factors approaches, such as usability evaluations or co-design studies, was reviewed and led to the development of the MOLDEM-US model (**MH**ealth for **OL**der adults with **DEM**entia – **US**ability) (Engelsma et al., 2021). This model provides high- level insights on potential barriers to mHealth use for those living with Alzheimer's disease and related dementias (ADRD). MOLDEM-US is based on the previously developed MOLD-US model (**MH**ealth for **OLD**er adults – **US**ability) as a base. MOLD-US captures barriers to mHealth use for the general aging population (Wildenbos et al., 2018). Applying this knowledge on barriers to mHealth use throughout the user-centred design process has the potential to increase the usability of mHealth. Both models will be further introduced in the next sections.

This chapter presents the application of design principles for people living with dementia and sets out guidance aimed at improving their experienced usability of mHealth. We gathered available suggestions to improve mHealth design through a similar literature-based human-factors approach. We have synthesised our findings into four categories: cognition, perception, frame of mind and speech and language.

The MOLD-US model

The MOLD-US model was created through a scoping literature review, by assembling scattered data on ageing-related human-factors across different clinical areas that introduce barriers to using mHealth applications. As described, these barriers can influence the usability and understandability of mHealth functionalities by older adults (Joe & Demiris, 2013; Gao et al., 2017) and pose user-errors that can lead to safety issues (Akbar et al., 2020). The medical domains associated with chronic diseases captured in the MOLD-US model include, among others, diabetes, stroke, multiple sclerosis, motor neurone disease, Parkinson's disease, glaucoma, depression and rheumatoid arthritis. MOLD-US relates the intricacies of these chronic diseases to their possible impact on the mHealth user-experience for older adults. These intricacies are classified into the following categories: cognition, motivation, perception and physical ability. Applying the MOLD-US model in the development, implementation and evaluation of mHealth applications can contribute to improving the safe use and adoption of these applications by older adults. In research, MOLD-US has been utilised to capture and classify usability problems resulting from usability testing with older patients suffering from chronic conditions such as heart failure and COPD (Wildenbos et al., 2019).

Expanding MOLD-US: MOLDEM-US

For the ageing population, general barriers to the use of mHealth are captured in the MOLD-US model. Dementia is one of the leading chronic diseases for the ageing population, characterised by specific symptoms that transcend those of the general aging population. Extensive research was in place to expand the MOLD-US model with an in-depth analysis of dementia-specific symptoms that can further pose particular barriers to mHealth use. Through a scoping review on usability studies with people living with dementia and clinical literature on dementia symptoms, additional barriers were identified that can potentially affect mHealth use by these people (Figure 21.1). This extended model is called MOLDEM-US. It distinguishes barriers that were (1) identified in usability studies with people living with dementia and dementia-related clinical literature *(ADRD-specific)*, (2) already captured in MOLD-US but *not* identified through the scoping review in contribution to the development of MOLDEM-US *(General* Ageing) and (3) *both* already captured in MOLD-US and also in usability studies with people living with dementia and dementia-clinical literature to expand MOLD-US to MOLDEM-US *(General ADRD Ageing)*. Sufficient dementia-specific barriers related to speech and language were identified to be organised in a new category. In addition, the motivation category was reformulated to 'frame of mind', as the identified barriers are not directly influenced by motivation but can cause motivational decline.

From barriers to design principles: the first steps

Design principles aiming to tackle the barriers to mHealth use for those living with dementia have been composed to promote inclusive mHealth designs (Figure 21.2). We have developed some context-specific guidance to apply these design principles with the aim of improving the usability of mHealth applications. These design guidelines were identified through literature, extracted and mapped onto the categories in MOLDEM-US. It is acknowledged that these design principles can be interdependent. To illustrate: a tutorial should be provided to users before an mHealth application is introduced to them. However, the development of a tutorial should also adhere to design principles related to cognition, perception, frame of mind and speech and language barriers. Another example concerns the implementation of rewards when a task has been completed successfully by a user, such as daily physical exercises, as this increases the willingness to use an application. This would address barriers from the frame-of-mind category. However, confirming that a task has been successfully completed could also help overcome cognitive barriers, as users should be able to track their task progress and completion.

Design principles and guidance to tackle cognitive barriers

Cognitive deterioration ranges in severity as dementia is a progressive disease. However, it includes issues with thinking speed, memory, reasoning, learning, planning and performing familiar tasks, spatial cognition, attention, making decisions and judgements, planning and organising thoughts or actions (Engelsma et al., 2021). Cognitive impairment may cause various issues with using mHealth, such as difficulties with learning and remembering how to use the mHealth application, posing interaction difficulties (Boman et al., 2014; Fardoun et al., 2017; Gonzalez-Palau et al., 2013; Span et al., 2015). Various hindrances, or usability issues, with respect to mHealth use include: experienced difficulty to perform or recollect a sequence of tasks (Boman et al., 2014; Meiland et al., 2012), being anxious in decision-making due to too complex instructions provided by the application (Riley et al., 2009) or failure to comprehend and recognise such things as symbols or buttons (Meiland et al., 2012).

For each principle, design guidance has been proposed based upon available literature (Table 21.1). First, users should be able to monitor their progress due to the previously mentioned cognitive barriers.This can be supported by implementing checklists, auto-prompts and configurable reminders. Second, users should be provided with tutorials throughout the app. This can support continuous understanding of performing sequences of actions in an app. Such tutorials should be provided at the start of app usage, beusage, step by step. To further support

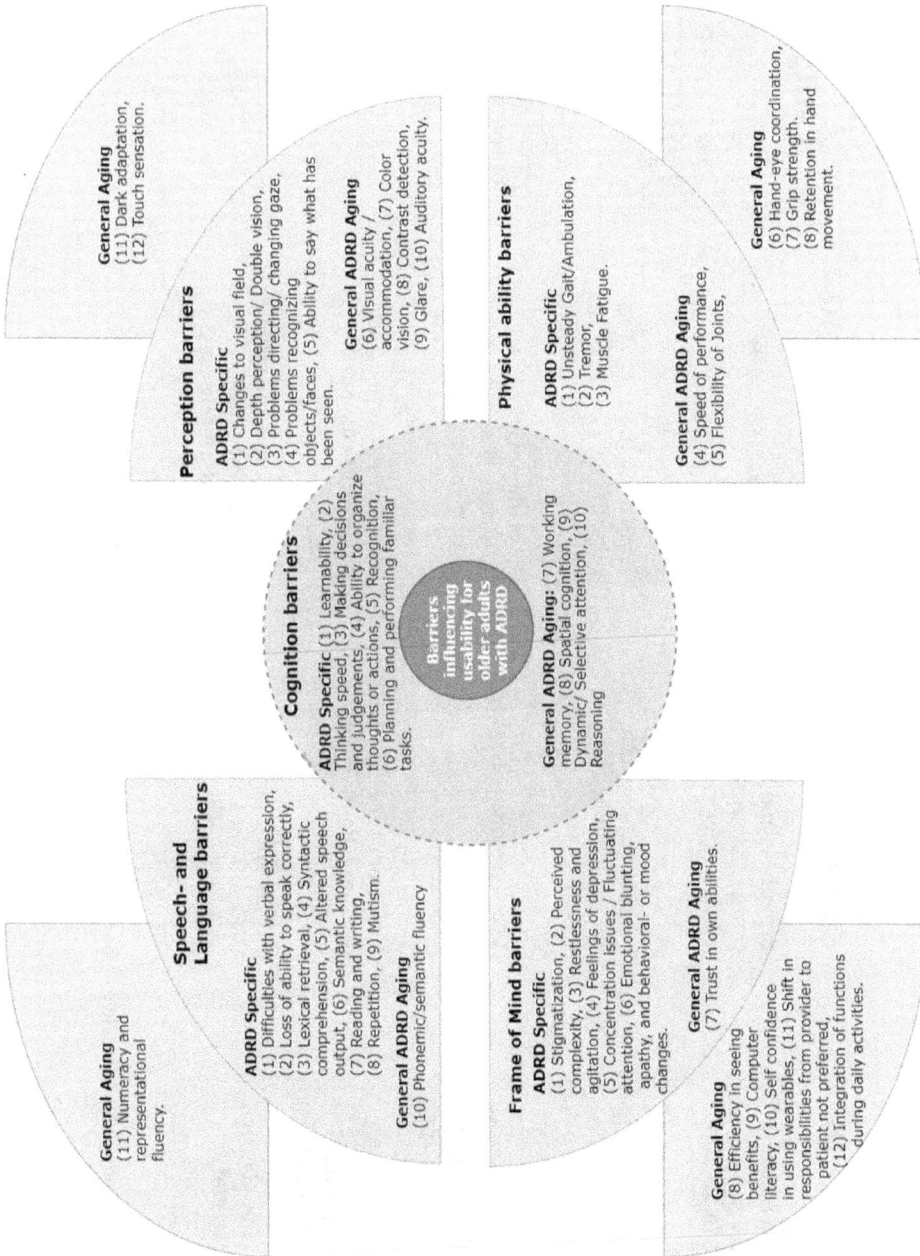

Figure 21.1 The MOLDEM-US model (Engelsma et al., 2021)

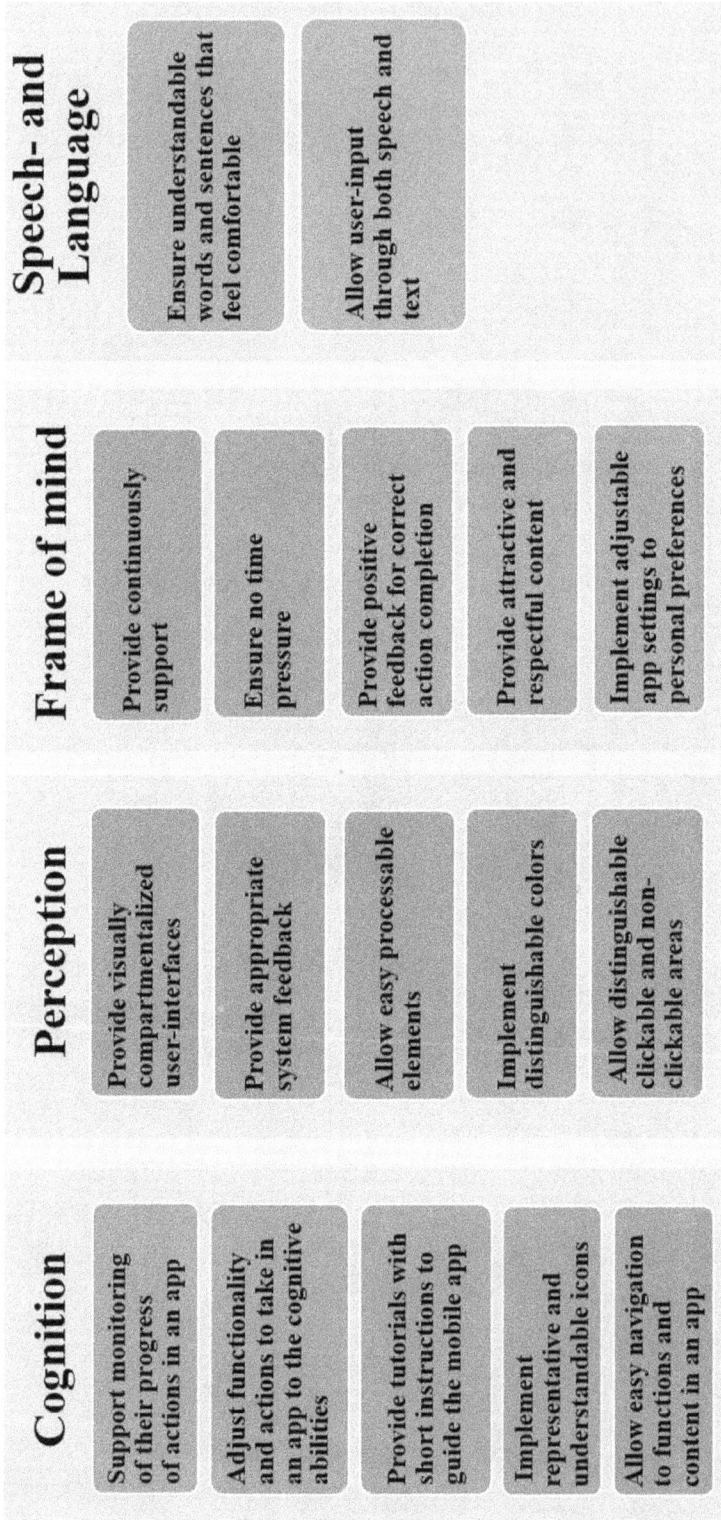

Figure 21.2 Design principles to tackle barriers to mHealth use for people living with dementia

Table 21.1 Design principles and actionable guidelines to tackle cognitive barriers

Design principle to tackle cognition barriers	Actionable Design Guidelines
Support monitoring of their action progress	• **Implement checklists** to support successful completion of daily actions such as symptom monitoring or medication reminders (Anderson et al., 2015; Øksnebjerg et al., 2019) • **Mark progress** by providing a step-by-step linear approach of actions to take (Boyd et al., 2021; Lazarou et al., 2021; Tak, 2021) • **Implement auto-prompt** feature to remind task completion (Joddrell & Astell, 2019) • **Implement configurable reminders** to support system use (Meiland et al., 2012; Lim et al., 2013) • **Minimise steps** for data entry to prevent cognitive overload and ease progress tracking • **Auto-save** functionality (Li et al., 2021) • **Confirm successful task completion** (Li et al., 2021)
Provide tutorials with short instructions to guide the mobile app	• **Tutorial at start** of mobile app usage for user-guidance (Zapata et al., 2015) • **Simple step-by-step tutorials throughout** (Li et al., 2021) • **Show limited information on a single screen** to prevent cognitive overload (Lim et al., 2013; Li et al., 2021; Zapata et al., 2015; Zmily et al., 2014; Ryan et al., 2020; Rai et al., 2020) • **Provide and repeat instructions** (Gonzalez-Palau et al., 2013; Zmily et al., 2014; Koo & Vizer, 2019) • **Break instructions into multiple simple steps** (Zmily et al., 2014) • **Filter irrelevant information** when a subset of functionalities is used (Li et al., 2021)
Provide adjustable functionalities and actions to user's cognitive abilities	• **Implement adaptation of task difficulty** (Gonzalez-Palau et al., 2013; Lazarou et al., 2021; Tak, 2021) • **Allow adaptation of sets of functionalities** to each individual's cognitive abilities (Boman et al., 2014; Joddrell & Astell, 2019; Malinowsky et al., 2014) • **Provide simple items** with potential to get more information on that item (Wesselman et al., 2018)
Allow easy navigation to functions and content in an app	• **Avoid strong hierarchical menu structures** (Li et al., 2021; Isaković et al., 2016) • **Allow to select one control method** (e.g. 'drag and drop' or 'tap') (Joddrell & Astell, 2019) • **Provide linear navigation** rather than a hypertextual structure (Rai et al., 2020)
Implement representative and understandable icons	• **Buttons should look like actual buttons** (Zapata et al., 2015) • **Provide visualisations** after successful task completion (Øksnebjerg et al., 2019) • **Consistent use** of generally intelligible symbols on buttons (Isaković et al., 2016) • **All icons should be visible on the home screen** to prevent scrolling (Li et al., 2021)

monitoring of progress, limited information should be shown on a single screen and instructions should be broken down into multiple steps. Third, functionalities should be adjustable to the user's cognitive abilities. This means that a variety of difficulty levels should be provided that can be easily set by the user or their supporter. Fourth, easy navigation should be ensured through linear navigation and avoidance of hierarchical structures. Moreover, users should be allowed to choose a preferred control method. For understandability, the function of icons should be clear, such as buttons representing the actual action of such icons.

Design principles to tackle perception barriers

Various issues relating to visual and other forms of perception may impair an individual's ability to use mHealth. The Alzheimer's Society mentioned potential hardships like changes to visual field and decreasing visual acuity (Alzheimer's Society, 2016). Other perception barriers that influence mHealth usability include impaired visual fields, double vision, problems with directing

Table 21.2 Design principles and actionable guidelines to tackle perception barriers

Design principle to tackle perception barriers	Actionable Design Guidelines
Provide visually compartmentalised user-interfaces	• **Use bold colours** to compartmentalise content in a user-interface (Boyd et al., 2021) • **Mix typography and iconography** (Boyd et al., 2021) • **Use headings and subheadings** (Li et al., 2021) • **Use standardized rules** (colours, sizes, text) for labelling buttons and icons (Li et al., 2021) • **Differentiate objects from other visual features** (Li et al., 2021)
Provide appropriate system feedback	• **Implement text-to-speech module** (Boman et al., 2014; Fardoun et al., 2017; Gonzalez-Palau et al., 2013) • **Provide audio-based cues** such as volume changes or button activation (Lazarou et al., 2021; Li et al., 2021; Lloyd et al., 2017; Quintana et al., 2020) • **Provide vibrations** for notifications (Lloyd et al., 2017) • **Provide text-based instructions** (Brown & O'Connor, 2020)
Implement distinguishable colours	• **Use clear, colour-neutral, distinguishable colours** to improve readability (Isaković et al., 2016) • **Avoid the use of excessively glaring colours** in images, graphics and depictions (Isaković et al., 2016) • **The colour of components should contrast** with the background (Zapata et al., 2015; Scase et al., 2018)
Allow distinguishable clickable and non-clickable areas	• **Provide simple intuitive distinction between click-sensitive and non-click-sensitive areas** (Isaković et al., 2016; Yi et al., 2021) • **Implement audible beeps** as system feedback to confirm an action on a click-sensitive area (Lloyd et al., 2017)
Allow easily processable elements	• **Options to magnify** elements such as buttons, graphics and text (Li et al., 2021; Yi et al., 2021) • **Use large font size** (Riley et al., 2009; Tak, 2021; Li et al., 2021) • **Implement "touch interface screen readers"** to hear elements like buttons, graphics, tables and text (Li et al., 2021) • **Automatic enlarging of captions and graphics** when user-screening occurs (Kerssens et al., 2015) • **Increase size of reminder pop-ups** to a quarter of the screen and increase when interacted with (Quintana et al., 2020) • **Implement auto-brightness of the screen** to enhance readability (Boman et al., 2014)

gaze, recognising objects, saying what has been seen, depth perception, colour vision, contrast detection, dark adaptation, glare, auditory acuity and touch sensation (Engelsma et al., 2021).

For each principle, design guidance has been developed based on available literature (Table 21.2). First, content in a user interface should be visually compartmentalised. Consider the use of bold colours, a mix of text and icons, and using headings and subheadings to make things clearer. Second, ensure system feedback to the user is provided in an appropriate manner in line with the user's perceptive abilities. This includes the implementation of a text-to-speech module, audio-based cues and vibrations. Third, due to difficulties with colour vision and glare, ensure the use of distinguishable colours that are clear and colour-neutral and are in contrast with the background colours. Fourth, due to potential decreasing touch sensation, the user interface should visually provide the user with cues to distinguish between clickable and non-clickable areas. Finally, elements in a user-interface need to be easily processed by the users. This may include, for example, using magnification user-interface elements, large font sizes, and potentially also "touch interface screen readers".

Design Principles to tackle frame of mind barriers

Changes to the frame of mind can profoundly impact the ability to use mHealth. Examples include: perceived complexity, (in)efficiency in seeing benefits, (less) trust in own ability, restlessness and agitation, limited computer literacy, concentration issues and stigmatisation (Engelsma et al., 2021). Assuming that a mHealth innovation is only created for a certain group can cause feelings of stigmatisation, which decreases one's motivation to use it (Rosenberg et al., 2012). Incorporating context-specific design principles, guidelines and rules for vulnerable populations within existing mHealth apps can improve the (positive) experience of using such apps (Joddrell & Astell, 2019). Barriers to using mHealth can arise if an app is seen to be too intricate to learn how to use it or if tasks to be performed seem to be highly complex (Meiland et al., 2012; Hattink et al., 2014; Howe et al., 2019). To increase willingness to use mHealth, a potential solution is to provide adjusted difficulty levels prior to using the application (Gonzalez-Palau et al., 2013). In addition, the degree of support should be appropriate for a user's abilities to understand or use mHealth (Malinowsky et al., 2014).

For each principle, design guidelines have been developed and founded through available literature (Table 21.3). First, continuous support should be provided to the users. This implies real-time support through, for example a helpdesk, but also implementation of mechanisms in the mHealth application that support users in recovering from errors. Second, the user should not feel pressured due to time. Time-based tasks should generally be avoided. If timers are included, or time to complete an action needs to be measured, timers should count up rather than down. Third, positive feedback should always be provided when an action has been completed successfully. This can be realised by providing failure-free content and allowing users to set goals to receive rewards. In addition, while performing actions, confirmations of successful tasks should be provided and brief encouragements when needed. Fourth, to improve the user's frame of mind, it is important to implement adjustable app settings that are in line with their needs and personal preferences. This can include adaptations based on cognitive or educational level, personalised privacy settings and giving users the options to turn on or off a series of app functionalities. Finally, users need to feel the content is both attractive and respectful. Appropriate language should be provided and stigmatisation throughout the app (titles, textual content and interactive functionalities) avoided.

Table 21.3 Design principles and actionable guidelines to tackle frame of mind barriers

Design principle to tackle frame of mind barriers	Actionable Design Guidelines
Provide continuous support	• **Ensure continuous support,** for instance through a helpdesk. This can be initiated through the action bar or a panic button (Meiland et al., 2012; Riley et al., 2009; Anderson et al., 2015; Howe et al., 2019; Espay et al., 2019; Pulido Herrera, 2017) • **Implement mechanisms to recover from errors** smoothly, such as an undo button (Li et al., 2021)
Ensure no time pressure	• **Allow ample time to respond or react** to improve acceptability and prevent stress (Zmily et al., 2014) • **Timers should count up instead of down** (Rai et al., 2020) • **Provide orientation to time** (Øksnebjerg et al., 2019) • **Implement time-based triggers** to ensure recognition of tasks that should be completed in a recurrent interval (Anderson et al., 2015)
Provide positive feedback for correct action completion	• **Provide failure-free content** (Riley et al., 2009; Alm et al., 2007) • **Allow to set goals and receiving rewards** to increase feelings of success (Lazarou et al., 2021; Li et al., 2021; Isaković et al., 2016; Lloyd et al., 2017) • **Confirm correct steps** to complete an action (Øksnebjerg et al., 2019; Wesselman et al., 2018) • **Provide brief encouragements** during task completion (Koo & Vizer, 2019)
Implement adjustable app settings to personal preferences	• **Pre-set difficulty levels of functionalities** based on educational and cognitive level (Gonzalez-Palau, 2013; Lazarou et al., 2021; Tak, 2021) • **Adjust or customise features** to individual's needs and wishes (Boman et al., 2014; Moehead et al., 2020) • **Implement functionality adaptations as a series of options** to enhance accessibility (Boman et al., 2014; Joddrell & Astell, 2019; Malinowsky et al., 2014) • **Implement personalised privacy settings** (Li et al., 2021)
Provide attractive and respectful content	• **Language should be appropriate,** taking into account age and (health) literacy appropriateness (Scase et al., 2018) • **Prevent stigmatisation** (Meiland et al., 2012; Joddrell & Astell, 2019) • **Use colours in the interface design and graphics** to attract interest (Lazarou et al., 2021)

Design principles to tackle speech and language barriers

Language deficiencies in Alzheimer's disease are present in the early, moderate and late phases (Szatloczki et al., 2015; Tang-Wai & Graham, 2008). Such deficiencies can prompt psychosocial burden (Ferris & Farlow, 2013) and depressive feelings (Potkins et al., 2003), both of which can decrease willingness to use mHealth. Deteriorations in speech and language include problems with syntactic and semantic fluency and comprehension and can pose barriers to mHealth use. Whenever there are components included in an mHealth application that require speech skills, it is critical to understand that a user might experience challenges with this, for example because of word-finding problems, repetitiveness or mutism (Cardarelli et al., 2010).

For each principle, design guidelines have been developed based on available literature (Table 21.4). First, it should be ensured that the difficulty levels of words and sentences are adjusted for the needs of the end users, and the focus should be on wording that makes the user

Table 21.4 Design principles and actionable guidelines to tackle speech- and language-barriers

Design principle to tackle speech- and language-barriers	Actionable Design Guidelines
Ensure understandable words and sentences that feel comfortable	• **Be explicit and consistent with word choice** (Boyd et al., 2021; Li et al., 2021) • **Explain difficult terms** and provide a glossary (Wesselman et al., 2018; Rathnayake et al., 2021) • **Avoid foreign language and technical terms** (Isaković et al., 2016) • **Use plain, appropriate language** with everyday words (Rai et al., 2020; Rathnayake et al., 2021) • **Use age-appropriate wording** (Scase et al., 2018)
Allow user input through both speech and text	• **Adhere to 'clear speech' recommendations:** '*speak slowly but loudly, insert breaks between phrases and sentences, stress keywords, enunciate each word precisely, and 'minimize background noise* (Li et al., 2021) • **Implement text-to-speech technology** to provide system feedback (Boman et al., 2014; Fardoun et al., 2017; Gonzalez-Palau et al., 2013; Li et al., 2021; Pulido Herrera, 2017; Ferrucci et al., 2021; Lancioni et al., 2020) • **Implement speech recognition and analysis** to allow speech input (Span et al., 2015) • **Avoid free text input**s when applicable, for example task completion through touch or slide (Zapata et al., 2015)

feel comfortable. Thus, word choices should be explicit and consistent, and the unavoidable use of difficult terms should be explained, for example, in a glossary. Moreover, the use of foreign language and technical terms should be avoided. Additionally, word choices should be plain and appropriate, using everyday and age-appropriate wording that conforms to the real world. The second principle focuses on the implementation of both textual and spoken user input. To do so, adherence to the clear speech recommendations should be ensured, and text-to-speech technology and speech recognition and analysis should be implemented.

Future steps to optimise mHealth design principles and guidelines

The sets of design principles and guidelines proposed in this chapter provide researchers and software developers with a foundation to further establish, implement and validate inclusive mHealth design principles and guidelines for people living with dementia. In addition, future steps need to be addressed.

First, symptoms related to physical abilities that are caused by dementia and ageing are well known; for example, tremors, decreasing grip strength and less flexible joints that may also influence mHealth application use. However, the approach described in this chapter has not identified any solutions for these potential barriers. In future research, the consequences of physical ability barriers on the use of mHealth applications should be studied from a human factors ergonomic perspective in order to develop design principles and guidelines to tackle these barriers as well.

Second, some design guidelines may become less effective if the user has multi-sensory impairments (both visual and auditory difficulties). When a person has visual impairment, it is usually recommended to implement auditory solutions. However, if both auditory and visual capabilities are severely impaired, these suggestions might not result in higher mHealth usability. Similarly, both auditory and visual solutions may be limited when the user experiences barriers related to speech and language. It should thus be further studied how to tackle these challenges with respect to optimal mHealth design and use.

Third, design principles and guidelines need to be tailored to the different functionalities that mHealth provides to its users. Since existing applications for people living with dementia often address different aspects of dementia, it is important to further specify the applicability of each design guideline to mHealth functionalities such as cognitive training and daily living, screening, health and safety monitoring, leisure and socialisation, or navigation (Yousaf et al., 2019).

In conclusion, through literature, mHealth design principles with context-specific design guidelines for people living with dementia have been composed aiming to tackle human factors that can influence their mHealth use. Validation of these principles and guidelines in future research and design practices are crucial to improve mHealth usability for this population.

References

Akbar, S., Coiera, E., & Magrabi, F. (2019). Safety concerns with consumer-facing mobile health applications and their consequences: A scoping review. *Journal of the American Medical Informatics Association JAMIA, 27*(2), 330–340. https://doi.org/10.1093/jamia/ocz175

Alm, N., Dye, R., Astell, A., Ellis, M., Gowans, G., & Campbell, J. (2007). Making software accessible for users with dementia. In J. Lazar (Ed.), *Universal usability: Designing computer interfaces for diverse user populations* (pp. 299–316).

Alzheimer's Society. (2016). Sight, perception and hallucinations in dementia. *Factsheet*, 527CP.

Anderson, S. M., Riehle, T. H., Lichter, P. A., Brown, A. W., & Panescu, D. (2015). *Smartphone-based system to improve transportation access for the cognitively impaired.* 2015 37th Annual International Conference of the IEEE Engineering in Medicine and Biology Society (EMBC). https://doi.org/10.1109/embc.2015.7320191

Boman, I.-L., Lundberg, S., Starkhammar, S., & Nygård, L. (2014). Exploring the usability of a videophone mock-up for persons with dementia and their significant others. *BMC Geriatrics, 14*(1). https://doi.org/10.1186/1471-2318-14-49

Boyd, K., Bond, R., Ryan, A., Goode, D., & Mulvenna, M. (2021). Digital reminiscence app co-created by people living with dementia and carers: Usability and eye gaze analysis. *Health Expectations, 24*(4), 1207–1219. https://doi.org/10.1111/hex.13251

Brown, A., & O'Connor, S. (2020). Mobile health applications for people with dementia: A systematic review and synthesis of qualitative studies. *Informatics for Health and Social Care, 45*(4), 343–359. https://doi.org/10.1080/17538157.2020.1728536

Cardarelli, R., Kertesz, A., & Knebl, J. A. (2010). Frontotemporal dementia: A review for primary care physicians. *American Family Physician, 82*(11), 1372–1377.

Constantine, L., & Lockwood, L. (1999). *Software for use: A practical guide to the models and methods of usage-centered design.* ACM Press/Addison-Wesley Publishing Co.

Cooper, A., & Reimann, R. (2003). *About face 2.0 the essentials of interaction design.* Wiley.

Engelsma, T., Jaspers, M. W. M., & Peute, L. W. (2021). Considerate mHealth design for older adults with Alzheimer's disease and related Dementias (ADRD): A scoping review on usability barriers and design suggestions. *International Journal of Medical Informatics, 152*, 104494. https://doi.org/10.1016/j.ijmedinf.2021.104494

Espay, A. J., Hausdorff, J. M., Sánchez-Ferro, Á., Klucken, J., Merola, A., Bonato, P., & Maetzler, W. (2019). A roadmap for implementation of patient-centered digital outcome measures in Parkinson's disease obtained using Mobile Health Technologies. *Movement Disorders, 34*(5), 657–663. https://doi.org/10.1002/mds.27671

Fardoun, H. M., Mashat, A. A., & Ramirez Castillo, J. (2015). Recognition of familiar people with a mobile cloud architecture for Alzheimer patients. *Disability and Rehabilitation, 39*(4), 398–402. https://doi.org/10.3109/09638288.2015.1025992

Ferris, S., & Farlow, M. (2013). Language impairment in Alzheimer's disease and benefits of acetyl cholinesterase inhibitors. *Clinical Interventions in Aging, 1007.* https://doi.org/10.2147/cia.s39959

Ferrucci, F., Jorio, M., Marci, S., Bezenchek, A., Diella, G., Nulli, C., & Castelli-Gattinara, G. (2021). A web-based application for complex health care populations: User-centered design approach. *JMIR Human Factors, 8*(1). https://doi.org/10.2196/18587

Gao, C., Zhou, L., Liu, Z., Wang, H., & Bowers, B. (2017). Mobile application for diabetes self-management in China: Do they fit for older adults? *International Journal of Medical Informatics, 101,* 68–74. https://doi.org/10.1016/j.ijmedinf.2017.02.005

Gerhardt-Powals, J. (1996). Cognitive engineering principles for enhancing human-computer performance. *International Journal of Human-Computer Interaction, 8*(2), 189–211.

Gonzalez-Palau, F., Franco, M., Toribio, J. M., Losada, R., Parra, E., & Bamidis, P. (2013). Designing a computer-based rehabilitation solution for older adults: The importance of testing usability. *PsychNology Journal, 11*(2), 119–136.

Hattink, B. J., Meiland, F. J., Overmars-Marx, T., de Boer, M., Ebben, P. W., van Blanken, M., & Dröes, R. M. (2014). The electronic, personalizable Rosetta system for dementia care: Exploring the user-friendliness, usefulness and impact. *Disability and Rehabilitation: Assistive Technology, 11*(1), 61–71. https://doi.org/10.3109/17483107.2014.932022

Howe, D., Thorpe, J., Dunn, R., White, C., Cunnah, K., Platt, R., & Wolverson, E. (2019). The CAREGIVERSPRO-MMD platform as an online informational and social support tool for people living with memory problems and their carers: An evaluation of user engagement, usability and usefulness. *Journal of Applied Gerontology, 39*(12), 1303–1312. https://doi.org/10.1177/0733464819885326

International Organization for Standardization. (2011). *ISO 26800:2011(en). Ergonomics – General approach, principles, and concepts.* https://www.iso.org/standard/42885.html

International Organization for Standardization. (2013). *ISO/TS 20282-2:2013(en), Usability of consumer products and products for public use — Part 2: Summative test method.* https://www.iso.org/standard/62733.html

Isaković, M., Sedlar, U., Volk, M., & Bešter, J. (2016). Usability pitfalls of diabetes mHealth apps for the elderly. *Journal of Diabetes Research, 2016,* 1–9. https://doi.org/10.1155/2016/1604609

Joddrell, P., & Astell, A. J. (2019). Implementing accessibility settings in touchscreen apps for people living with dementia. *Gerontology, 65*(5), 560–570. https://doi.org/10.1159/000498885

Joe, J., & Demiris, G. (2013). Older adults and mobile phones for health: A review. *Journal of Biomedical Informatics, 46*(5), 947–954. https://doi.org/10.1016/j.jbi.2013.06.008

Kerssens, C., Kumar, R., Adams, A. E., Knott, C. C., Matalenas, L., Sanford, J. A., & Rogers, W. A. (2015). Personalized technology to support older adults with and without cognitive impairment living at home. *American Journal of Alzheimer's Disease and Other Dementias, 30*(1), 85–97. https://doi.org/10.1177/1533317514568338

Koo, B. M., & Vizer, L. M. (2019). Examining mobile technologies to support older adults with dementia through the lens of personhood and human needs: Scoping review. *JMIR mHealth and uHealth, 7*(11). https://doi.org/10.2196/15122

Lancioni, G. E., Singh, N. N., O'Reilly, M. F., Sigafoos, J., D'Amico, F., De Vanna, F., & Pinto, K. (2019). Smartphone technology for fostering goal-directed ambulation and object use in people with moderate Alzheimer's disease. *Disability and Rehabilitation: Assistive Technology, 15*(7), 754–761. https://doi.org/10.1080/17483107.2019.1686075

Lazarou, I., Stavropoulos, T. G., Mpaltadoros, L., Nikolopoulos, S., Koumanakos, G., Tsolaki, M., & Kompatsiaris, I. (2021). Human factors and requirements of people with cognitive impairment, their caregivers, and healthcare professionals for mHealth apps including reminders, games, and geolocation Tracking: A survey-questionnaire study. *Journal of Alzheimer's Disease Reports, 5*(1), 497–513. https://doi.org/10.3233/adr-201001

Li, C., Neugroschl, J., Zhu, C. W., Aloysi, A., Schimming, C. A., Cai, D., & Sano, M. (2021). Design considerations for Mobile Health Applications Targeting Older Adults. *Journal of Alzheimer's Disease*, *79*(1), 1–8. https://doi.org/10.3233/jad-200485

Lidwell, W., Holden, K., & Butler, J. (2010). *Universal principles of design*. Rockport Publishers.

Lim, F. S., Wallace, T., Luszcz, M. A., & Reynolds, K. J. (2013). Usability of tablet computers by people with early-stage dementia. *Gerontology*, *59*(2), 174–182. https://doi.org/10.1159/000343986

Lloyd, G., Munro, S. D., & Arnott, J. L. (2017). Mobile delivery of health information for people with mild cognitive impairment. *Studies in Health Technology and Informatics*, *242*, 31–37.

Malinowsky, C., Nygård, L., & Kottorp, A. (2014). Using a screening tool to evaluate potential use of e-health services for older people with and without cognitive impairment. *Aging &. Mental Health*, *18*(3), 340–345. https://doi.org/10.1080/13607863.2013.832731

Meiland, F. J. M., Bouman, A. I. E., Sävenstedt, S., Bentvelzen, S., Davies, R. J., Mulvenna, M. D., & Dröes, R.-M. (2012). Usability of a new electronic assistive device for community-dwelling persons with mild dementia. *Aging &. Mental Health*, *16*(5), 584–591. https://doi.org/10.1080/13607863.2011.651433

Moehead, A., DeSouza, K., Walsh, K., & Pit, S. W. (2020). A web-based dementia education program and its application to an Australian web-based Dementia Care Competency and training network: Integrative systematic review. *Journal of Medical Internet Research*, *22*(1). https://doi.org/10.2196/16808

Nielsen, J. (1994, April 24–28). Enhancing the explanatory power of usability heuristics. Proceedings of the ACM CHI'94 conference, Boston, MA, pp. 52–158.

Øksnebjerg, L., Woods, B., & Waldemar, G. (2019). Designing the react app to support self-management of people with dementia: An iterative user-involving process. *Gerontology*, *65*(6), 673–685. https://doi.org/10.1159/000500445

Potkins, D., Myint, P., Bannister, C., Tadros, G., Chithramohan, R., Swann, A., & Margallo-Lana, M. (2003). Language impairment in dementia: Impact on symptoms and care needs in residential homes. *International Journal of Geriatric Psychiatry*, *18*(11), 1002–1006. https://doi.org/10.1002/gps.1002

Pulido Herrera, E. (2016). Location-based technologies for supporting elderly pedestrian in "getting lost" events. *Disability and Rehabilitation: Assistive Technology*, *12*(4), 315–323. https://doi.org/10.1080/17483107.2016.1181799

Quintana, M., Anderberg, P., Sanmartin Berglund, J., Frögren, J., Cano, N., Cellek, S., & Garolera, M. (2020). Feasibility-usability study of a tablet app adapted specifically for persons with cognitive impairment—SMART4MD (support monitoring and reminder technology for mild dementia). *International Journal of Environmental Research and Public Health*, *17*(18), 6816. https://doi.org/10.3390/ijerph17186816

Rai, H. K., Schneider, J., & Orrell, M. (2020). An individual cognitive stimulation therapy app for people with dementia: Development and usability study of Thinkability. *JMIR Aging*, *3*(2). https://doi.org/10.2196/17105

Rathnayake, S., Moyle, W., Jones, C., & Calleja, P. (2020). Co-design of an mHealth application for family caregivers of people with dementia to address functional disability care needs. *Informatics for Health and Social Care*, *46*(1), 1–17. https://doi.org/10.1080/17538157.2020.1793347

Riley, P., Alm, N., & Newell, A. (2009). An interactive tool to promote musical creativity in people with dementia. *Computers in Human Behavior*, *25*(3), 599–608. https://doi.org/10.1016/j.chb.2008.08.014

Rosenberg, L., Kottorp, A., & Nygård, L. (2011). Readiness for technology use with people with dementia. *Journal of Applied Gerontology*, *31*(4), 510–530. https://doi.org/10.1177/0733464810396873

Ryan, A. A., McCauley, C. O., Laird, E. A., Gibson, A., Mulvenna, M. D., Bond, R., & Ferry, F. (2018). 'There is still so much inside': The impact of personalised reminiscence, facilitated by a tablet device, on people living with mild to moderate dementia and their family carers. *Dementia*, *19*(4), 1131–1150. https://doi.org/10.1177/1471301218795242

Scase, M., Kreiner, K., & Ascolese, A. (2018). Development and evaluation of cognitive games to promote health and wellbeing in elderly people with mild cognitive impairment. *Studies in Health Technology and Informatics*, *248*, 255–262.

Shneiderman, B., Plaisant, C., Cohen, M., Jacobs, S. M., & Elmqvist, N. (2017). *Designing the user interface: Strategies for effective human-computer interaction*. Pearson Education Limited.

Span, M., Smits, C., Jukema, J., Groen-van de Ven, L., Janssen, R., Vernooij-Dassen, M., & Hettinga, M. (2015). An interactive web tool for facilitating shared decision-making in dementia-care networks: A field study. *Frontiers in Aging Neuroscience, 7.* https://doi.org/10.3389/fnagi.2015.00128

Szatloczki, G., Hoffmann, I., Vincze, V., Kalman, J., & Pakaski, M. (2015). Speaking in Alzheimer's disease, is that an early sign? importance of changes in language abilities in Alzheimer's disease. *Frontiers in Aging Neuroscience, 7.* https://doi.org/10.3389/fnagi.2015.00195

Tak, S. H. (2021). In quest of tablet apps for elders with Alzheimer's disease. *CIN: Computers, Informatics, Nursing, 39*(7), 347–354. https://doi.org/10.1097/cin.0000000000000718

Tang-Wai, D. F., & Graham, N. L. (2008). Assessment of language function in dementia. *Geriatrics, 11*(2), 103–110.

Wang, C.-M., & Huang, C.-H. (2015). A study of usability principles and interface design for mobile e-books. *Ergonomics, 58*(8), 1253–1265. https://doi.org/10.1080/00140139.2015.1013577

Wesselman, L. M. P., Schild, A., Coll-Padros, N., van der Borg, W. E., Meurs, J. H. P., Hooghiemstra, A. M., … Sikkes, S. A. M. (2018). Wishes and preferences for an online lifestyle program for Brain Health – A mixed methods study. *Alzheimer's &; Dementia: Translational Research &; Clinical Interventions, 4*(1), 141–149. https://doi.org/10.1016/j.trci.2018.03.003

Wildenbos, G. A., Jaspers, M. W. M., Schijven, M. P., & Dusseljee- Peute, L. W. (2019). Mobile health for older adult patients: Using an aging barriers framework to classify usability problems. *International Journal of Medical Informatics, 124*, 68–77. https://doi.org/10.1016/j.ijmedinf.2019.01.006

Wildenbos, G. A., Peute, L., & Jaspers, M. (2018). Aging barriers influencing mobile health usability for older adults: A literature based framework (Mold-US). *International Journal of Medical Informatics, 114*, 66–75. https://doi.org/10.1016/j.ijmedinf.2018.03.012

Yi, J. S., Pittman, C. A., Price, C. L., Nieman, C. L., & Oh, E. S. (2021). Telemedicine and dementia care: A systematic review of barriers and facilitators. *Journal of the American Medical Directors Association, 22*(7). https://doi.org/10.1016/j.jamda.2021.03.015

Yousaf, K., Mehmood, Z., Saba, T., Rehman, A., Munshi, A. M., Alharbey, R., & Rashid, M. (2019). Mobile-health applications for the efficient delivery of health care facility to people with dementia (PWD) and support to their carers: A survey. *BioMed Research International, 2019*, 1–26. https://doi.org/10.1155/2019/7151475

Zapata, B. C., Fernández-Alemán, J. L., Idri, A., & Toval, A. (2015). Empirical studies on usability of mHealth Apps: A systematic literature review. *Journal of Medical Systems, 39*(2). https://doi.org/10.1007/s10916-014-0182-2

Zmily, A., Mowafi, Y., & Mashal, E. (2014). Study of the usability of spaced retrieval exercise using mobile devices for Alzheimer's disease rehabilitation. *JMIR mHealth and uHealth, 2*(3). https://doi.org/10.2196/mhealth.3136

22 Flexibility and customisation

Starting from ASD to design sensory healthcare environments for people's wellbeing

Elena Bellini and Alessia Macchi

Introduction

People's quality of life is related to the physical environment. It is well known that the hospital environment has a direct and indirect impact on people (Setola et al., 2019). Since the 1990s, evidence-based design (EBD) aims to develop evidence of the therapeutic role of spaces in terms of patients and staff's satisfaction (Ulrich et al., 2008). Converting the healthcare experience into something positive can be done through the integrated design of spaces that are able to be welcoming and make you feel 'at home', in a familiar, non-threatening place. These spaces can positively distract patients and family members and accompany them even for a few moments in scenarios full of imagination and creativity, far from the suffering condition in which they find themselves.

Nature, art and playing games have a particular role in generating this distraction and regenerating sensation in the patient and their family (Bellini, 2022). These expedients favour the healing process and its duration, as well as emotions and positive responses, stimulating the patient and their family, fighting boredom and depression, anxiety and worries, perception of pain and suffering.

According to Attention Restoration (Kaplan, 1995; Korpela & Hartig, 1996) and Supportive Design (Ulrich et al., 2001; Ulrich & Gilpin, 2003) theories, the patient's regeneration occurs through 'positive distraction', which reduces stress and generates positive feelings and thoughts through this world of surprise, magic and imagination. Boredom, on the other hand, brings a feeling of depression in the patient, making them perceive that time never passes, leading to a sense of dissatisfaction and discomfort (Bishop, 2012).

Autism and sensory sensitivity: is it possible to talk about 'design for all'?

Autism spectrum disorders (ASD) are pervasive neurodevelopmental disorders which affect social communication and interaction, as well as restricted or repetitive behaviours or interests (APA, 2013). People with ASD can present a particular sensory sensitivity, in terms of hyper- or hyporeactivity to sensory stimuli. The world in which we live can be overstimulating, confusing and stressful. This sensitivity often causes a sensory overload. It is common to talk about problem behaviours in autism, but it is not often considered that these 'socially inappropriate' behaviours are only a reaction to the sensory overload. Sensory overload can be expressed as an alteration of perceptions and the inability to filter sensory information by the environment. These aspects can generate confusion and the environment can become 'frightening' and 'hurting'.

Everything we know about the world starts from the senses (Bogdashina, 2003). We are able to understand the context around us by interacting with the environment and through sensory processing. If our perceptions are altered, we are unable to 'make sense' of our surroundings.

DOI: 10.4324/9781003318262-28

A different perception of the environment leads to a different understanding of the world. Such sensory alterations can affect comprehension and the development of abilities throughout life.

The word 'spectrum' well defines the huge variety in people with ASD. Each person is different and presents a different level of sensory sensitiveness and perception. For this reason, it is impossible to define universal rules of wellbeing in ASD. However, it is possible to improve knowledge about people with autism and to understand when and why they present different afflictions or, on the contrary, different sensory preferences that can promote wellbeing and relaxation.

For example, many studies express that people with autism are often hypersensitive to hearing. This represents one of the biggest challenges in autism and often causes stress and pain (it can also hurt!) (Bellini, 2019).[1] Noise is one of the most common stressful experiences, especially loud and sudden noises; background buzz; reverberation; buzzing and whistles of neon lights, electrical sockets, the ticking of a clock, etc.; high and acute frequencies, such as some people's voices. Hearing disorders can affect orientation, comprehension, attention, communication and learning ability. On the contrary, some sound stimulations are much appreciated, such as music or sound vibrations, and can be an effective way to relax.

Light and glare can profoundly affect visual sensitivity. Colour and texture preferences may differ from one person to another but can be an important source of disease or wellbeing. For example, some people consider a white environment very relaxing as it promotes attention and concentration. On the contrary some people would consider it cold and aseptic. Bright colours can be loved by someone, and contrasts can support comprehension and way-finding, but can be overloading for other people, who may become over-activated and excited. Pastel and neutral colours are suggested for public environments so as not to be overwhelming. The visual overload can also be represented by the necessity to control the environment, such as a rigid order in the home environment. Of course, it is not possible to control this aspect in public environments. Art, pictures, video and multimedia are usually much appreciated and represent a positive distraction to relax. Sensory restoration can also be promoted by dim light, and some people express the necessity to have a completely dark environment to sleep well.

Scents can be at the same time appreciated or hated, causing distress. For this reason, it is better not to use aromas in public spaces if they can be avoided.

Tactile sensitivity can affect a person's choice of clothes, as some fabrics may cause discomfort, such as toothache or nausea. On the other hand, tactile stimulation can be very good for relaxation, such as touching rough or smooth textures, being enveloped by soft and wrapping elements, etc. For example, Temple Grandin (Grandin, 1995) often talks about her 'squeeze machine' which is able to offer a sensation of containment, often appreciated by people with autism.

Sensory sensitivities can also be stronger if they occur in combination, and this can generate overloading, stress and ill-health. Sensory deprivation is not always the right answer, also because sensory stimulation can represent a unique source of wellbeing and relaxation. The solution is not sensory deprivation, but sensory regulation, in terms of customisation.

Affordances describe the relationships that exist between organisms and their environments (Gibson, 1977). We are constantly changing, adapting and controlling the environment to design and express new affordances. What if we are not able to control the environment around us? (Gaudion et al., 2015). How is it possible to design an environment that can be completely flexible and adaptable?

It is difficult to define general rules that can satisfy all the different needs of the population within the spectrum. In conclusion, the state of the art and the case studies about designing for autism express the inability to define evidence-based design policies in this field, as guidelines

320 Elena Bellini and Alessia Macchi

cannot be representative for all. Therefore, does the phrase 'design for all' make sense for people with ASD?

A customised design adapts the environment to each person's sensory preferences. As designers, we should change our point of view and create empathy with people with autism and their caregivers, who can interpret and express their needs. But how can we design public spaces?

It is necessary to find new ways of designing to create dynamic and collaborative solutions. What we propose in this chapter is flexibility and customisation. Sensory design represents a design solution that takes into account people's sensory preferences making professionals able to design public spaces for all. Thanks to assistive technologies, this design approach supports space flexibility and environment adaptation to different users. In the healthcare environment, which represents one of the biggest challenges in cases of ASD, the application of this design has been experienced through sensory rooms.

Snoezelen and multisensory rooms in healthcare environments

Sensory rooms[2] are spaces designed both to stimulate and to help self-regulate all the senses, with the aim of generating positive sensations and emotions, reducing stress, promoting relaxation and a sense of choice and control acquisition or recovery (Cavanagh, 2020; Unwin et al., 2021).

They have particular relevance, especially for fragile or sensitive users, since environmental flexibility and customisation allow users to self-regulate and rebalance according to their sensory preferences. Flexibility and customisation can be provided not only by designing the environment and its components, but also by automation technology, allowing simplified stimulation control.

In sensory rooms, users can experience different sensory stimulations, which activate them and create interest in the surrounding environment; on the contrary, sensory deprivation can lead to negative outcomes such as stress, anxiety, depression and poor motivation, which affect the quality of life (Cavanagh et al., 2020).

Sensory interventions are based on two types of stimuli: external ones derived from the relationship of the organs of sight, touch, smell, hearing and taste with the outside world, giving information on the surrounding context and one's own safety; and the somatic senses, such as pressure on the skin, awareness of one's own body (proprioception) of space and balance (vestibular) which can communicate instead a sense of internal security. The somatic senses, in particular, can promote calm. Stimulations for reducing anxiety and stress are defined: relaxing sounds or classical music, coloured lights (to watch and adjust), fish or air bubbles moving in the water, manipulation objects, massages through dedicated chairs, or a deep pressure on one's body produced by elements such as very heavy blankets (Sutton, 2013; Novak et al., 2012; Champagne & Stromberg, 2004).

Sensory solutions promote the containment of emotional experiences, aiming to reduce stress levels and therefore aggression and adaptive behaviours (Sutton, 2013), especially for those who are often unaware of their sensory needs and stress responses. Hypo- or hypersensitivity to sensory stimuli often causes problems in independently regulating arousal levels (Bowman & Jones, 2016). Often, these people are unable to adjust their senses according to the 'sensory diet' that each individual modifies – even in an unconscious way – at different times of the day to adapt to the external environment and context stimuli (Champagne & Stromberg, 2004). A study performed in Serbia involving persons with ASD associated with intellectual difficulties reported that the continual sessions in a Snoezelen-Multisensory room had effects on reducing the severity of ASD and repetitive and stereotyped behaviours on the CARS scale (Novakovic et al., 2019). Furthermore in the last few years, there have been a growing number of investigations into the implementation of multisensory rooms in persons with cognitive deterioration from neurodegenerative disorders, including Parkinson's disease, Alzheimer's disease and other types of dementia, Huntington's disease and bipolar disorder, among others (Berkheimer et al., 2017; Duchi et al., 2019; Hayden et al., 2022).

Many studies have demonstrated the positive impact of sensory rooms in healthcare settings. Their therapeutic effect is related to the experienced sensation of finding oneself in a completely different world, living a 'travel and sensory experience' provided by the integrated design of the environment, an immersive situation that cannot be created through the use of individual objects or elements of stimulation.

An innovative design approach to healthcare environments able to support both persons with autism or users with temporary sensory fragility is the provision of multisensory rooms as dedicated waiting spaces or as environments for relaxation. Hospital wards where patients undergo invasive or painful procedures (such as burn dressings) the sensory environment can be supportive, lowering anxiety and fear levels, and it can be provided both in the room where clinical procedures are performed and in a dedicated environment, even before surgery (Del Nord, 2006). For example, it was found to be favourable for children who frequently have blood samples taken.

Sensory rooms have been used in cases of trauma – even psychological ones connected to physical violence – and rehabilitation (Dorn et al., 2020) but also to counteract the effects of isolation for patients with acute psychiatric disorders (Champagne & Stromberg, 2004; Novak et al., 2012). Since sensory environments are able to calm users and prepare them by encouraging other therapeutic approaches, these solutions are often used within psychiatric wards. . In general, these rooms have been used in situations that impact one person's emotional perception, sensory sensibility, behaviour and relationships and in places where sensory regulation provision can promote a sense of personal control, security, stability and calm (Champagne & Stromberg, 2004; Sutton, 2013; Bowman & Jones, 2016) including labour moments for childbearing women. Furthermore, sensory rooms facilitate communication and relationships, in particular with health professionals, supporting users' self-awareness and self-control (Sutton, 2013).

In addition, there are many examples of sensory rooms in children's hospitals around the world, particularly in the UK, Denmark and Northern Europe, the USA, Canada and Australia. Distraction and relaxation strategies were used in the Royal Alexandra Children's Hospital in Brighton, where a multisensory room was created in 2016. In Italy, a Snoezelen environment was created for the Physical Medicine and Rehabilitation Unit of Hospital Gaslini in Genoa, dedicated to sensory integration and stimulation for the rehabilitation of children with severe cognitive, sensory and motor disabilities. A similar use of sensoriality is also seen in the Synesthesy Room of the Department of Neurorehabilitation of the Bambino Gesù Paediatric Hospital in Rome, where sound, visual and tactile stimulations are integrated for a cognitive rehabilitation activities, aimed mostly at children with severe disabilities. Nemours Children's Hospital (Orlando, USA) was selected for the humanisation system of the hospital environment with the integration of sensoriality and play, but above all, for the REACH – Respecting Each Awesome Child Here – (2016) programme, created to support accessibility in the emergency room for children with autism or other behavioural and developmental conditions.

Recently, some examples have emerged of sensory rooms related to the birth care environment. The Snoezelen environment offers childbearing women distraction, relaxation, comfort and environmental control within the safety of a hospital environment (Hauck, 2008). Distracting senses in the Snoezelen room during labour and birth moments decrease mother's pain intensity, the length of labour and the incidence of episiotomy (Manesh et al., 2015). In

January 2016, an experimental labour and birth room was inaugurated called 'Delivery room of the future' in the existing maternity ward of the regional hospital in Herning, Denmark, bringing nature into the room to reduce stress and promote physiological birth. Findings from a qualitative study of women's experiences of giving birth in the alternative delivery room support the use of principles of healing architecture and Snoezelen in birth environments (Nielsen et al., 2020). In 2019, an adaptable birthing room was realised at one of three labour wards at Sahlgrenska University Hospital (SUH) Gothenburg, Sweden, during the *Room4Birth* research project (Berg et al., 2019). A randomised controlled trial was run, and conclusions of the study reported that when planning and designing hospital-based birthing rooms, it is crucial to offer possibilities to adapt the room and physical features according to personal wishes (Skogström et al., 2022).

As we can see from these examples, the use of sensory rooms is growing in different contexts because of their capacity to answer different user needs, providing flexibility and customisation to spaces dedicated to people's care and wellbeing. This aspect assumes particular relevance related to healthcare settings, where policies have recently become more orientated towards humanisation of hospital environments and patient-centred care. The introduction of sensory rooms in hospitals is today's challenge that strictly relates to co-design processes to define new spaces and practices for users' healthcare and wellbeing.

Co-design experience: three case studies in hospitals

Careggi ED sensory waiting room

People with an ASD and an intellectual disability who need to attend hospital may experience high levels of discomfort and present challenging behaviours due to stress-related hyperarousal, sensory sensitivity, novelty-anxiety, communication and self-regulation difficulties. Increased agitation and acting out can disturb the diagnostic and therapeutic processes, and affect the healthcare climate. Architectural design disciplines aim at reducing distress in hospitals or creating autism-friendly environments, considering the physical environment as an important point of intervention. The right setting can help enhance confidence and self-esteem and can have a profound impact on people's health and wellbeing.

A sensory environment where people are able to self-regulate through sensory stimulation could reduce stress and anxiety, especially in the Emergency Department (ED) where things are done faster, there are sudden and loud noises, unpleasant smells, and very bright lights that can increase the risk of agitation and aggressive behaviours resulting from the increase in physiological arousal.

Environmental psychology has evaluated the perceived quality of care, looking at the design of hospital rooms, paths and circulation, waiting rooms, services and devices. Furthermore, many studies have investigated the influence of the hospital environment on patients, in terms of stress-reduction and therapeutic intervention speed, but also on health professionals and their work. Careggi's Emergency Waiting Room in Florence has been built to satisfy this challenge (Bellini, 2019).

It is an application of the use of sensory rooms in the ED of one of the biggest hospitals in Italy and represents one of the main interventions of the accessibility hospital policy. It comes from a collaboration between Tuscany Health Trust, Florence Municipality, Careggi Hospital, Committee of Disabled People, PAMAPI[3] Autism Centre, the Department of Architecture at the University of Florence and DU IT,[4] an innovative start-up expert in sensory environments. It leads to the hospital accessibility plan, called 'H code', to develop an intervention protocol to promote the accessibility of health services for people with disabilities.

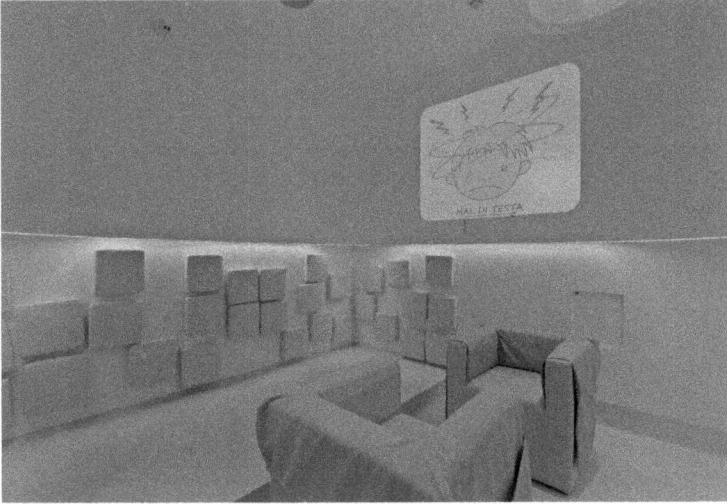

Figure 22.1 Photo of the Careggi ED waiting room

A preferential path has been created to reduce waiting times and allow the family members to always be present to support the patient with a disability. Their support is fundamental to interpreting the reactions and signals transmitted by patients, especially if they are not able to communicate verbally; for example, when they are overwhelmed and stressed by the environment.

A special training programme for health staff has been promoted to make them welcoming, supportive and able to relate and communicate with people with autism.

Finally, a sensory waiting room (Figure 22.1) has been provided to facilitate waiting for medical intervention, as this represents the most critical moment for the patient.

The methodology of the focus group involved architects, psychologists and professionals through a transdisciplinary research, centred on the links between the spatial characteristics and clinical state of people with ASD. The relationship between architectural space and quality of life is studied to pay maximum attention to users' needs to promote sensory integration and relaxation. This autism-friendly space is able to contain the patient's emotional experiences, reduce stress and promote a state of calm, through the transformation of the sensory aspects of the physical environment, thanks to assistive technology.

This prototype is the first example in Italy of a multisensory environment in the ED and one of the few internationally. It represents a repeatable module thanks to its wide flexibility given by the technological structure, but also by the modular wooden structure, and can be installed in a few days.

The wooden structure also contains acoustic insulation that reduces noise from the ED and makes the space more comfortable. All the facilities and the medical equipment are hidden inside the wall, to make the environment less frightening, but accessible by an opening panel, locked with a key. It is a protected room that maximises comprehension and predictability. The curved shape makes people feel contained and wrapped by the environment, increasing the idea of safety and security. It is a welcoming and home-like environment, different from the typical hospital waiting room. The sensory waiting room is a neutral space, where stimuli can be activated and regulated by the patient itself or by the caregiver/healthcare staff using a specific technological system that supports requests, choices and self-determination in order to fit sensory stimulation to personal preferences.

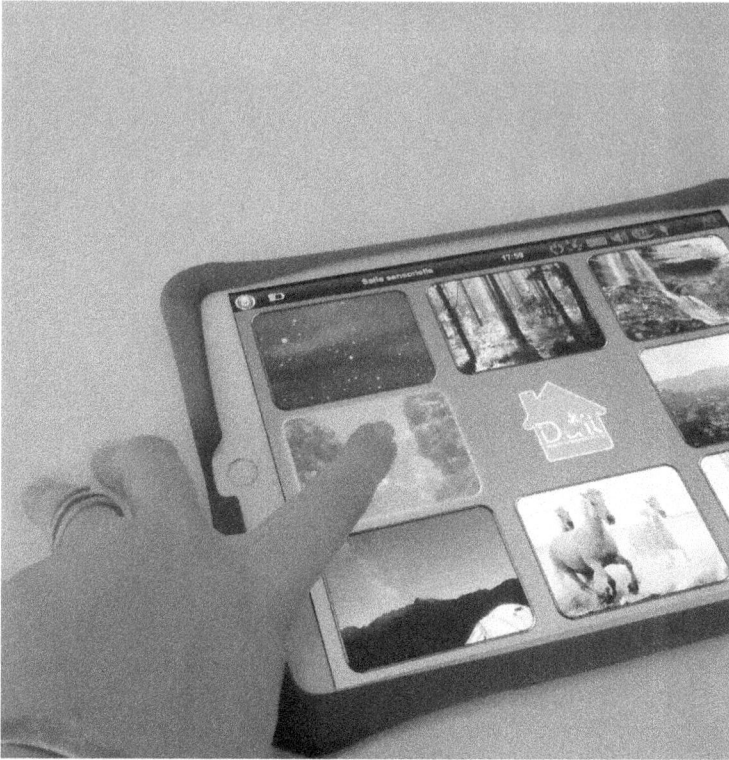

Figure 22.2 The user manages the environment by an iPad. In this photo, the i-Pad screen presents some pictures which represent the scenarios that people can choose inside the sensory room

In terms of positive distraction, this environment supports people using different strategies of relaxation. A software programme permits the management and regulation of the sensory stimulations (Figure 22.2): people can choose a video on a personal USB (it is very important to bring something familiar that could be very effective in relaxation, especially for people with autism) or on the web, projected onto the wall; they can select music or sounds that are coordinated with tactile vibration and can change volume and frequencies; they can play with colours and change the intensity of the lights, etc. The technological system is managed by a tablet, a device that is familiar to people with autism, and the graphics are designed specifically by DU IT with the contribution of PAMAPI (Figure 22.2). In the first screen, there are some pictures that people can use as facilitators for the communication of primary needs even if they can't use verbal language: expressing pain, asking for water; asking for going to the toilet, etc. When they press an icon, the picture is projected onto the wall and the staff can understand their needs. Then, they can 'play' with the room, changing the environment and enjoy the sensory stimulations to be distracted and relaxed.

Every element in the room is intended to promote relaxation. A soft area is characterised by a wooden platform that diffuses the tactile vibration where it is possible to build your own customised spot thanks to the mobile, wall-mounted furniture cushions. Two 'cocoon' rocking armchairs make people feel hugged, as expressed by Temple Gradin in the idea of containment. This comfortable and positive place promotes people's dialogue and empathy and it could be an opportunity to develop a safe relation between patients, families and staff.

Finally, some cameras give the possibility of leaving people inside alone, to have a moment to be alone with themselves and feel a sense of relaxation, and at the same time of controlling the room from the staff desk to promote safety.

All these characteristics should ensure better regulation of arousal, fewer behaviour problems, improved treatment accessibility, safety and effectiveness.

The sensory emergency waiting room was designed for people with ASD, but also with the idea of offering specific care for vulnerable people: elderly people, people with dementia, etc. . In fact, the sensory room was also used for victims of violence (women and children) to make them feel secure and confident. It was really appreciated as a safe and protected environment, isolated from the rest of the hospital, especially from the entrance that could represent the idea of danger. Women could be hugged in the armchair, feeling safe and comfortable. Children can play in the soft area and thus be distracted while their mothers talk with the staff. This dialogue itself may be promoted by the welcoming environment.

The sensory room is also very helpful in managing health professionals' burnout, which is always very high in the Emergency Department, as reported during the interviews with the staff in the post-occupancy evaluation of the sensory room after several months of use. Overall, this flexibility makes the room an autism-friendly facility, but also a secure space 'for all' that promotes wellbeing and mental health.

PISTA: sensory birth space

Another application of sensory rooms in hospital environments is PISTA,[5] a project that aimed to prototype a multi-sensory architectural environment based on childbearing women's sensory-perceptive needs to be placed in the new Birth Centre and LDR unit at Grosseto Hospital, Italy. Through assistive technologies, the prototype is designed to support women's individual biopsychological needs. Most maternity facilities are currently clinical spaces that emphasise a medical approach to birth, though many women desire less medicalised, more emotionally sensitive birth experiences. A dynamic and flexible sensory environment contributes to this step, influencing at the same time women's psychological and physiological outcomes, operating directly on relaxation and stress levels.

The PISTA project was initiated in 2018, running an inclusive design process through collaboration with the hospital health board and professional staff in the research and development process. The methodology included focus groups and interviews with midwives and medical staff, prototype design and technology co-development process.

The prototype is a compact free-standing nest that provides complete sensory regulation through combination of ergonomic design and innovative technology for automation and customisation. Women and staff can interact with advanced domotic systems to adapt the environment to users' sensory preferences, changing lights, colours, music and sounds, tactile sound vibrations and aromas. Women can lie down inside the nest or stand up hanging on handrails and choose one or more scenarios, depending on the labour stage. Prototype ergonomics are designed to enhance relaxation and movement in a secure and protective nest. An acoustic curtain can answer users' need for privacy. The project integrates the complete free-standing sensory nest into existing birth spaces, fitting within standard hospital room dimensions, providing women and maternity staff with highly customisable sensory solutions to enhance relaxation in labour moments, easy to access and self-manage.

The prototype validation process is currently part of a PhD thesis, with the aim of evaluating new technology solutions for future birth spaces pursuing flexibility as a continuous and dynamic response to specific users' needs. Furthermore, the sensory design approach was introduced in the economic technical feasibility plan for the renovation process of the whole Woman and Child Centre of Grosseto Hospital – that includes the Birth Centre and LDR unit – providing sensory requirements also for emergency spaces, patient rooms, surgery rooms and staff relaxation rooms.

Sensory psychological services in a French hospital

Le Nid Sensoriel (sensory nest) is a care and assistive service for people who have 'fallen' from their familiar, social or human nest. The aim is to improve socio-emotional skills and mental health conditions by creating bonds between people and dealing with difficulties together.

The sensory environment was built in Polyclinique Lyon Nord, a hospital in Rillieux-la-Pape (Lyon, France). It was designed by DU IT in collaboration with the medical staff of *Le Nid Sensoriel*, composed of a psychologist, an educator, a psycho-pedagogue, a neuro- and psychomotor therapist, a hypnotherapist and a sophrologist (relaxation practitioner). The aim of the sensory environment was to welcome all people, of any age and at any stage of their life, to satisfy their specific needs and requirements and to create psychological support in relation to their families. It is a place where people can feel comfortable and relaxed. It promotes cognitive development, relaxation, awakening and communication through the senses.

Le Nid is the first example of psychological consulting in a public hospital by a sensory environment. It is composed of a waiting room, in which it is possible to sit in soft curved alcoves, hidden in the wall, coloured by customised lights; a consulting room, a wooden central cabin where it is possible to create a private and empathic dialogue with the staff and prepare before the treatment; and the sensory room for treatments.

The sensory room is designed for both adults and young people, to provide maximum of flexibility. There is an area dedicated to psychomotricity; an area for relaxation through sound, with a vibrating wooden platform/chaise-longue and a large water mattress; some elements that stimulate the senses such as a bubble column or optical fibres; and some elements that introduce the concept of biophilic design, such as wooden surfaces and a coloured backlit tree ceiling. The sensory software allows for the opportunity to manage the environment and enables complete flexibility.

At present, the psychological service is offered to pupils from local schools and pregnant women by the maternity area of the hospital, but the intention is that eventually it will benefit every person in the hospital.

It represents an interesting example of healthcare policy, promoted by a public/private consortium to offer a new service to improve mental health through sensory environments. The staff will start the evaluation process to understand the impact of the use of this treatment in the everyday life of the hospital.

Method and policy: how to design sensory environments?

> Health is a state of complete physical, mental and social well-being and not merely the absence of disease or infirmity. The enjoyment of the highest attainable standard of health is one of the fundamental rights of every human being without distinction of race, religion, political belief, economic or social condition.
>
> (WHO, 1946, up. 2005)

In a hospital, the state of the environment is fundamental to promote comfort and satisfaction not only for patients, but also for their families and for staff. A patient is a vulnerable person and their physical condition is strongly related to mental health. The sensory environment is one of the strategies that can be promoted to enhance wellbeing.

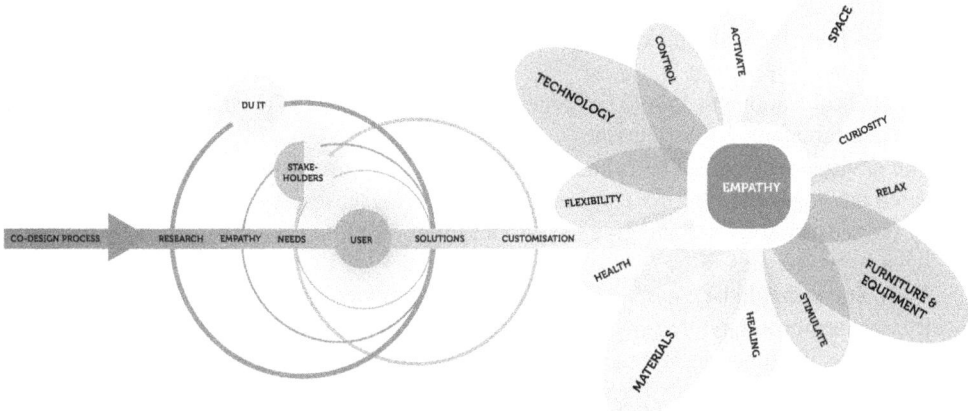

Figure 22.3 Diagram of the co-design process

he case studies presented above have described the opportunity for developing a new meth-odology to 'design for all'. The Careggi sensory waiting room represented the first prototype of a sensory module that DU IT has been developing during the years, defining a methodology. This is based on different principles: multidisciplinarity, co-design, empathy, innovation, auto-mation and customisation. DU IT's team is composed of architects, psychologists and auto-mation developers. The psychologists express people's needs in terms of mental health, the architects design the space and the equipment to comply with the requirements and integrate the system of automation that make the environment flexible and customised. As we can see from Figure 22.3, we can say that the first part of the co-design process is inside DU IT, where differ-ent professionals work together to define the project of the sensory space.

The second step of the co-design process involves the stakeholders, expressing needs to be solved by the project itself. The aim is to develop empathy to understand people's needs, but also to develop a therapeutic process by the space and the technology. The use of different mate-rials, specific furniture or equipment could support in response to the requirements.

It is a user-centred design process, but it also develops a user-centred final product thanks to the assistive technology. This phase of the design process will last for the life of the product. In fact, users will change the environment and adapt it constantly. The users promote their own wellbeing by regulating the sensory environment and finding the right balance between relaxation and stimu-lation. Similarly, the sensory environment represents a tool for the staff to customise the treatment for each patient and promote healing environments and a better quality of care in hospitals.

Starting from these different experiences, DU IT has developed some principles to design sen-sory environments:

SPACE

• It is important to create an 'escape space', different from daily-life environments, to stimu-late curiosity and interaction and promote positive distraction.
• The environment should be welcoming and friendly to promote the relations between users. Furniture could support these feelings.

- A 15–25 m² room is suitable to provide the idea of containment. A bigger space could be useful if there space for several people.
- Curved lines for walls make the environment more welcoming and promote the idea of protection.
- All medical equipment should be hidden and integrated inside the walls to create a familiar and non-threatening environment.
- The environment should be calming and neutral. All sensory stimulations should be activated and controlled by the user/caregiver/staff. The sensory system should be managed by the sensory software and give the possibility of adapting each stimulation by the user's sensory preferences.
- The colours should be clear, not too bright and not reflecting.
- It is better not to have too many contrasts. Contrasts can be used to highlight something with a specific function, so that it is easy to recognise (e.g. a button to press).

FURNITURE AND EQUIPMENT

- Soft elements and furniture (rocking armchair, pouf, chaise longue, etc.) are suggested to promote relaxation.
- Specific furniture and equipment could be designed to stimulate senses and promote the idea of playing and enjoy the sensory experience.
- A vibrating platform for lying down on can help people enjoy the music by tactile stimulation and promote the floortime.
- The furniture and all the equipment should be safe, cleanable and fireproof.
- Safety is particularly important for vulnerable people, e.g. people with autism who often present alterations in perception, proprioception and orientation. Furniture and equipment should be stable, durable and able to resist stress in case of a crisis.
- Furniture and equipment should be friendly, so that the necessities of healthcare do not affect the general idea of welcoming.
- All the elements (furniture, equipment, colours, scenarios, etc.) should promote nature to develop the idea of biophilic design and promote wellbeing, calm and relaxation.

MATERIALS

- Soft materials are suggested to promote relaxation, especially for the floor surface.
- Specific materials could be designed to stimulate senses and promote the idea of playing and enjoying the sensory experience (e.g. tactile materials).
- The materials should be cleanable and fireproof.
- Materials should be stable and durable, also able to resist stress, e.g. in case of crisis and episodes of stereotypical behaviour.
- It is preferable to use natural and non-toxic materials without chemical agents, such as formaldehyde, that can cause irritation.
- Materials should be friendly, so that the sense of welcome is maintained despite the clinical environment.

TECHNOLOGY

- Sensory scenarios that integrate video, music, sounds, colours, lights, aroma, vibrations, etc. should be composed to generate calming and sensory stimulating environments. The user should have the possibility to turn on and turn off every stimulus and adapt it according to their preferences.

- It must be possible to regulate the colour and intensity of light because visual over-stimulation can often cause distress.
- Similarly, sound (volume, frequencies, typology of music/sound) also needs to be regulated, to avoid causing distress through acoustic stimulation.
- Aromas also need to be customised because the olfactory stimulation may be distressing.
- The system of sensory control should be very easy to use and the graphics should be designed to facilitate comprehension, use. and communication.

As our literature review has shown, there are no guidelines for designing sensory environments. A few cases have been developed and experimented, but there is no scientific evaluation of the impact of design on people. This evaluation is very important as it could promote the use of sensory environments as policies for an accessible, health-promoting and supportive hospital.

Notes

1 In her doctoral thesis, Elena Bellini conducted interviews and questionnaires with people with ASD and their families to understand their sensory profiles and how the environment could affect everyday life.
2 Also called 'snoezelen rooms' (Hulsegge and Verheul, 1987).
3 P.A.M.A.P.I. – Parenti e Amici Malati di Autismo e Psicosi Infantile, Centro Abilitativo per Disturbi dello Spettro Autistico.
4 DU IT – Design for User Innovation Technology, was founded as an innovative startup in 2015 in Florence (Italy) www.duitfor.com
5 Sensory-perceptive integrated design approach for birth spaces.

References

American Psychiatric Association (APA). (2013). *DSM-5: Diagnostic and statistical manual of mental disorders* (5th ed.). APA Press.

Bellini, E. (2019). *Ambienti sensoriali "terapeutici" che rendano Abili. Un percorso di vita integrato per persone con Disturbi dello Spettro Autistico.* Firenze University Press.

Bellini, E. (2022). Ambientazione e scenari per la fantasia. In P. Felli & M. C. Torricelli (Eds.), *L'ospedale pediatrico: Una comunità accogliente. La cura* (pp. 268–291). La Nave di Teseo.

Berg, M., Goldkuhl, L., Nilsson, C., Wijk, H., Gyllensten, H., Lindahl, G., et al. (2019). Room. 4Birth-the effect of an adaptable birthing room on labour and birth outcomes for nulliparous women at term with spontaneous labour start: Study protocol for a randomised controlled superiority trial in Sweden. *Trials, 20*(1), 629.

Berkheimer, S. D., Qian, C., & Malmstrom, T. K. (2017). Snoezelen therapy as an intervention to reduce agitation in nursing home patients with dementia: A pilot study. *Journal of the American Medical Directors Association, 18*(12), 1089–1091.

Bishop, S. L., & Seltzer, M. M. (2012). Self-reported autism symptoms in adults with autism spectrum disorders. *Journal of Autism and Developmental Disorders, 42*(11), 2354–2363.

Bogdashina, O. (2003). *Sensory perceptual issues in autism and Asperger syndrome.* Jessica Kingsley.

Bowman, S., & Jones, R. (2016). Sensory interventions for psychiatric crisis in emergency department - A new paradigm. *Journal of Psychiatry and Mental Health, 1*(1). http//doi.org/10.16966/jpmh.103

Cavanagh, B., Haracz, K. L., & James, M. C. (2020). Receptive arts engagement for health: A holistic and trans-disciplinary approach to creating a multisensory environment. *SAGE Open, 10*(4). https://doi.org/10.1177/2158244020978420

Champagne, T., & Stromberg, N. (2004). Sensory approaches in inpatient psychiatric settings innovative alternatives to seclusion & restraint. *Journal of Psychological Nursing, 42*(9), 34–44.

Del Nord, R. (2006). *Lo stress ambientale nel progetto dell'ospedale pediatrico. Indirizzi tecnici e suggestioni architettoniche*. Motta Architettura.

Dorn, E., Hitch, D., & Stevenson, C. (2020). An evaluation of a sensory room within an adult mental health rehabilitation unit. *Occupational Therapy in Mental Health, 36*(2), 105–118.

Duchi, F., Benalcázar, E., Huerta, M., Bermeo, J. P., Lozada, F., & Condo, S. (2019). Design of a multisensory room for elderly people with neurodegenerative diseases. In. *Singapore: World Congress on Medical Physics and Biomedical Engineering* (pp. 207–210). Springer.

Gaudion, K. H., Myerson, A., Pellicano, J., & L. (2015). Design and wellbeing: Bridging the empathy gap between neurotypical designers and autistic adults. In M. Mani & P. Kandachar (Eds.), *Design for sustainable well-being and empowerment* (pp. 61–77). IISc Press and Delft: TU.

Gibson, J. J. (1977). The theory of affordances. In R. Shaw & J. Bransford (Eds.), *Perceiving, acting and knowing: Toward an ecological psychology* (pp. 67–82). Erlbaum.

Grandin, T. (1995). *Thinking in pictures: And other reports from my life with autism*. Doubleday.

Hauck, Y., Rivers, C., & Doherty, K. (2008). Women's experiences of using a Snoezelen room during labour in Western Australia. *Midwifery, 24*(4), 460–470.

Hayden, L., Passarelli, C., Shepley, S. E., & Tigno, W. (2022). A scoping review: Sensory interventions for older adults living with dementia. *Dementia, 21*(4), 1416–1448.

Kaplan, S. (1995). The restorative benefits of nature: Toward an integrative framework. *Journal of Environmental Psychology, 15*(3), 169–182.

Korpela, K., & Hartig, T. (1996). Restorative qualities of favourite places. *Journal of Environmental Psychology, 16*(3), 221–233.

Manesh, M. J., Kalati, M., & Hosseini, F. (2015). Snoezelen room and childbirth outcome: A randomised clinical trial. *Iranian Red Crescent Medical Journal, 17*(5), e18373.

Nielsen, J. H., & Overgaard, C. (2020). Healing architecture and Snoezelen in delivery room design: A qualitative study of women's birth experiences and patient-centeredness of care. *BMC Pregnancy and Childbirth, 20*(1), 283.

Novak, T., Scanlan, J., McCaul, D., MacDonald, N., & Clarke, T. (2012). Pilot study of a sensory room in an acute inpatient psychiatric unit. *Australasian Psychiatry, 20*(5), 401–406.

Novakovic, N., Milovancevic, M. P., Dejanovic, S. D., & Aleksic, B. (2019). Effects of Snoezelen— Multisensory environment on CARS scale in adolescents and adults with autism spectrum disorder. *Research in Developmental Disabilities, 89*, 51–58.

Setola, N., Naldi, E., Cocina, G. G., Eide, L. B., Iannuzzi, L., & Daqly, D. (2019). The impact of the physical environment on intrapartum maternity care: Identification of eight crucial building spaces. *HERD: Health Environments Research and Design Journal, 12*(4), 67–98.

Skogström, L. B., Vithal, E., Wijk, H., Lindahl, G., & Berg, M. (2022). Women's experiences of physical features in a specially designed birthing room: A mixed-methods study in Sweden. *HERD: Health Environments Research and Design Journal, 15*(3), 193–205.

Sutton, D., Wilson, M., Van Kessel, K., & Vanderpyl, J. (2013). Optimising arousal to manage aggression: A pilot study of sensory modulation. *International Journal of Mental Health Nursing, 22*(6), 500–511.

Ulrich, R. S. (2001). Effects of healthcare environmental design on medical outcomes. In A. Dalani (Ed.), *Design and health: The therapeutic benefits of design* (pp. 49–59). Swedish Building Council.

Ulrich, R. S., & Gilpin, L. (2003). Healing arts: Nutrition for the soul. In S. B. Frampton, L. Gilpin, & P. A. Charmel (Eds.), *Putting patients first: Designing and practising patient-centred care* (pp. 117–146). John Wiley & Sons.

Ulrich, R. S., Zimring, C., Zhu, X., et al. (2008). A review of the research literature on evidence-based healthcare design. *HERD: Health Environments Research & Design Journal, 1*(3), 61–125. doi:10.1177/193758670800100306

Unwin, K. L., Powell, G., & Jones, C. R. (2021). The use of multi-sensory environments with autistic children: Exploring the effect of having control of sensory changes. *Autism, 26*(6), 1379–1394.

World Health Organization. (1946). *Constitution of the world health organisation*.Geneva: World Health Organization.

23 Sensory-friendly LED lighting for healthcare environments

Co-producing design regulations to meet autistic needs

Jill Corbyn, Alexia Gkika and Jane Cannon

Introduction

Many autistic and otherwise neurodivergent people experience heightened sensory sensitivity, including photophobia – increased sensitivity to light. Recent legislative changes, including the banning of fluorescent bulb sales, and the national and organisational zero carbon initiatives have instigated significant changes to lighting across the United Kingdom National Health Service (NHS) estates. The installation of LED lighting equipment has caused additional sensory problems for some neurodivergent people who are accessing or spending a considerable time at hospital facilities.

A collaboration led by autistic people from the National Development Team for Inclusion (NDTi), inclusive designers, lighting designers and engineers from Buro Happold, as well as researchers, lecturers and engineers from educational bodies, is seeking to address these challenges and influence future policy developments. Our work and influence ambitions have included:

- Developing an advisory technical guidance note (NHSE, 2022) shared online and embedded in NHS England (NHSE) projects, including sensory friendly ward guidance, sustainable lighting toolkit and health building note specifications.
- Positively engaging NHSE colleagues to support understanding of the issues and influence change across NHS estates.
- Developing a research collaboration with University College London (UCL).
- Sharing our work on 'All in the Mind' on BBC Radio 4.
- Technical guidance produced is referenced in British Standards Institution PAS 6463: 2022 'Design for the Mind – neurodiversity and the built environment – guide'.
- Publishing editorial and journal articles about our work and the need for sensory considerations in lighting in professional lighting journals such as the *Lighting Journal* issued by the Institute of Lighting Professionals and the Light Lines issued by CIBSE's Society of Light and Lighting.
- Developing a white paper with CIBSE, to ensure this work can be referenced in the revised CIBSE document 'Lighting for Healthcare Premises' LG02, the guidance document for lighting in all healthcare settings when it is published in 2024.

Lighting, net zero carbon initiatives and legislative changes

Responding to the climate emergency and crisis, the report 'Delivering a Net Zero National Health Service' for NHS England (NHSE) updated in July 2022 delivers a clear commitment towards improving NHSE's carbon footprint and reducing the environmental impact of the

DOI: 10.4324/9781003318262-29

services. As part of this combined effort, one of the targeted early steps to decarbonise is to upgrade lighting to LED technology across the entire NHSE. It is estimated that the cost of delivering 100% LED lighting will be recovered in savings from reduced energy costs in under four years, and will save over £3 billion in operational costs over the next 30 years (NHSE, 2020, p. 21).

LED lighting has been the dominant light source for the past decade, gradually leading to the phasing out of conventional light sources such as tungsten filament bulbs and fluorescent tubes. The rapidly advancing LED technology and lighting controls offer great benefits in terms of energy consumption and the management of electrical services performance. However, caution needs to be taken regarding aspects relating to the sensory stimulation and the visual comfort of all users, with particular attention to people who are hypersensitive to light. This is often the case for many people with sensory processing differences, including autistic individuals and those with other neurodivergent and neurodegenerative conditions.

Universal design principles and good design practice are to ensure that environments are accessible and comfortable for all users. This reduces or eliminates the need to make specific adjustments to meet the needs of individuals, often benefiting others who use the space. As well as reducing the cost of adaptation and retrofitting, accessibility has a social benefit, particularly in healthcare environments. This is supported on a national level through the *Equality Act 2010* set by the UK Government.

Autism

Understanding, diagnostic criteria and conceptualisation of autism have continued to evolve since it was first used by Sukhareva in 1925 (Zeldovich, 2018) and described by Kanner in the 1940s. Although autism is a form of neurodivergence and not a mental health condition or neurodegenerative disease, this project has focused on the impact of sensory environments on wellbeing in mental health settings. Autistic people experience higher rates of anxiety and depression and are significantly more likely to think about, attempt and die by suicide than the general population (Conner et al., 2020; Hand et al. (2020).

Understanding the sensing and perceptual world of autistic people is central to understanding autism.

> Our five senses are how each of us understands everything that isn't us. Sight, sound, smell, taste, and touch are the five ways – the *only* five ways – that the universe can communicate with us. In this way, our senses define reality for each of us… What if you're receiving the same sensory information as everyone else, but your brain is working differently? Then your experience of the world around you will be radically different from everyone else's, maybe even painfully so. In that case, you would literally be living in an alternate reality – an alternate *sensory* reality.
>
> (Grandin & Panek, 2014, p. 70)

Tolerance for sensory input is variable and can be impacted by a range of other factors, including individual wellbeing and other users in the space. The impact of the environment is cumulative, and it is helpful to consider the overall sensory environment. For example, loud noises from banging doors or alarms might reduce overall tolerance to bright overhead lighting.

Parmar et al. (2021) found that autistic people experience a range of visual hypersensitivities, including to light, motion, patterns and particular colours, which contributed to distraction and were frequently part of a wider multisensory issue. Such experiences had significant negative impacts on personal wellbeing and daily life with participants describing fatigue, stress and hindrances on day-to-day activities (e.g., travel and social activities).

Incandescent bulbs such as tungsten are the preferred artificial light source for many autistic people. However, as part of an energy saving initiative, legislative changes in the UK have phased out sales of tungsten, halogen and some types of fluorescent bulbs, with the production of the latter being gradually banned in the next years. For the past decade, LED lighting is the dominant light source being introduced in new or regeneration projects.

Typically, key complaints expressed by people with some level of light sensitivity are:

1. Control of lighting operation and intensity. In hospitals, much of the lighting is automatically operated. The lack of user control intensifies the experience as people are dependent on others to make change, and may feel trapped in a painful or challenging environment.
2. Brightness and glare: overhead lighting which often grants direct view of the light source is very likely to be perceived as glary and discomforting. This is something that is commonly noticed with LED lighting.
3. Colour of light: hospitals are clinical environments. The use of cool white light contributes to the institutional feel, increasing emotional and psychological stress in visitors, staff and long term users of the space. During the first years of wide use of LED lighting, the efficiency of the cooler white light was considerably higher than warmer white light. Therefore, the use of cooler white light rapidly expanded in order to prove and maximise the benefits of using LED lighting in terms of energy saving and systems efficiency.
4. Flicker: one of the key complaints received by people with light sensitivity continues to be the detection of flicker and its negative effects. This is notable in fluorescent lighting and can also be seen in LED lighting where component compatibility issues occur.

Co-production, participation or citizen control

Arnstein's ladder of participation (1969) (Figure 23.1) illustrates the range of involvement of people with lived experience from non-participation, through tokenism, to citizen control. In more recent years, co-production has been cited as the gold standard for working with people with lived experience of issues. Typically, projects are led by the services, working in partnership alongside people with lived experience, but it is the service that determines the project agenda.

In contrast, the identification of the need to understand LED lighting and to develop sensory-friendly guidance has not been led by services but by people with lived experience of photophobia. This work represents the culmination of input by people with lived experience and by professional partners who volunteered their time and expertise to drive and support the ambitions for change, engaging with services only when the guidance was complete.

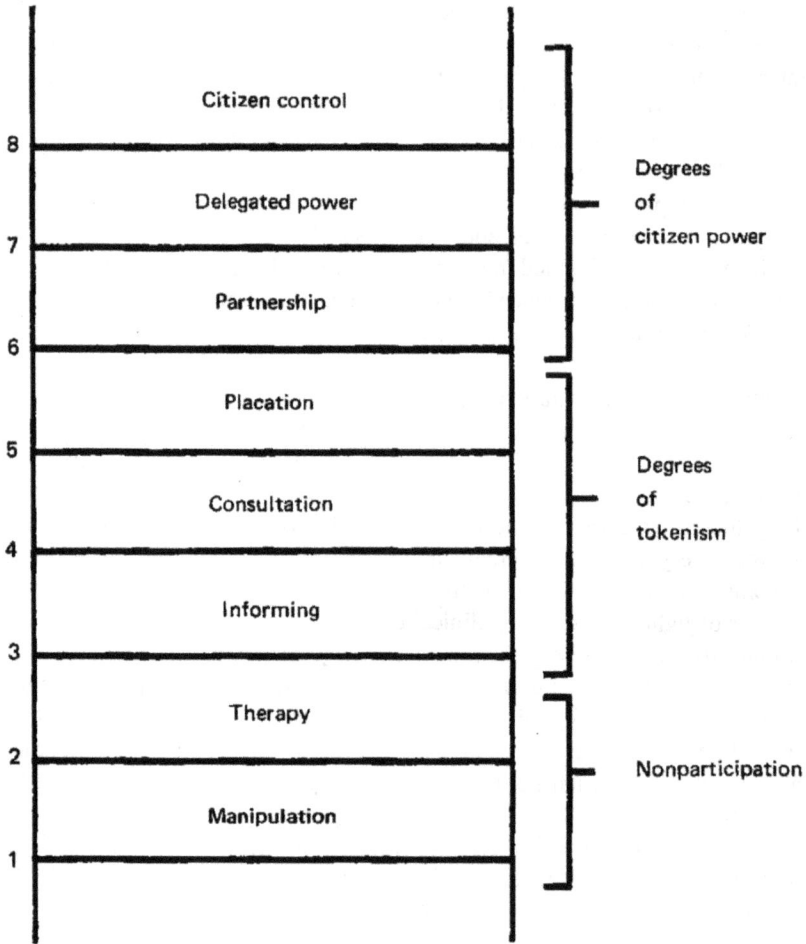

Figure 23.1 Arnstein, S. (1969) Ladder of Participation, *The Journal of the American Planning Association*

The origins of the work

The 'Sensory Friendly Ward' work at National Development Team for Inclusion (NDTi) that preceded the lighting guidance started with autistic team members not being able to access hospital buildings as part of their work on care, education and treatment reviews (CTRs and CETRs) because of the challenging sensory environments. CTRs were developed in 2015 by NHSE as part of their commitment to improving the care and treatment of autistic people and people with a learning disability. The policy aims to reduce admissions to mental health inpatient services and reduce the length of stay following the abuse uncovered in the Winterbourne View scandal in 2012.

Data from the Mental Health Data Set, analysed by the CQC (2022) shows that since Assuring Transformation data collection commenced in 2015, the number of people with a learning disability in hospital has almost halved, while the number of autistic people recorded as being in hospital has increased by over 60%.

The number of autistic people admitted to hospital has increased in recent years. In addition to this, their length of stay in mental health settings is considerable. In December 2021, 55% of autistic people or people with a learning disability in a mental health hospital at the end of December 2021 had a total length of stay in hospital of more than two years. Around 355 people (17% of autistic people and people with a learning disability in inpatient services) had a total length of stay in hospital of more than 10 years.

We were curious about what the sensory environment would be like for the growing numbers of autistic children and adult inpatients if the autistic Experts by Experience were not able to tolerate the space for a one-day meeting. Inspired by the experience of autistic team members, NDTi sought and received a commission to review the sensory environment of some inpatient services. The work was delivered by the autistic team members who had uncovered the initial issues. With samples of experiences collected by NDTi, Buro Happold Lighting and inclusive teams with members who have lived experience were brought on board to provide professional input and lead the composition of the technical note with the view to raise awareness and address the issues through guidance.

Sensory environment reviews

The NDTi autism programme was developed, and inpatient sensory environment reviews continued to be commissioned. The reviews consist of two team members, at least one of whom is autistic, walking through all of the areas that patients access and reviewing the sensory inputs in every room. The team shares their experiences during the 'walk through' and share findings in a written report following the visit. These highlight areas of good practice, identify comfortable sensory spaces and make recommendations for change and potential future good practice adaptations.

Not only is it good practice to make accommodations that will support positive outcomes for autistic people, but it is also a legal requirement under the *Equality Act 2010*. All healthcare providers have a duty to make reasonable adjustments, including adjustments to the spatial environment. The CQC report into restraint, seclusion and segregation (2020, p. 12) found that

> people were not having their needs met. Environments they were living in were not adapted to their sensory needs and they were not being offered support to communicate. Some providers were not making reasonable adjustments legally required under the Equality Act 2010.

Sensory environments are critical to autistic health and wellbeing. The CQC report (2020, p. 13) goes on to say that:

> Being placed in an inappropriate environment can be damaging and creates a pattern of distress, restraint and seclusion, which often cannot be broken. In many cases, we found that the impact of the environment on people, such as the noise, heating and lights of the wards, had not been considered. In many cases staff did not understand people's individual needs and the distress that being in the wrong environment could cause, particularly for people with sensory needs. This could lead to people expressing their distress in a way that others find challenging, leading to staff resorting to using restrictive practices.

After multiple visits to a range of mental health inpatient services including general wards, psychiatric intensive care units and low and medium secure wards, it was evident that there are some common sensory challenges and solutions that could be identified across all locations. The NDTi team approached the National Quality Improvement Taskforce for Children and Young People's Mental Health Inpatient Services and the National Learning Disability and Autism Team. The former commissioned a report on sensory environments to be co-produced with autistic young people who had been in hospital. The report is titled 'It's not Rocket Science' (NDTi, 2021). The latter commissioned Sensory Friendly Ward Principles. The Sensory Friendly Ward Principles were developed with autistic children and young people as part of the 'It's Not Rocket Science' report and were reviewed and revised following consultation with autistic adults.

The 'It's Not Rocket Science' report and the original Sensory Friendly Ward Principles were published in 2021 and included recommendations to replace fluorescent lighting with LED lighting alternatives. Halogen and tungsten bulbs had already been banned, and fluorescent lights cause visible strobe-like flickering that is visible and painful to many neurodivergent and photophobic people. The team was hopeful that LED lighting would improve the lit environment for patients. However, during subsequent visits to hospitals where LED lighting had been installed, the autistic team members were more negatively impacted than they had been by fluorescent overhead lighting.

One of NDTi's team members, Chris, described his experience at one hospital for children and young people as follows:

There was a mix of lighting around the hospital. I remember being impressed with the classrooms. They had big windows allowing in natural light, and blinds so this could be controlled. The overhead lights, although not diffused, were all dimmable. They dimmed without flickering or making any noise, which was really good to see. They were all on one circuit which limited the amount of control possible if people in one room had different needs and preferences, but it was better than we often see. Some of these rooms were carpeted, which really improved the soundscape. Overall, the classrooms were a pretty good sensory environment.

When we went to the residential part of the hospital, it was a different story. It was so much louder and brighter. I had a real moment of realisation when we visited one of the bedrooms. I walked into the en-suite and the overhead light came on automatically. It was blindingly bright and was on a motion sensor that didn't have a manual control.

I remember it being so bad. The light was reflecting on the glossy white surface on the walls, as well. It was like being surrounded by light. What made it even worse was that the automatic lights are on a timer, and it stayed on for five minutes after movement was detected. That's a long time when lights hurt. The en-suite didn't have a door, so I could imagine someone using the facilities at night under the bright glare and the light then flooding their room for another five minutes. It's so disruptive. I don't think I'd be able to get back to sleep in that scenario.

It's a nightmare for me, the thought of being trapped in a building like that. How are people supposed to get well and access therapy and support? I spent the whole visit on automatic. It's like I'm holding my breath. I just can't think, my brain is full of light and noise and there's no space left for thoughts. Then I get outside away from it all, and it all feels a bit calmer. It takes me a day or two to get over the shock and for my body to regulate after a visit. It's really physically demanding.

In response to this, the team sought lighting guidance available in the industry to share with hospitals to ensure that their luminaires were appropriate to the setting and did not negatively impact those using the space. Shocked to find that there was not any clear or comprehensive guidance related to LED lighting installations to ensure a best practice and autism-informed approach, we shared our frustration with others and the foundations of our working group with the Buro Happold Lighting team emerged.

Coming together to understand the problem and identify solutions

Within the group, autistic team members shared their experiences of photophobia. The lighting designers, inclusive designers and electrical engineers shared their knowledge of lighting systems and the guidance that informs hospital lighting installations. A shared understanding was established, and it became clear that many of the questions we asked as a group had not been considered and did not yet have sufficient answers due to a lack of research. Challenges we sought to address include:

- There is general guidance for lighting installation in hospitals, but it is not specific to LED lighting. Current version of guidance does not make any specific recommendations related to people with a degree of photosensitivity.
- It is difficult to specify or establish clear guidance because some of the available documentation/guides are quite generic and not associated to particular needs of users under neurodivergent or neurogenerative groups. For instance, one of the key observations and feedback from lived experience is related to light intensity. Average light levels included in available guidance to date seem to lead to overstimulation for neurodivergent users.
- The smooth uninterrupted operation of LED lighting installations relies primarily on the compatibility between the LED luminaire and the electronic drivers that are required to convert mains voltage (230V), alternating current to low voltage, direct current. They also keep the voltage and current flowing through an LED circuit at its rated level. Despite their considerable benefits in adjusting the ambience of the space, manual/digital dimmers and their associated issues with minimum and maximum capacity add to the complexity.
- There is no known research on photophobia or light sensitivity, and limited research about how neurodivergent individuals experience LED lighting (or any other type). Without this evidence base, it is challenging to set a baseline to support the need for change.
- The need to encourage the lighting supply industry to produce appropriate products using as baseline the highest-sensitivity users. These would need to satisfy and provide a balanced performance between glare and efficiency criteria and their ability to dim up/down without visible flicker.
- The very nature of an LED lighting assembly typically comprising of the luminaire body, the driver and/or power supply and the lighting control systems, all produced by different entities can meant that incompatibilities are only experienced post-completion of the installation and during the operational/in-use phases of the project, where liability shifts hands from the contractor to the facilities management team.
- Luminaire product design is now largely governed by the need to adopt sustainable processes and generate a product that is as energy efficient as possible. Energy efficiency is determined by the initial output of the raw LED light source inserted in the luminaire compared with the delivered output of the product accounting for internal light losses and absorptions from materiality or other components. The more concealed and well controlled the optics of the luminaire, the more comfortable the luminaire is to look at, preventing glare. However, in doing so, the energy efficiency of the assembly drops, leading to a conflicting issue between glare and energy efficiency.

Following the 'It's Not Rocket Science' report, it was felt that a more in-depth analysis of some technical characteristics affecting lighting performance and visual perception was needed in order to relate to the design and construction teams' language when commissioned to perform upgrades in existing healthcare environments. The technical note, co-authored by Buro Happold Lighting and NDTi (2022) and reviewed by other members of the working group, addresses key principles related to daylight and artificial lighting. Where deemed appropriate, area-specific criteria are outlined for consideration. Current regulations and technical guidance documents are summarised to enable easy review by readers and encourage opportunities for discussion on the need for further research on the impact of lighting on people who experience hypersensitivity to lighting. The baseline was built upon good practice guidance, including specific and wider considerations that affect spatial experience and our behavioural reaction to our environment. Furthermore, the methodology employed for the composition of this technical note is the collection of qualitative observational data through a series of meetings with NDTi members, consisting of people with mixed levels of light sensitivity. We held monthly meetings aimed to pass real user feedback gathered through conversations with inpatients in hospitals, such as a medium-secure CAMHS inpatient facility and useful insights on spatial experience in varying factors, including but not limited to lighting conditions.

The group engaged with other professionals, including Jemima Unwin Teji, who leads the MSc Light and Lighting programme at University College London, and Nicholas Bukorovic, the technical author and chair of CIBSE's Lighting for Healthcare Guidance taskforce.

Jemima shared her experience of research and engaged one of the Masters students to undertake a research study relevant to the topic under discussion as their thesis project. The research project involved a small group of individuals with various representative neurodivergent profiles. A physical experiment took place based on a simple set-up of an office environment using artificial lighting only. A series of scenarios was tested varying the intensity of the light and the duration over which the intensity shift occurred. Even though there was no statistically significant difference between neurotypical and neurodivergent participants in their ability to detect dimming, the most evident result of the experiment was the clear preference of neurodivergent users for much lower light levels than neurotypical users in the working environment. This result underpins the importance of having user-control and dimming enabled in the various spaces where we expect variety of cognitive profiles to co-exist and share. This requirement, in turn, makes the need for eliminating flicker in dimming a key priority. This pilot study used a small sample; therefore the findings are not generalisable to the wider population; however, the study does provide a starting point for further research about the perceptual differences and preferences between neurotypical and neurodivergent individuals.

We have also developed guidance to support providers, ward staff and facilities teams in inpatient settings to adapt the lighting to ensure an autism-informed approach that reduces harm to patients and supports better outcomes for individuals.

In summary, the key outputs and impacts of this work are as follows:

- Developing an advisory technical guidance note shared online and embedded in NHSE projects including sensory friendly ward guidance, green-light toolkit and health building note specifications.
- Positively engage NHSE colleagues, to support understanding of the issues and influence change across NHS estates.
- Develop a research collaboration with UCL

- Share our work on 'All in the Mind' on BBC Radio 4.
- Referenced in British Standards Institution PAS 6463: 2022 'Design for the Mind – neurodiversity and the built environment – guide'
- Articles about our work and the need for sensory considerations in lighting in professional lighting journals such as the *Lighting Journal* issued by the Institute of Lighting Professional and the Light Lines issued by CIBSE's Society of Light and Lighting.
- Exploration of a white paper with CIBSE, and intention to include reference to this work and recommendations in the revised CIBSE document 'Lighting for Healthcare Premises' LG02, the guidance document for lighting in all healthcare settings.

Our next steps will include:

- A meeting has been scheduled with our Net Zero NHSE contact.
- Influence and encourage further research.
- Get involved in NHS Framework to become advisors to the design/contractor teams that undertake new installations and refurbishment projects.
- Discuss with CIBSE the publication of the technical guide as a fact sheet or its incorporation into LG2: Lighting for Healthcare environments.

Conclusion and recommendations

Our aim in starting this work was to identify best practices and to share them with hospitals and facility teams. It turned into a much bigger project than we had imagined when we found that detailed guidance was not available, and we took on the challenge of developing it ourselves. As the work has evolved, our understanding has developed, the group has grown, and we have continued to extend our aims and seek improvement for neurodivergent and otherwise photophobic individuals. The feedback that we have received shows that the changes we recommend also benefit neurotypical users of the space, including staff, patients and visitors. We are strong believers that lighting that caters to neurodivergent people will also improve the lives of neurotypical groups.

Whether it constitutes co-production, citizen power or collaboration, the joint enterprise involving autistic people and lighting, engineering and research professionals has enabled this work to flourish. The involvement and leadership of autistic individuals and those who directly experience adverse impact from lighting have been central to this work. The collaboration from lighting professionals has been equally important in understanding what is needed, what is possible and how to pursue practical change.

The work has been facilitated by a joint ambition to understand the challenges and provide evidence and solutions to support improvement. The shared contacts and connections have enabled the group to extend its influence across the lighting sector, getting articles in the two national journals for lighting professionals, and engaging with two of the members that oversee the lighting for healthcare guidance, as well as gaining support to influence across NHS estates and mental health services. We advocate for this collaborative and user-led approach. We encourage services to be open to approaches and to engage with and support user-led initiatives.

Further recommendations

- More research!
- Environmental impact, carbon efficiencies and cost are important, but must not overshadow user experience and potential negative impact on people using the space.

- Implement technical guidance and guidelines from the PAS in new builds and retrofits. Although not mandatory, user controls, diffused lighting, quality component parts, warm colour tones and reduced glare all align with universal design principles and will improve the user experience.
- Get feedback from those using the space after fitting new lighting. User experience should be central to success.
- These principles and suggestions can be applied to other sectors too, most notably the educational and cultural sectors with the view of providing equitable spaces for all.
- Collaborate and show care for the environments we live and operate in.

Acknowledgements

The authors wish to thank:

Buro Happold.

The CAMHS Quality Improvement taskforce at NHS England (NHSE) requested funding for original work and ongoing support;

The Learning Disability and Autism team at NHSE for supporting Sensory Friendly Ward principles;

University College London;

Nic Bukorovic and the Chartered Institution of Building Service Engineers (CIBSE); and The National Development Team for Inclusion (NDTi) for hosting guidance notes on their website.

References

Arnstein, S. (1969). A ladder of citizen participation. *Journal of the American Planning Association, 35*(4), 216–224.

British Standard's Institution. (2022). *PAS 6463 design for the mind. Neurodiversity and the built environment. Guide.* Retrieved May 19, 2023, from https://knowledge.bsigroup.com/products/design-for-the-mind-neurodiversity-and-the-built-environment-guide/standard

Bukorovic, N. (2019). *Lighting guide 2: Lighting for healthcare premises (2019).* Retrieved May 19, 2023, from https://www.cibse.org/knowledge-research/knowledge-portal/lighting-guide-02-lighting-for-healthcare-premises-2019

Buro Happold and NDTi. (2022). *Sensory friendly led lighting for healthcare environments.* Retrieved May 19, 2023, from https://www.ndti.org.uk/assets/files/Sensory-friendly-LED-lighting-for-healthcare-environments_Final.pdf

Care Quality Commission. (2020). *Out of sight – Who cares? A review of restraint, seclusion and segregation for autistic people, and people with a learning disability and/or mental health condition.* Retrieved May 19, 2023, from https://www.cqc.org.uk/sites/default/files/20201218_rssreview_report.pdf

Care Quality Commission. (2022). *Restraint, segregation and seclusion review: Progress report.* Retrieved May 19, 2023, from https://www.cqc.org.uk/publications/themes-care/rss22_03_hospital

Conner, C., Golt, J., Righi, G., Shaffer, R., Siegel, M., & Mazefsky, C. A. (2020). A comparative study of suicidality and its association with emotion regulation impairment in large ASD and US census-matched samples. *Journal of Autism and Developmental Disorders, 50*(10), 3545–3560.

Grandin, T., & Panek, R. (2014). *The autistic Brain: Exploring the strength of a different kind of mind.* Rider Books.

Hand, B., Benevides, T., & Carretta, H. (2020). Suicidal ideation and self-inflicted injury in medicare enrolled autistic adults with and without co-occurring intellectual disability. *Journal of Autism and Developmental Disorders*, *50*(10), 3489–3495.

NDTi. (2021). *It's not rocket science*. Retrieved May 19, 2023, from www.ndti.org.uk/assets/files/Its-not -rocket-science-V6.pdf.

NHS England. (2017). *Care (education) and treatment review – Policy and guidance*. Retrieved May 19, 2023, from https://www.england.nhs.uk/wp-content/uploads/2017/03/ctr-policy-v2.pdf

NHS England. (2020). *Delivering a net zero national health service*. Retrieved May 19, 2023, from https:// www.england.nhs.uk/greenernhs/wp-content/uploads/sites/51/2020/10/delivering-a-net-zero-national -health-service.pdf

Parmar, K. R., Porter, C. S., Dickinson, C. M., Pelham, J., Baimbridge, P., & Gowen, E. (2021). Visual sensory experiences from the viewpoint of autistic adults. *Frontiers in Psychology*, *12*, 633037. https:// doi.org/10.3389/fpsyg.2021.633037

Zeldovich, L. (2018). How history forgot the woman who defined autism. *Spectrum Magazine*. Retrieved May 19, 2023, from https://www.spectrumnews.org/features/deep-dive/history-forgot-woman-defined -autism/

24 Conclusions

Designing for a better life

Kristina Niedderer, Geke Ludden, Tom Dening and
Vjera Holthoff-Detto

Taking stock

In this final chapter, we want to take stock and reflect on the insights and messages of the three parts of the book with their corresponding chapters, and of the book as a whole. In this book, we have set out to bring together an overview of design for dementia, mental illness and neuro-diversity in an assumption that there are commonalities between design approaches, interventions and policy in these three areas that warrant such an approach. We therefore now want to reflect on what commonalities, and differences, the contributions reveal, what we can learn from design for the different conditions and illnesses, and how these insights can inform the design across the different areas to allow for the development of a common design approach for mental health and wellbeing.

In terms of commonalities, importantly all the work reported in chapters across Parts 1, 2 and 3 shares the wellbeing values – emotional and social wellbeing and agency – each in their distinct ways, providing illustrative examples from different perspectives. Examples presented in the chapters range from a focus on ethics and citizenship to participation, co-design, arts-based, compassionate and mindful design interventions, concerns for evaluation, guidance and regulation for designs and designers, all the way to concerns relating to the wider 'eagle eye' perspective of policy. What holds this diversity of accounts and perspectives together is a deep conviction in the need for humane mental health care that is fuelled by compassion and mindfulness in order to promote people's wellbeing and gift as good a quality of life as is possible.

Although we define wellbeing in the book's introduction and there is generally a good understanding of wellbeing as a whole, in real-life situations it is apparent that wellbeing can mean many things and take many faces. A key tool, then, to find out and create consensus in local settings is co-design, which enables everyone involved to learn about people's individual perceptions and experiences by working together and sharing their experiences. In addition, it allows people with lived experience to make a contribution and take ownership in the development of the services, environments and products that are being developed to support them, giving participants a sense of value and agency. This ethos of inclusion, of teamwork and of mutual acceptance and respect can have a measurable impact on people's wellbeing (Rodgers, 2018; Zeilig et al., 2019). It means the co-design process itself can help build wellbeing and also resilience. This makes co-design and cognate participative and collaborative creative approaches an immensely valuable set of tools that is starting to become more commonly recognised now also in health and care. While this is the aim, it is not necessarily a given. Designers as well as policymakers need to be aware of when and how people with lived experience could and should be involved in design processes. Otherwise, involvement can become tokenistic through limited

DOI: 10.4324/9781003318262-30

numbers, or biased, involving a selected group of people who are willing and able to participate. Likewise, it is important to consider the burden put on participants (van Velsen et al., 2022), and to determine any needs and wishes regarding involvement together with participants to ensure that any co-design is truly collaborative.

In addition, the use of co-design allows for the development of tailor-made outcomes – whether this be products, environments, services, regulations or policy. It allows to develop them from the multiple perspectives of different stakeholders, to review criteria for their development from the experience of first-hand knowledge and, if necessary, to negotiate different needs and requirements to find the best possible solution for all concerned in terms of relevance and suitability. This can transform the design process and produce novel and exciting results. Involvement of people with lived experience in the vetting and certification of specifications for, and the implementation of, services is already being used, though further work to ensure truly user-appropriate and user-friendly designs in all areas is still needed. However, before drawing further conclusions and highlighting future scenarios and the need for further work, we want to reflect on the core insights from the three parts of the book.

A book of three parts: reflections on the findings

Part 1 has brought together seven chapters reflecting the diversity of co-design approaches and techniques as well as the aim to define the field. They have led the reader from considerations of the ethics of collaborative working with people with lived experience, via a review and comparison of current approaches of co-design, to three chapters offering guidelines on different aspects, finishing with two case studies.

One of the key insights from across these different contributions is the emphasis and importance of *the creative component in co-design*. Surfacing in a number of the chapters, but especially in the review of Chapter 3, the approach to co-design from the creative disciplines ('creative co-design', e.g. Nakarada-Kordic et al., 2017; Niedderer et al., 20202022; Rodgers et al., 2018; Slattery et al., 2020; Wallace et al., 2021; Wang et al., 2019; Zeilig et al., 2019) is significantly different to health and care-related approaches, such as experience-based co-design (EBCD, Mulvale, 2016). While as ever there will be no hard borders but rather a continuum between these two approaches, there are some clear differences that lie in the flexibility and multitude of tools available for the creative approach as compared to the more stringently defined EBCD process. This difference in approach points to a shift in balance: whereas EBCD looks at identifying people's experiences of a specific issue or situation, this does not necessarily lead to, or support, the development of tangible solutions, whereas the creative approach tends to focus on solution finding, perhaps at times at the expense of seeking to fully understand participants' experiences about a situation first. The synthesis framework in Chapter 3, then, reveals the need to cover the various areas and how to approach them methodologically.

Complementing the high-level framework perspective of Chapter 3, the adjacent chapters, especially Chapters 2, 4, 5 and 6, have looked in more detail at what is or should be happening at the local level of co-designing. They reveal two further key insights about co-designing: the need to appreciate people's *co-production values and understanding of wellbeing* and that this understanding will always be defined at the local level. Further, this local understanding is usefully framed within the wider understandings of definitions of wellbeing and co-production values to provide perspective to local differences. Therefore, taking care to understand the local setting, and people's local understandings, experiences, aims, aspirations and values, and to reflect on these within the larger context, is paramount to successful co-design.

The third key issue that reflects ongoing discussions across the different fields is that of the *ethics of collaboration*. This includes the values of co-production and an understanding and acknowledgement of the power-relationships to create a healthy balance between researchers, healthcare partners and lived experience participants. There are some key lessons here. Since there is a wide spectrum of collaborative processes, the need for transparency and agreement as early as possible in the process on who is involved, at what stage and in what capacity, what the joint and/or individual aims are for the collaboration, and how input and decisions are made in the process and by whom. This may depend on the nature of the collaboration. For example, research projects may be different from community projects or healthcare-services-driven projects. Traditional research tends to include participant involvement as research subjects in a hierarchical relationship, with participants providing information, but with no further involvement in shaping the study or its outcomes. At the other end of the spectrum, we find fully collaborative research projects, which may be directed by the community, perhaps with the researcher as a facilitator, but where the community participants direct the aim and decision-making. Whoever receives the funding is thereby bestowed with a degree of power over other collaborators. This raises issues about how the project will operate as a whole, and to what extent, and how community participants and other stakeholders will be involved. There appears to be a general consensus by now that stakeholder and lived experience participants should be involved as early as possible, ideally from the conception and application stage of any project onwards. This is increasingly reflected by funder requirements, including funding review panels with relevant stakeholder representatives. While this is the case now in many countries, such as Australia, the Netherlands or the UK, this is not yet the norm everywhere, and much more work needs to be done at all levels with regard to the understanding of co-design, the development and implementation of design interventions and through policy directives.

Looking at the design and application of design interventions in the mental health and care context, the key issues raised in Part 1 are also reflected in Part 2. Here, the recognition of *value-sensitive design* is important for how it enables integrating ideas from people's values about care in design. This recognises that design is not a neutral entity. Quite the opposite: design strongly embodies values at various levels and by various means. For example, through its visual aesthetic, or through the story it tells. Based on semiotic theories, this ability of design to attract, communicate and tell stories has long been used by design companies in all areas whether this is advertising or the design of tableware, such as by the Alessi company (Ciccolo, 1996). Further, values can be embedded in the functional aspects of products, services, systems and environments through product semantics (Krippendorff, 1993). This directs the way we handle and make sense of design products, or how we interact with services and environments: are they suggesting a certain way for us to behave, to do something or to interact (Norman, 2002)?

This leads to another insight, which is the *culturally sensitive adaptation* of interventions. Part 2 emphasises the differences in cultures around care and how different cultures can learn from each other and find inspiration in how they organise care differently. It also highlights where things are not transferrable or where they need culturally sensitive adaptation to ensure that an intervention is suitable and appropriate to be used in a new cultural environment, even if the problem it seeks to address is the same. The importance of involving a local culture throughout a design process becomes apparent, for example in Chapter 11, where the starting point for creating a support tool for informal carers of people with dementia was the lack of awareness of the illness in India. This generated the aim to raise awareness for families because, in India, the person with dementia is at home and cared for by family members in a multi-generational family setting. This creates different challenges for family members than, e.g. in Western countries where people often live with their spouse, or alone, cared for by children, friends or relatives who live remotely. Therefore, different settings may require different approaches.

There is further a call for *evidence-based evaluation* of interventions, which goes hand in hand with questions about who sets the criteria for any evaluation. Any evaluation raises questions as to who sets the evaluation criteria, whose outcomes and whose benefits count, and what impact is measured. It becomes clear that evidence-based evaluation, while being regarded as desirable on the whole, has a local, or rather experiential, component that must be considered. When talking about evidence-based evaluation, the outcomes too often focus solely on health-related outcomes, geared towards health-related methodologies, often quantitative, with the gold standard being randomised clinical trials (Burns et al., 2011). However, such trials rarely consider the experiential, design or wellbeing experiences of patients or other stakeholders (Smits et al., 2022). This means that such methodologies regularly overlook and therefore exclude 'soft measures' that help assess important benefits for people's wellbeing and quality of life. Such benefits may, for example, consist of getting easily and stress-free to an appointment because of having clear directions and finding one's way easily or being able to select a health support service that is easy and a joy to use because it has clear wellbeing benefits. Or people may feel heard and valued if a doctor or care professional actually looks them in the eye and listens and enables the person they support to organise their own care. Such measures can also offer valuable feedback to designers to further improve a product, service, system or environment. Therefore, it is important to look at evaluation holistically to include a variety of methodologies and outcome measures to capture the most relevant and meaningful information to truly understand the benefit of an intervention.

Part 3, then, has provided an overview of ways in which policy drives the development of innovation and interventions of and for care. A key issue emerging from the discussions is how policy can be most effective, and how this requires *perspective* – looking up at policymakers and decision-makers, but also looking down at stakeholders to root any decisions in real-world needs and realities. This means the inclusion of stakeholders and collaborative working at policy level is equally important, and the inclusion of community and stakeholder representation in think tanks and/or governmental consultations or policy groups is becoming increasingly common.

One interesting observation, which we feel warrants drawing attention to, is the issue of policy design. While policy design may be regarded as not being part of the traditional canon of design disciplines, and generally is not taught in design schools, but rather as part of business and management, it is now visible in design and design research circles where higher level discussions are desired. It is also evident that policy designers draw on various design tools, especially those from co-design and behaviour change (Kimbell & Bailey, 2017). This demonstrates once again the importance and influence of design as a practice and creative thinking tool with regard to making a difference, not just in health and care, but any area where policy development and change is desired. However, when it comes to policy *for* design, there is little there yet. What there is tends to be focused on business development rather than on the development of value-based design. Hence, this is an area that would benefit from more attention and development.

If policy design is closely linked to design, the implementation of policy is even more closely related to design. There is a need for guidance and regulations to facilitate the desired implementation of policy *for* design by translating it into real-world interventions, whether in the form of services or products, etc. This is the area that is perhaps least developed, or at least where the different interdisciplinary voices are least integrated. In policy implementation, we encounter

Table 24.1 Key design issues revealed by the three lenses of the book: co-design, interventions and policy

Part 1: Co-design	Part 2: Interventions	Part 3: Policy
Creative co-design	Culturally sensitive adapting	Policy for design for health and wellbeing
Ethics of collaboration	Value sensitive design	Integrating top-down and bottom-up perspectives
Valuing local experiences	Experience-rich evidence-based evaluation	Experiential and value-based guidance and regulations

once more a strong reliance on an evidence base that is numerically driven and that tends to ignore the qualitative importance of the values and experiences of interventions. However, these are essential to provide not just a satisfactory or good user experience but a delightful one (Guimarães, 2007), which may itself add to wellbeing and quality of life. In other cases, such as in Chapter 22, Bellini and Macchi observe that little to no standards or guidance is available to guide designers in the development of interventions to support, for example, children with autism. This is why research is important to establish standards and guidance as demonstrated in Chapter 21 with regard to the development of mHealth design principles and guidelines for people living with dementia or in Chapter 23 with regard to the development of guidance for LED lighting to meet the needs of people with autism and other neurodivergent conditions.

In summary, all three parts raise a set of related issues. As these issues emerge, from one to the next, they transform in line with the different lens each part takes on design for mental health and wellbeing (Table 24.1). They bring to the fore the creative power of design, fuelled by its ability to support and embed cultural and ethical values through its collaborative practice and in its experientially derived outcomes.

Final words: looking towards the future

Overall, the discussions in this book have shown three key points: they have demonstrated the benefit of bringing together design for mental health and wellbeing in the context of dementia, mental illness and neurodiversity in one volume. They have further highlighted the importance and ways of including user perspectives and values, especially those with lived experience, and making them paramount in collaborative working to leading to successful outcomes. This includes nuances and different meanings of such values as well as the notion of wellbeing and how they shape the power relationships within collaborations to make them truly inclusive and equitable, but most of all transparent and mutually agreed.

A limitation of such a broad-brush approach is, of course that this single volume can only scratch the surface of the many issues these discussions have raised. Conversely, we hope that in raising these issues, it will help other researchers to follow in our footsteps and to investigate the individual areas of dementia, mental illness and neurodiversity from a design point of view in more depth. We hope that this will result in more advanced interventions in each of the areas that are both founded in experiential and evidence-based development and evaluations to assess their impact.

However broad, this book, of course, had to exclude many areas, such as the area of education and training in collaborative practices for designers and other stakeholders involved in the process of developing design interventions and policy for mental health and wellbeing. There is now an emerging landscape of interdisciplinary educational provision that includes a number of relatively novel Masters courses that promote and teach creative collaborative approaches for health and wellbeing. We hope that this new generation of interdisciplinary and collaborative design, health and care professionals and scholars will become the new generation that will continue the work of this book.

Last, but not least, the discussions have highlighted that policy for design in relation to mental health and wellbeing is only emergent and that the development of value-based design is an area that would benefit from more attention and development, including, for example, in the areas of education but also standards and regulations. Therefore, we believe this book is a start to developing the area of design for mental health and wellbeing, and that more breadth, more depth relating to the specific areas and generally more work is needed. So, this work is not yet done, and we hope this volume offers a direction and start for our readers to follow.

References

Burns, P. B., Rohrich, R. J., & Chung, K. C. (2011). The levels of evidence and their role in evidence-based medicine. *Plastic and Reconstructive Surgery*, *128*(1), 305–310. https://doi.org/10.1097/PRS .0b013e318219c171

Ciccolo, E. (1996). *L'oggetto dell'equilibrio. Centro studi Alessi 1990–1996 [Object of equilibrium. Alessy Study Centre 1990-1996]*. Alessi.

Guimarães, J. E. R. (2007). *The Kano Model as a tool to identify attractive features of Inclusive Design among users* (PhD Thesis). Staffordshire University.

Kimbell, L., & Bailey, J. (2017). Prototyping and the new spirit of policy-making. *CoDesign*, *13*(3), 214–226. https://doi.org/10.1080/15710882.2017.1355003

Krippendorff, K., & Butter, R. (1993). Where meanings escape functions. *Design Management Institute Journal*, *4*(2), 30–37.

Mulvale, A., Miatello, A., Hackett, C., & Mulvale, G. (2016). Applying experience-based co-design with vulnerable populations: Lessons from a systematic review of methods to involve patients, families and service providers in child and youth mental health service improvement. *Patient Experience Journal*, *3*(1). https://pxjournal.org/journal/vol3/iss1/15

Nakarada-Kordic, I., Hayes, N., Reay, S., D., Corbet, C., & Chan, A. (2017). Co-designing for mental health: Creative methods to engage young people experiencing psychosis. *Design for Health*, *1*(2), 229–244. doi:10.1080/24735132.2017.1386954

Niedderer, K., Holthoff-Detto, V., van Rompay, T. J. L., Karahanoğlu, A., Ludden, G. D. S., Almeida, R., Losada Durán, R., Bueno Aguado, Y., Lim, J. N. W., Smith, T., et al. (2022a). This is Me: Evaluation of a board game to promote social engagement, wellbeing and agency in people with dementia through mindful life-storytelling. *Journal of Aging Studies*, *60*. https://doi.org/10.1016/j.jaging.2021.100995

Niedderer, K., Harrison, D., Gosling, J., Craven, M., Blackler, A., Losada, R., & Cid, T. (2020). Working with experts with experience: Charting co-production and co-design in the development of HCI based design. In G. Kenning & R. Braenkert (Eds.), *HCI and design in the context of dementia* (pp. 303–320). Springer. https://doi.org/10.1007/978-3-030-32835-1_19

Norman, D. A. (2002). *The design of everyday things*. Basic Books.

Rodgers, P. A. (2018). Co-designing with people living with dementia. *CoDesign*, *14*(3), 188–202. https://doi.org/10.1080/15710882.2017.1282527

Slattery, P., Saeri, A. K., & Bragge, P. (2020). Research co-design in health: A rapid overview of reviews. *Health Research Policy and Systems*, *18*(17). https://doi.org/10.1186/s12961-020-0528-9

Smits, M., Kim, C., van Goor, H., & Ludden, G. (2022). From digital health to digital well-being: Systematic scoping review. *Journal of Medical Internet Research*, *24*(4), e33787. https://doi.org/10 .2196/33787

van Velsen, L., Ludden, G., & Grünloh, C. (2022). The limitations of user-and human-centered design in an ehealth context and how to move beyond them. *Journal of Medical Internet Research*, *24*(10), e37341. https://doi.org/10.2196/37341

Wallace, N., David, A., & Gwilt, I. (2021, June 21). Wellbeing through participation: Creativity and co-design as processes of 'welldoing'. *Non-Traditional Research Outcomes*, *35*. Retrieved July 7, 2023, from https://ualresearchonline.arts.ac.uk/id/eprint/17864/1/Wellbeing%20through%20participation .pdf

Wang, G., Marradi, C., Albayrak, A., & van der Cammen, T. J. M. (2019). Co-designing with people with dementia: A scoping review of involving people with dementia in design research. *Maturitas*, *127*, 55–63. https://doi.org/10.1016/j.maturitas.2019.06.003

Zeilig, H., Tischler, V., van der Byl Williams, M., West, J., & Strohmaier, S. (2019). Co-creativity, well-being and agency: A case study analysis of a co-creative arts group for people with dementia. *Journal of Aging Studies*, *49*, 16–24. https://doi.org/10.1016/j.jaging.2019.03.002

Index

For Product Safety Concerns and Information please contact our EU
representative GPSR@taylorandfrancis.com
Taylor & Francis Verlag GmbH, Kaufingerstraße 24, 80331 München, Germany

9 781032 331171